Handbook of
Blood Transfusion
Therapy

Handbook of Blood Transfusion Therapy

SECOND EDITION

J. A. F. NAPIER

National Blood Transfusion Service (Wales), Cardiff, UK

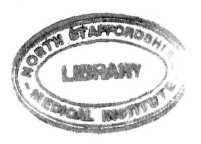

JOHN WILEY & SONS

Chichester · New York · Toronto · Brisbane · Singapore

Other Wiley Editorial Offices

John Wiley & Sons, Inc., 605 Third Avenue,
New York, NY 10158-0012, USA

Jacaranda Wiley Ltd, 33 Park Road, Milton,
Queensland 4064, Australia

John Wiley & Sons (Canada) Ltd, 22 Worcester Road,
Rexdale, Ontario M9W 1L1, Canada

John Wiley & Sons (SEA) Pte Ltd, 37 Jalan Pemimpin #05-04,
Block B, Union Industrial Building, Singapore 2057

Library of Congress Cataloging-in-Publication Data

Napier, J. A. F.
    Handbook of blood transfusion therapy / by J.A.F. Napier. — 2nd
ed.
        p. cm.
    Rev. ed. of: Blood transfusion therapy. c1987.
    Includes bibliographical references and index.
    ISBN 0-471-95378-4 (alk. paper)
    1. Blood—Transfusion.   I. Napier, J. A. F. Blood transfusion
therapy. II. Title.
    [DNLM: 1. Blood Transfusion.   WB 356 N199h 1995]
    RM171.N36   1995
    615'.39—dc20
    DNLM/DLC
    for Library of Congress   95-19767
                                                                  CIP

British Library Cataloguing in Publication Data

A catalogue record for this book is available from the British Library

ISBN 0-471-95378-4

Typeset in 10/12pt Palatino by Acorn Bookwork, Salisbury, Wilts
Printed and bound in Great Britain by Bookcraft (Bath) Ltd
This book is printed on acid-free paper responsibly manufactured from sustainable foresta-
tion, for which at least two trees are planted for each one used for paper production.

Contents

Preface

The practice of blood transfusion has changed so much since publication of the first edition that a substantial revision of most of the chapters has been necessary.

Although blood transfusion has never been safer than it is today, concerns about safety and the corresponding need for information about risks and benefits are greater than ever before. The increasing demand for health care resources has put pressure on the need to treat wisely and economically; quality standards increase, as does the possibility of litigation should practice be shown to be substandard. For all these reasons, a more informed and discriminating approach to the use of blood transfusion is now required. Alternatives to what may be regarded as conventional (allogeneic) transfusion are increasingly considered. Technical approaches towards autologous blood salvage and reutilization have become cheaper and more reliable, and a variety of pharmacological methods for reducing surgical blood loss are under investigation. Recombinant haemopoietic growth factors are poised to influence blood product use profoundly over the next few years. In various other less obvious ways, attitudes to management of transfusion problems have also changed—even areas in which basic facts and therapeutic modalities have not substantially advanced. The impact of new genetic technology has begun to influence profoundly the supply of therapeutic materials and of reagents as well as the design and accuracy of diagnostic procedures. As an example, HLA genotyping for transplantation purposes has been given new precision with techniques that can be applied routinely and rapidly for typing and direct cross-matching procedures.

I have tried to accommodate these various developments without substantially altering the layout and presentation of the first edition.

I am grateful for the assistance of a number of people in the preparation of this edition. Mr Andrew Dawson kindly provided help with Figure 3 of chapter 21. Dr C. Poynton and Mrs Tracey Rees provided critical advice with regard to the revision of the chapter on organ transplantation and matching. Dr Martin Guttridge also gave help with regard to Figures 4 and 5 of chapter 22 on DNA genotyping. Similarly, Dr Diana Westmoreland provided source material for Figure 6 of chapter 24. Finally, for the enormous work of coping patiently with what must have seemed endless changes to the manuscript, redrawing numerous figures, or chasing errant references I am grateful to Mrs Judith Brooks.

Preface to the First Edition

In compiling this book I have tried to produce the sort of reference source that I first sought at the start of my serious involvement with the practice of blood transfusion. This specialty of medicine might seem to many to be relatively discrete and free from complication and disagreement. Transfusion practice does, however, interrelate closely with many other clinical specialties, for example those of surgery, medicine, obstetrics and gynaecology, haematology, anaesthetics and intensive care, and it therefore behoves the transfusion specialist to understand and take an interest in the problems of his clinical colleagues. Perhaps it should come as no surprise to learn that controversy surrounds the value of many areas of transfusion therapy. Established practices for the management of particular problems often show considerable differences when international or intercontinental boundaries are crossed, despite the plethora of published information in many periodicals. Fiscal differences and national enthusiasms and prejudices clearly have a large part to play in the evolution of these variations. However, there are also genuine differences in the donor population as well as in the transfusion needs of superficially similar groups of patients throughout the world which, for valid reasons, must affect the details of their management.

Transfusion is costly and resources in both human and financial terms are finite, so economy in the use of transfusion materials should never be far from the minds of those engaged in transfusion practice. Transfusion can be hazardous just as much as it can be beneficial, so the decision to transfuse should also take into account a risk–benefit analysis appropriate to each individual patient. The recent and quite unexpected appearance of AIDS (acquired immuno-deficiency syndrome) must serve to displace any feelings of complacency about the safety of transfusion that may have arisen.

I have tried, I hope without causing confusion, to reflect the diversity of viewpoints covering various topics. There are some subjects in which sufficient facts are not yet available to permit reconciliation. In these instances the conclusions I have reached will reflect local practices coloured by or influenced by my own prejudices and may at times appear unjustifiably dogmatic or even didactic. I hope, however, that in the main these will be representative of the most considered opinions available.

In the selection of references and bibliographies, I have not chosen on the basis of historical precedence but, instead, quoted relatively recent publications on the basis of their ability to provide an introduction to more detailed examination of the current literature. The selection of references may also appear unbalanced, some topics being more intensively covered than others. In so far as I have selected references that seemed most clinically pertinent from major periodicals I hope the selection represents, reasonably accurately, the level of clinical interest in the various topics. I have attempted to devote various chapters to particular topics of clinical concern although unavoidably a degree of overlap and repetition occurs with the contents of other chapters, for example those devoted to blood components and principles of transfusion physiology. I hope that cross-referencing and brevity in appropriate places has partially overcome this problem.

In preparing this manuscript I have made use of, and am grateful for, innumerable discussions with colleagues as well as benefiting subconsciously from the information and stimulation of others who have written in both this and related fields. I have been particularly helped by many of my colleagues who have read portions of the manuscript and made constructive criticisms. Errors of interpretation or of fact I hope are few and for those I must accept sole responsibility.

In conclusion, I wish to express my thanks for secretarial help, in particular to Mrs Ticia Holland and Mrs Elizabeth Campbell for their patience during the endless revisions and rearrangements involved in the preparation of the manuscript.

Part A
BLOOD COMPONENTS AND PRODUCTS

1

Blood Components and Products: A Brief Guide to Their Uses

The following table lists the materials most commonly available from transfusion services, their principal characteristics and their clinical uses:

Blood Components and Products: Materials most commonly available from transfusion services; their principal characteristics and clinical uses

Blood component	Volume and composition	Principal indications for use	Risks	Shelf life	Comments
Red cells (concentrates)	Approx. 180 ml RBCs + 75 ml plasma. Haematocrit 0.55–0.75. Provides red cell replacement only	Correction of anaemia. Replacement of blood loss (in combination with plasma expanders)	All risks of transfusion except reduced risk of volume overload. Compatibility testing required	Depends on choice of anticoagulant. Usually 35 days	The standard red cell replacement material
Red cell suspensions in optimal additive solutions	Approx. 180 ml RBCs, 20 ml plasma, 100 ml preservative solution. Haematocrit 0.50–0.70	As for red cell concentrates	As for red cell concentrates	35–49 days, depending on type of preservative solution	Excellent flow properties
Stored whole blood	450 ml donor blood + 63 ml anticoagulant. Provides RBCs, plasma proteins and coagulation factors (except V and VIII). Haematocrit 0.35–0.40	Use only when both RBCs and plasma protein must be replaced (e.g., rapid massive blood loss)	All risks that may be associated with transfusion	Depends upon choice of anticoagulant— usually 35 days	Very rarely specifically indicated. Component therapy preferred
Frozen red cells	Approx. 150 ml RBCs + 100 ml saline	Rare blood group transfusions	As for red cell concentrates but no leucocyte or plasma reactions	10 years. 24 hours following thawing	Expensive. Transportation from banks and preparation may take a long time

Product	Content	Indications	Risks	Shelf life	Comments
Leucocyte-depleted red cells	Approx. 180 ml RBCs <5 × 10^6 leucocytes	Used to avoid sensitization at start of transfusion programmes or to prevent febrile reactions in already sensitized patients	As for red cells	24 hours (unless prepared under sterile conditions)	Ward use filters available
Platelet concentrates (random donor)	50 ml plasma containing 55–70 × 10^9 platelets	May be presented as a pool of 4–5 donations. May be presented leucodepleted (see ch. 5:4.4) (1) Prophylactic use when platelet counts are below 10–20 × 10^9/l (2) Bleeding due to thrombocytopenia (counts below 50 × 10^9/l) (3) To cover surgery during thrombocytopenia, e.g. counts of 50–100 × 10^9/l	Most transfusion risks. Alloimmunization reducing effectiveness of future transfusions is a particular problem	Usually 5 days	(1) Use identical ABO groups when possible. Any ABO groups, however, can be used provided red cell counts are low (2) Rh D sensitization is possible
Single-donor platelets (apheresis donations)	Usually 300 ml plasma containing 3–5 × 10^{11} platelets. Can be leucodepleted (see ch. 5:4.4)	As above	Reduced donor exposures compared to pooled platelets	5 days provided that the collection procedures is 'closed'	Particularly useful for HLA matched or cross-match-compatible donations
Single-donor (apheresis) granulocytes	1–5 × 10^{10} granulocytes in 300–600 ml plasma and variable numbers of platelets and RBCs	Neutropenia (less than 0.5 × 10^9 l) and evidence of infection unresponsive to antibiotic therapy. At least 5 days' consecutive therapy is usually required	Risks of transfusion generally. CMV infection and GVHD are a particular concern	6 hours	The preferred granulocyte product

continues

Blood component	Volume and composition	Principal indications for use	Risks	Shelf life	Comments
Granulocytes (random-donor buffy coats)	$>1 \times 10^9$ granulocytes in a volume of 50 ml (10–20 donations may be required). Haematocrit 0.5 unless red cells are removed	As above	As above	6 hours	Now rarely used. Ensure ABO and Rh D compatibility. Red cell-contaminated products need compatibility confirmation with negative antibody screen results
Fresh frozen plasma (FFP)	150–250 ml anticoagulated plasma. Contains all coagulation factors at >70% normal levels	(1) Haemorrhage due to broad-spectrum coagulation factor deficiency (dose 12–15 ml/kg) (2) Specific coagulation factor deficiencies where concentrates are unavailable	Occasional severe anaphylactoid reactions. Virus transmission	12 months frozen. 2 hours following thawing	Give ABO-compatible donations. Effective replacement dosage is limited by the large volumes required
Cryoprecipitate	10–20 ml plasma enriched for Factor VIII >70 IU/pack, fibrinogen >140 mg/pack	Disseminated intravascular coagulation and hypofibrinogenaemia	Virus transmission	12 months in frozen state. 2 hours following thawing	Formerly used for mild bleeds in haemophilia A and for von Willebrand's disease

Product	Presentation and dose	Indication	Safety	Shelf life	Comments
Factor VIII concentrate	Freeze-dried presentation. 250–1000 IU. Dose 10–40 IU/kg according to clinical severity	(1) Haemophilia A (2) von Willebrand's disease	Plasma-derived products now believed to be virtually virus free	1–3 years at 4°C	Numerous products of differing specifications available. Use according to specialist advice
Factor IX concentrate	Freeze-dried presentation. Specifications vary according to products. Factors II and X also present. Dose 20–50 IU/kg according to clinical severity	Haemophilia B	Plasma-derived products now believed to be virtually virus free. Most products have some thrombogenic potential	1–3 years at 4°C	Thrombotic risk of conventional products precludes their use for 'liver' factor deficiencies. High-purity products now available
Crystalloids, synthetic plasma volume expanders (e.g., saline, dextrans, gelatins)	A wide variety of products available (see ch. 10)	Initial treatment of hypovolaemia and hypotension following blood or plasma loss. Selection should consider: (1) Oncotic activity (2) Intravascular/extra-vascular distribution (3) Duration of plasma volume expansion required	Very safe products. Dextrans have antithrombotic effects. All synthetic colloids have very rare allergic effects	Prolonged (years)	Should always be selected in preference unless a human blood product has proven advantages
Albumin 4–5%	>95% albumin in saline. Various volumes available (e.g., 100, 250, 500 ml)	Hypovolaemia and hypotension following substantial plasma loss. Use in combination with other volume expanders and red cells	Very safe, virus free and pasteurized. Some preparations have had hypotensive effects	Usually 3 years	Use where prolonged plasma expansion is necessary, particularly in presence of hypoproteinaemia

continues

Blood component	Volume and composition	Principal indications for use	Risks	Shelf life	Comments
Albumin 20–25%	>95% albumin in saline. 100 ml volume	(1) As above, particularly in presence of hypoproteinaemia. (2) Reabsorption of oedema and expansion of plasma volume to enable diuresis			Useful in combination with diuretics to gain control over hypoproteinaemia and oedema. Not for treatment of chronic hypoproteinaemia
Immunoglobulin preparations: Human normal Ig	Freeze-dried or ready-to-use solution for i.v. use presented in 1–6 g vials	(1) For prophylaxis or therapy in congenital or acquired antibody deficiency syndromes (2) Passive immunity where specific Ig is not available (3) Autoimmune thrombocytopenia	Viral transmission risk very low (occasional batches have transmitted PTH). Uncommon allergic reactions	Prolonged (years)	Various products available, differing according to preparative methods and Ig subclass composition
Specific antimicrobial immunoglobulins	Various formulations for i.m. or i.v. use	Conferring passive immunity following exposure to infection	Viruses are not transmitted by i.m. products. Uncommon allergic reactions	Prolonged (years)	
Anti-D immune globulin (see ch. 21)	Ready-to-use vials 250–500 IU (UK). 1500 IU standard dose in USA and some European countries	Prevention of Rh haemolytic disease: (1) During risky events in pregnancy, i.e. amniocentesis, abortions (2) After giving birth to Rh D-positive babies	No virus transmission from i.m. products	Prolonged (years)	Should be given to all unsensitized Rh D-negative mothers. Test for fetomaternal haemorrhage advised

Part B
BLOOD GROUP ANTIGENS
AND ANTIBODIES

2
Blood Group Antigens and Antibodies

1 INTRODUCTION

Human red cells display extensive antigenic polymorphism; the various blood group systems together contribute to a total of over 400 characterized antigens. It is therefore fortunate that most of these are such weak antigens that they rarely cause clinical problems. Traditional nomenclature for red cell antigens has been used throughout this text. It should be noted however, that blood group terminology which for historical reasons is somewhat confusing and inconsistent has now been standardized[1] on an alphanumeric basis to enable computer coding. The blood group antigen systems that attract frequent clinical notice number less than a dozen and of these only two, the ABO and Rhesus (Rh) systems, require routine prospective matching prior to blood transfusion. The remaining blood group differences present problems for only a small number of patients in whom a previous antigenic challenge, usually from pregnancy or an earlier transfusion, has stimulated the formation of antibodies which then necessitate selection of more accurately matched blood. Unravelling the complexities of antigens and their genetic, immunological and biochemical characteristics will continue to provide an endless source of research interest. Their clinical significance for routine serologists is of a much more restricted nature, although even within this practical area of serology there are many clinically pertinent questions which remain unanswered.

The following account attempts to cover only those aspects of red cell serology which are likely to affect clinical practice and illustrates the difficulties faced by blood bank workers attempting to provide compatible blood when serological problems arise. The serological presentation is accordingly brief and no attempt has been made to discuss serological aspects that are unlikely to require the attention of those working outside the blood bank.

1.1 General Features of Red Cell Antigens

The *ABO blood group system* is by far the most important system that needs to be considered during blood transfusion. Red cells selected for transfusion are usually from donations *ABO-identical* to those of the recipient, but occasionally non-identical but *ABO-compatible* blood is given and in these instances the donor red cells lack antigens possessed by the recipient. Examples of this include use of group A blood for AB patients and the use of group O blood for recipients of any blood group. Blood carrying ABO antigens lacking in the recipient cannot be transfused because of the almost universal presence of the complementary ABO isoantibodies which cause prompt and dangerous destruction of the incompatible red cells.

The *Rh blood group system* ranks next in clinical importance. Naturally occurring antibodies to Rh antigens do not usually occur so transfusion of antigenically dissimilar blood does not have immediate adverse consequences. However, the Rh D antigen is a potent immunogen and transfusion of Rh D-positive blood to individuals who are Rh D negative stimulates formation of an immune anti-D that can complicate the management of future transfusions or pregnancies. It is customary, therefore, to ensure that Rh D-negative recipients, especially women of childbearing age, are only transfused with Rh D-negative blood. The Rh D antigen well exemplifies some aspects of the clinical concept of immunogenicity. In blood transfusion terms the most important 'antigens' are:

(1) Immunochemically distinct from their common alleles. They are thus easily recognized as foreign antigenic material. (The product of the gene allelic to that for the Rh D antigen, however, has not yet been defined.)
(2) Prevalent in a sufficient number of the donor population to ensure a high chance of antigen-positive units being transfused.
(3) Absent in a significant proportion of recipients, who therefore represent the population that is susceptible to immunization.
(4) Capable of producing antibodies causing destruction of incompatible transfused red cells.

The remaining antigens of the Rh system, together with those of the Kell, Duffy, Kidd, Lutheran, MNSs, Lewis and P systems, do occasionally cause problems during transfusion but not with such frequency that they merit use of fully matched blood in order to avoid immunization. Their immunogenicity appears to be considerably less than that of the Rh D antigen and matched antigen-identical blood is only needed when clinically significant alloantibodies have been formed.

Certain rare developmental abnormalities of blood group antigens create particular difficulties when transfusion is required. Failure to develop the common ABO antigens (e.g., the Bombay phenotype), the Kell antigens (e.g., the Ko phenotype) or the Rh null phenotype (lacking the entire expression of Rh antigens) is usually associated with the formation of antibodies reactive against the corresponding normal antigenic structures which are present on virtually all other human red cells. A similar though slightly less serious problem occurs when individuals lacking *high-frequency antigens* form antibodies against those antigens. For example, 0.04% of people have the genotype Kp^aKp^a and lack Kp^b antigen; if they form anti-Kp^b they must only be transfused with the rare Kp(b−) blood.

Antigens of very low frequency do not often create clinical transfusion problems but may present as abnormal laboratory results which may take a considerable time to resolve. The chance mixing of red cells carrying a *low-frequency antigen* with the equally uncommon sera containing the corresponding antibody can create unexpected difficulties during routine red cell typing or compatibility testing.

1.2 Red Cell Antibodies: General Characteristics

Antibodies against red cell antigens can be grouped into broad categories according to the circumstances of their occurrence and their likely biological significance.

Antibodies of the ABO system are almost invariably present in the blood of individuals lacking the corresponding antigen. ABO antibodies are said to be *naturally occurring* since their formation does not appear to depend on any single clearly identifiable stimulus. These antibodies are dangerously haemolytic and accordingly blood transfusions must always be ABO compatible.

Alloantibodies against antigens of the remaining major blood group systems do not generally appear unless the individual has been challenged by previous trans-fusion, pregnancy or, on some occasions, by microorganisms or parasites bearing similar antigens. Once an antibody has been identified, and if it is judged to be of potential clinical significance (see section 5), future transfusions must not carry the corresponding antigen. In many cases the incidence of compatible donors is suffi-ciently high that the occurrence of alloantibodies does not cause blood banks undue difficulty. However, it frequently happens that further antibody specificities appear, and under these circumstances the development of each new antibody progressively reduces the chances of obtaining compatible red cell units.

Once alloantibodies appear it is usual to proceed in the following way :

(1) The specificity must be defined.
(2) The patient must be shown to lack the antigen (a logical prerequisite).
(3) Blood which is negative for the antigen concerned must be selected for future transfusions.
(4) These donations must be shown to be cross-match compatible thereby con-firming the accuracy of the serological conclusions.

Autoantibodies by definition react with the patient's own red cells, but will usually also react with most other red cells, including of course those used as reagent red cells for blood group determination, for antibody screening and the donor red cells used in compatibility tests. Autoantibodies can therefore be a cause of errors in blood grouping and can also create difficulties during the provision of compa-tible blood of which experienced blood bank workers are fully aware. A particular problem is that of excluding the presence of coexisting *alloantibodies* which, in con-trast to autoantibodies, usually do have a defined specificity and may cause greater haemolysis of transfused red cells. Autoantibodies may be associated with overt haemolytic anaemia or may, on the other hand, be clinically insignificant. Into this latter category fall autoantibodies reacting only by enzyme techniques, and the ubiquitous low-titre cold agglutinins, which are mainly noteworthy for the nuisance they create during routine serology testing.

The practical difficulties posed by antibodies against very high frequency anti-gens have been referred to earlier. It may be necessary to resort to autologous transfusion (chapter 15) or to obtain donations from rare donor panels when patients with these antibodies must be transfused.

2   THE ABO BLOOD GROUPS

The discovery of the major ABO groups in 1900 and the classification of pheno-types into A, B, O and AB permitted for the first time the use of blood transfu-sion as a safe and practicable form of treatment. A B and H (O) antigens were later identified as oligosaccharide structures synthesized under the control of spe-cific glycosyltransferases. Ninety years after the original discovery, DNA cloning and sequencing has revealed the very small genetic differences coding for the transferases that produce such a fundamental immunological distinction between the major human blood types.[2]

The most common ABO phenotypes in populations of European origin are

Table 1 The ABO blood group system

Phenotype	Incidence (%)	Alloantibodies
O	44	Anti-A, B
A_1	33	Anti-B
A_2	9	Anti-B, up to 9% have Anti-A_1
B	10	Anti-A
A_1B	3	–
A_2B	1	22–35% have anti-A_1

shown in Table 1. Group O individuals constitute about 50% of most populations, followed closely by group A, with groups B and AB showing much lower incidences.

Amongst many non-European populations group B shows higher frequencies (reaching 26% in Chinese) while the incidence of group A shows a corresponding decline.

Since the complementary ABO alloantibodies are almost invariably present ABO blood grouping is performed both by typing red cells and by examining the serum for the appropriate antibodies. The security of this procedure is thereby enhanced since results from both must agree before the ABO group can be assigned.

Group A or B individuals can be genetically *AO, AA* or *BO, BB* respectively. Heterozygous parents can of course have group O children.

2.1 ABO Antigen Variants: Subtypes of A and B

For practical purposes most blood samples are grouped and identified as group A, B, AB or O alone; only when problems emerge is it necessary to make the distinction between the group A or B subtypes.

(1) The A_2 subgroup is by far the commonest and most important of these variants. The antigen on A_2 red cells appears to differ both quantitatively (fewer antigen sites are present) and qualitatively from the A antigen of most other group A individuals (which is designated A_1). This has two practical consequences.

(a) Group A_2 individuals can produce anti-A_1. This can be discovered during ABO grouping when an 'A' individual also appears to have anti-A in the serum. If the anti-A_1 is not detected at this stage it may, in prospective transfusion recipients, be discovered when group A donations are found to be incompatible during compatibility testing. Anti-A_1 is most easily detected during 'cold' (i.e., room temperature) testing, but can on very rare occasions have sufficient activity at 37 °C to be capable of destroying transfused A_1 cells. Once anti-A_1 is detected, A_2 cells are sometimes requested for transfusion, although it has been well established that purely cold-reacting anti-A_1 can be disregarded.[3] Clearly, if an anti-A_1 antibody is suspected it is axiomatic that the person concerned must be shown not to be group A_1. A plant lectin (from *Dolichos biflorus*) serves as an excellent specific anti-A_1 typing reagent and is used in this situation.

The majority of group A_2 individuals who have not formed anti-A_1 remain unrecognized as A_2 and are therefore grouped as A. They are transfused uneventfully with group A red cells which similarly consist of unidentified group A_1 or A_2 donations.

(b) The expression of the A_2 antigen may be so weak on A_2B cells as to escape detection if tests are not performed carefully. The presence of anti-A_1 in the serum will then produce blood typing results typical of a group B individual. This will not matter much for transfusion recipients since transfused group B blood may be well tolerated. A_2B blood donors must, on the other hand, be reliably identified because these cells will undergo accelerated destruction if given inadvertently as group B blood to a group B recipient.

(2) *Rare subgroups of A*: rather less than 1% of group A people possess red cells carrying even weaker expressions of the A antigen than are shown by the A_2 subtype. A_3, Ax and Am, as well as some other even less common subtypes have been distinguished. As transfusion recipients they may be mistakenly grouped as O but will not be harmed by transfusion of group O blood. It is more important to identify them correctly when presenting as donors for the reasons discussed above.

(3) *'Bombay' phenotypes* represent a well-known but exceptionally rare genetic abnormality in the biosynthetic pathway for ABO antigen formation. Most frequently there is failure to form 'H substance'—an essential carbohydrate precursor necessary for the subsequent manufacture of A and B antigens. Lack of this material, which is normally ubiquitous on human red cells, and absence also of A and B substances, is associated with the appearance of powerfully haemolytic anti-H, anti-A and anti-B in the serum. The presence of these antibodies of course means that blood of all normal ABO phenotypes is incompatible. The red cells and serum of these people type as group O; fortunately the anti-H shows its presence during antibody screening (it will react with all group O cells, but is not an autoantibody) and also during compatibility testing.

2.2 Antibodies of the ABO System

Anti-A and anti-B are predominantly naturally occurring IgM antibodies. They agglutinate cells particularly well at low temperature but also do so at 37 °C. *In vivo* they also cause agglutination; the agglutinates characteristically become trapped by hepatic reticuloendothelial cells, and most importantly fix complement, resulting in intravascular haemolysis. The biological potency of ABO alloantibodies is such that transfusions must always be ABO compatible. The aggressive destruction of transfused ABO-incompatible cells is the major cause of transfusion morbidity and mortality. ABO-incompatible transfusions mainly arise from organizational mishaps (see chapter 25, section 2) but serological errors can also occur.

The mechanisms underlying antibody-mediated haemolysis are discussed in section 5. IgG anti-A and anti-B also occur as immune antibodies, particularly in group O subjects. They are probably of most importance as a cause of mild haemolytic disease of the newborn because, unlike IgM anti-A and anti-B antibodies, placental transfer can occur.

2.3 Transfusion Amongst ABO Groups

It would be safest and least confusing to all concerned to restrict transfusions of red cells solely to those in which the donor and recipient ABO group are identical. In that way simple instructions could be laid down to ensure the safety of transfusion procedures. Unfortunately, the scarcity of some ABO groups means that these rules cannot always be adhered to and clinical and serological common sense must therefore be brought to bear on the situation.

Group O red cells are suitable for all recipients but the anti-A, B in the plasma could, if given in large doses, potentially destroy the red cells of group A or group B recipients. This risk should be borne in mind particularly when group O donations from donors of African origin are used. High-titre haemolysins (causing complete lysis of A and/or B cells) have for example been reported in over 30% of Nigerian donors.[4]

In practice:

(1) Most transfusion centres screen and identify those donations with high-titre antibodies which could have haemolytic effects in non-group O recipients (e.g. Apheresis platelets, transfusions for neonates). Such donations should only be used for group O recipients.
(2) The antibody content of the first few units of blood will be both diluted and neutralized by secreted A and B substance in the recipient plasma.
(3) Donor plasma containing the offending antibodies will have already been removed from many currently available red cell components.

Transfusion of group O red cells to recipients of other groups should not, however, be used too liberally. If this happened to any great extent, the supplies to group O recipients, particularly those who are Rh negative, would be prejudiced. Use of group O blood is most likely to be required (in European populations) for:

(1) Transfusion of group B patients where group B blood is unavailable.
(2) Where transfusion is urgent and or where there are serological uncertainties regarding the patient's ABO status, i.e. group A variants.

Group A blood should be given to group AB patients if AB blood is lacking. Group O or preferably group B red cells could be given to A_2B recipients.

If blood of the patient's own ABO group is available it is probably best to use this initially. If changeover is required it is advisable to continue using the substituted group until the transfusion episode is over. *The transfusion set must be changed when blood of an alternative group is started.*

2.4 Problems Encountered during ABO Grouping

In the majority of cases ABO grouping is straightforward and the results are clear and unequivocal. The cell and serum grouping results must agree, and confirmation of this provides extra security to the procedure. Most ABO grouping problems are uncovered when cell and serum grouping results show discrepancies. A fascinating variety of ABO grouping anomalies have been described[5] and these include the following:

(1) *ABO antigen expression can be reduced.* Examples include the weak inherited variants of A and B antigens. Weakened expression of A or B antigens is typical of neonates and sometimes also occurs in the elderly; it is found occasionally in myeloid leukaemias, in which instance it probably reflects disordered erythroid cell development.

(2) *Alteration of ABO antigens* can occur as an acquired abnormality and this may be sufficiently pronounced to cause an apparent change in the ABO group. Acquired B antigens sometimes appear in leukaemia and they may also result from the actions of enzymes released from intestinal bacteria in certain bowel disorders. In these latter instances the bacterial enzymes appear to produce B substance from ABH precursor material in a similar manner to the normal B transferases of group B individuals.

(3) ABO alloantibodies are lacking in neonates (apart from those of maternal origin) and can be reduced in the elderly and in many acquired states of immunodeficiency.

(4) There may be *unexpected agglutinins* in sera directed against other blood group systems and these can produce false positive serum grouping tests. The cold agglutinins of anti-I specificity are a common example of this problem. The occurrence of other saline antibodies, e.g. anti-M reacting against reagent cells which happen to be M positive, can also be misinterpreted as ABO reactions.

(5) There may be *mixed red cell populations* as, for example, following transfusion of group O blood to non-O recipients. Rare causes of mixed cell populations being produced by the bone marrow include *mosaics* and *chimeras.*[6,7] In the former both cell populations are derived from a single zygote either as an inherited anomaly or arising sometime later as a result of somatic mutation. The appearance of red cells showing altered ABO groups or Tn polyagglutinability (see section 4.9) sometimes found in leukaemia are examples of mosaics arising from somatic mutation. Chimeras represent the haemopoietic output from two separate zygotes and may arise naturally from stem cell exchanges between the circulatory systems of dizygotic twins or, in a more modern fashion, following bone marrow transplantation.

(6) Erroneous ABO grouping results may be obtained with sera which promote *rouleaux* (e.g. in myeloma and chronic inflammatory states) and sometimes *following bacterial contamination* of blood samples. The presence of Wharton's jelly on cord cells can cause unexpected agglutination results; the problem is less likely if blood samples are collected using a syringe and needle.

(7) *Polyagglutinable red cells* are produced in some patients with bacterial infections, particularly those due to *Clostridium* species (see section 4.9). These red

cells appear to have been altered by the action of bacterial neuraminidase in such a way that a normally hidden antigen (T antigen) is exposed. The antibody to this antigen is present in virtually all adult sera; thus cells from such patients become agglutinated by any serum to which they are added. The red cells therefore group as AB during routine grouping tests but unlike AB cells they will also be agglutinated by AB serum. Monoclonal ABO grouping reagents are of course serum free and will provide accurate results with poly-agglutinable cells.

3 THE RH BLOOD GROUPS

3.1 Rh Antigens

All blood donors and recipients are classified according to their Rh D antigen status. The Rh D antigen stands out as the most conspicuously immunogenic of all the non-ABO blood group systems and for this reason Rh D-positive blood is not given to Rh D-negative individuals unless the risks associated with immunization are outweighed by other circumstances. In many countries (e.g. China, where only 0.2% are rr) the majority of the population are Rh D positive and Rh immunization and Rh D haemolytic disease are therefore rare.

The Rh D antigen is the product of one of a series of three closely linked alleles. The products of the principal allelic pairs are designated:

C and c
D and d ('d', the original presumed antithesis to Rh D, has now been shown not to exist)
E and e

The Rh phenotype is of course determined by the product of haplotypes of maternal and paternal origin. Each haplotype will include one gene of each from the three allelic pairs. Thus *CDe* and *cde* are examples of genetic haplotypes; a person inheriting one of each of these will be typed serologically positive for C, c,

Table 2 Rh system: major genotype frequencies

Genotype	Fisher–Race notation	Incidence (%)
Rh positive		
CDe/cde	R^1r	32
CDe/CDe	R^1R^1	18
CDe/cDE	R^1R^2	12
cDE/cde	R^2r	11
cDE/cDE	R^2R^2	2
cDe/cde	R^0r	2*
Rh negative		
cde/cde	rr	15

*42% in African populations.

D and e antigens. Although D is strongly immunogenic the antigenic nature of d has not been demonstrated; C, c, E, e are also but to a much lesser extent immunogenic to recipients lacking the respective antigens. There is no 'dominance' or 'recessiveness' for the genes C, c, E or e as might be implied by the nomenclature. A shorthand notation devised by Fisher and Race is used in referring to Rh haplotypes and genotypes and use of this shorthand notation is invaluable during routine spoken and written communication. The common European Rh genotypes are listed in Table 2. with their frequencies and the conventionally used shorthand notation. It should be clear from consideration of how haplotypes are inherited that Rh-negative children are perfectly possible even when both parents are Rh D positive, provided that they are heterozygous for the gene expressing D antigen.

3.2 Rh Antibodies

Rh antibodies (e.g. anti-D, -C, -c, -e) are usually stimulated as a result of transfusion or by fetomaternal leaks during pregnancy. These are usually IgG antibodies reacting well by enzyme and antiglobulin techniques. They can cause both haemolytic transfusion reactions and haemolytic disease of the newborn. Occasionally 'naturally occurring' IgM saline agglutinins occur; anti-E is the most frequent example. Further details of Rh antibodies are given in Table 8. The frequency of immunization to Rh antigens other than D is so low that it is unnecessary to match donors and recipients for these antigens during routine transfusions.

3.3   Weakened or Incomplete Expression of the D Antigen: Rh D^u/D Variants

In European populations approximately 85% type as Rh D positive and 15% as Rh D negative. About 0.2% (1.5% of Rh D negatives) may have a weak D antigen which is detected by the more sensitive D grouping techniques (e.g. antiglobulin methods) but may be missed by some routine methods.

Weakened or variant D antigens encompass a spectrum of unusual conditions in which there are either fewer D antigen sites on the cell surface (D^u) or, less commonly, a portion of the D antigen complex is missing (D variant). There is some potential clinical importance in the distinction because those deficient in a portion of the D antigen can, and occasionally do, make an antibody against the part they lack. These are discovered by the paradoxical finding of an apparent anti-D antibody in an Rh D-positive individual. On analysis the anti-D is found to react only against a portion of the antigen structure. Anti-D^B is one such example formed by people lacking a portion (B) of the full D antigen and forming anti-D^B when confronted by appropriate antigenic challenge. This terminology has been replaced by one in which D variants are classified into six categories D^{I-VI}, category D^{VI} being almost equivalent to D^B.

In practice decisions have to be taken whether to regard individuals in whom the D antigen is weakly expressed as Rh D positive or negative. D^u red cells have traditionally been defined as being D positive by antiglobulin tests (or other tests of equivalent sensitivity, e.g. automated grouping methods).

Although D^u red cells are much less immunogenic than D red cells (and probably also less so than other Rh antigens such as C or c), it is customary to regard D^u blood donors as Rh D positive and their donations are not used for Rh D-negative recipients. Accelerated destruction of D^u cells has been shown to take place after transfusion to patients with anti-D.

There is no need to make special efforts to determine the D^u status of hospital patients. They may well be typed as Rh D negative by the grouping methods in routine use. Their D^u status would only be discovered if it were customary practice for the laboratory concerned to perform confirmatory antiglobulin D testing on apparently D-negative patients. This distinction is in fact unnecessary since patients will come to no harm if regarded as D negative; *it is in fact far more important for the blood bank to ensure that all D-positive groups are confirmed as correct.* It seems in fact to be clinically immaterial whether D^u patients receive Rh D-positive or negative blood, since they will not be capable of anti-D formation. Mothers that have for some reason (e.g. previous blood donations) already been identified as D^u do not need anti-D prophylaxis; the anti-D would probably be absorbed on to the D^u cells in any case. On the other hand, the time and expense required to identify the D^u mothers from amongst those who were at first thought to be Rh negative is hardly justified by the savings in anti-D administration.

3.4 Less Common Rh Antigens and Antibodies

Although most individuals possess one of the common Rh genotypes shown in Table 2, the Rh blood group system is in fact highly complex and a large number of rare variants have been discovered amongst the products of the Rh genes. These usually come to light when unexpected antibodies are found during compatibility testing and which are subsequently shown to have specificities directed against unusual Rh antigens.

Certain of these antibodies, for example anti-C^W against an uncommon allele, C^W, at the C/c locus and anti-V and -VS, found most frequently in negroes against a ce-like antigen, may be missed if the corresponding antigens are not present on the cells used for antibody screening. These antibodies are therefore sometimes discovered only during the cross-match.

Anti-C+D sometimes causes confusion when it appears in pregnancies in which the only expected antigenic source is D positive but C negative. The antibody is in fact anti-G which reacts against an immunochemical configuration shared by both the C and D antigens.

3.5 Practical Problems in Rh D Grouping

Laboratory errors in which Rh D-negative patients are erroneously grouped as Rh D positive are potentially serious and not as infrequent as they should be. This is discussed in chapter 25, section 2.2. Some of these errors stem from mistakes in reading or recording results. In other cases false positive results occur, with red cells showing positive direct antiglobulin results such as might occur in warm autoimmune haemolytic anaemias or with cord cells in cases of haemolytic disease.

3.6   The 'Rh-negative' Blood Donor

Confusing inconsistencies have arisen as a result of the various practices for assigning Rh-negative status to blood donors.[8] In some countries, donations must be not only D negative but would also be tested and shown to be C negative and E negative as well. This latter requirement (to be C− and E−) is now being dropped in the UK and the Rh-negative donor is more specifically designated as Rh D negative. In most countries donors should be unreactive in tests for D^u— this entails antiglobulin D typing unless modern monoclonal reagents are used. Most automated blood-grouping systems can be made sufficiently sensitive to identify D^u as D positive. Generally, use of two D grouping reagents is mandated and these should be reactive with most commonly found D variants (see section 3.3).

4   OTHER BLOOD GROUP SYSTEMS

4.1   Kell Blood Groups

Two relatively common alleles denoted by K (Kell) and k (Cellano) at one locus account for the most important antigens in this system (Table 3). K is a potent antigen; the corresponding antibody (anti-K) is an important cause of transfusion reactions and also causes haemolytic disease of the newborn.

Transfusion of K+ blood carries around a 5% chance of eliciting anti-K (anti-Kell in common parlance) formation in *kk* 'Kell-negative' recipients. Since only one in 10 randomly selected units of (European) blood will be K+, the formation of anti-K, once recognized, does not cause difficulties in finding compatible blood. In contrast, the formation of anti-Cellano (k) in the rare *KK* individuals is more problematic; fewer than one in 500 random donor units will be compatible. The incidence of Kell immunization in normal practice is not high enough to warrant routine matching prior to transfusion. K− group O Rh-negative units should, however, be selected for emergency obstetric transfusions because anti-K is one of the more common clinically important antibodies found in pregnancy.

The Kell system also includes several closely linked allelic antigens which occasionally give rise to transfusion problems. Kp^a, for example, is an uncommon antigen found in less than 2% of Europeans and is extremely rare in black populations. The allelic gene product Kp^b is conversely very common in Europeans and is universally present in negroid bloods. Provision of Kp(a+b−) blood for Kp(b−) patients with anti-Kp^b is correspondingly difficult. Anti-Kp^b is a good example of an antibody against a 'high frequency antigen' for which the assistance of rare donor panels may be required (see chapter 25, section 7). Js^a and Js^b are also allelic

Table 3 Common Kell phenotypes

Genotype	Phenotype	Frequency (%)	Antithetical antibodies
kk	'Kell negative'	90 (Europeans) 98 (black Africans) 100 (Indo-China)	Anti-K (Kell)
Kk	'Kell positive'	Approx. 10 (Europeans) 2 (black Africans)	
KK	'Kell positive'	0.2 (Europeans) 0.1 (black Africans)	Anti-k (Cellano)

gene products of the Kell locus which occasionally present a somewhat similar problem. Around 1% of the negroid population (but virtually no Europeans) are Js(b−) and homozygous for the Js^a antigen. Clearly, it is only worthwhile screening black donor samples for compatible blood. These people have the capacity to form anti-Js^b following the stimulus of transfusions or pregnancy.

Individuals of the rare Ko phenotype lack all known Kell antigens and as a consequence develop antibodies (anti-Ku) reactive against all red cells except those of the same Ko group.

Kell antibodies are usually 'immune' non-complement-fixing IgG antibodies, although a minority do fix complement. In either case they are detected best by the antiglobulin test. Unfortunately a small proportion of anti-K antibodies, usually those of low titre, may not be detected by automated antibody screening systems.

4.2 The Duffy Blood Groups

Two Duffy antigens, Fy^a and Fy^b, represent the products of the common alleles. Anti-Fy^a can cause serious transfusion reactions and also occasional cases of haemolytic disease of the newborn. In contrast anti-Fy^b seems to be a much less potent antibody. Duffy antibodies are typically immune IgG non-complement-fixing antibodies; some, however, are complement fixing: they are detected well by antiglobulin methods.

The Duffy antigen site appears to be essential for enabling malarial parasites (particularly *Plasmodium vivax*) to enter and parasitize red cells. This may explain the high frequency of the relatively plasmodium-resistant Fy(a−b−) phenotype in African populations.

4.3 Kidd Blood Groups

The Kidd system comprises the principal alleles Jk^a and Jk^b; their frequencies and the most frequently encountered antithetical antibodies are listed in Table 5.

Table 4 Duffy antigens and antibodies

Phenotype	Frequency (%)	Antithetical antibody
Fy(a+b−)	Europeans 17 African blacks 10[*]	Anti-Fy^b (rare)
Fy(a−b+)	Europeans 34 African blacks 20[*]	Anti-Fy^a
Fy(a+b+)	Europeans 40 African blacks 1[*]	
Fy(a−b−)	Europeans very rare African blacks 69[*]	Anti-Fy^3

[*]Duffy antibodies are formed much less frequently in blacks than in Europeans.

Kidd antibodies (principally anti-Jk^a) are notorious causes of delayed, but nevertheless serious, haemolytic transfusion reactions. They are typically IgG complement-fixing antibodies causing intravascular haemolysis of incompatible transfused red cells. Four main problems hinder the prevention of these haemolytic transfusion reactions:

(1) The antibodies *in vivo* tend to fall to undetectable levels but nevertheless are boosted rapidly following transfusion to cause destruction of incompatible cells.
(2) The antibodies are most reliably detected by the antiglobulin reaction and best when reagents are used which contain anti-complement activity. The patient's serum is also best tested soon after collection before complement levels fall. The difficulties in detection of Kidd antibodies form one of the major justifications for including an anti-complement component in antiglobulin reagents for compatibility testing.[9]
(3) Kidd antibodies appear to deteriorate during serum storage.
(4) Reactions against heterozygous cells may easily be missed.

Table 5 Kidd blood group system antigens and antibodies

Phenotype	Frequency	Antithetical antibody
Jk(a+b−)	27	Anti-Jk^b
Jk(a+b+)	50	
Jk(a−b+)	23	Anti-Jk^a
JK(a−b−)	Very rare	

The Kidd blood group system also has a 'null' type, Jk(a−b−), present in close to 1% of Chinese and Polynesians, a proportion of whom form anti-Jk^{a+b} (anti-Jk3).

Table 6 Antigens of the MNSs
blood group systems

Genotype	Frequency (%)
MM	30
MN	50
NN	20
SS	10
ss	46
Ss	44

This is a further example of an antibody against a high frequency 'public' antigen implicated in transfusion reactions and haemolytic disease of the newborn. In areas where this problem is found (which include Australia and New Zealand) inclusion of Jk(a−b−) cells within cell panels is useful.

4.4   MNSs and U Blood Groups

M and N are allelic gene products; S and s also represent alleles closely linked to the MN locus. The U antigen is apparently associated with the Ss alleles since most U-negative people are also S and s negative. The U antigen is found in all individuals of white races but is lacking in around 1% of black people. Anti-U has caused transfusion reactions and haemolytic disease of the newborn.

Anti-M, anti-N and anti-S are usually non-haemolytic IgM naturally occurring cold agglutinins of little or no clinical significance. Warm-reacting antibodies should, however, be taken seriously; these are often immune, complement-fixing IgG antibodies. The rare anti-s usually comes into this latter category. Anti-N is also an uncommon antibody but has, intriguingly, been found most often in renal dialysis patients. It appeared that residual formalin used during sterilization of dialysis equipment, altered the MN antigens of the patient's red cells to create a different immunogenic 'N-like' antigen and as a result stimulated production of an anti-'N-like' antibody. This reacted with the N antigen present or with normal N+ red cells, including the patient's own cells if these were N+.

4.5   P Blood Groups

The various antigens of the P blood group system are rarely of practical clinical importance. In the laboratory cold-reacting anti-P_1 antibodies are very common causes of difficulty during compatibility testing but clinically destructive examples reacting at 37 °C are extremely rare. Anti-P_1 is formed in the 20% or so of the population who are P_1 negative (these are mostly P_2); the antibodies give variable reactions with P_1 cells, which are classed thereby as P_1 (strong) or P_1 (weak). Once a patient is identified as having anti-P_1 it is sufficient to transfuse randomly selected units which are cross-match compatible but have not, as is usual with most other antigen systems, been selected as previously typed and shown to be P_1 negative. 'Cold' anti-P_1 antibodies do not appear to be boosted by transfusion to form clinically haemolytic antibodies.[10]

The rare antibodies against variants of the P blood group system do appear to be clinically important. Individuals of a phenotype designated 'p' can form an immune IgG clinically haemolytic antibody sometimes labelled anti-Tj^a (after the first identified patient) or alternatively anti-P+P_1+p^k (the various identifiable antigenic products of the P locus). This antibody or the similar anti-P has been associated with early spontaneous abortions in mothers with the p or p^k blood groups respectively, presumably as a result of transplacental passage of IgG antibody lethal to the embryo.[11,12] Patients with *paroxysmal cold haemoglobinuria* appear to have an anti-P-like autoantibody (Donath–Landsteiner antibody) which shows an unusual biphasic serological activity. Antibody is bound *in vitro* at low temperatures but complement fixation and red cell lysis follow rewarming of the cell serum mixture. The clinical symptoms of this condition can probably be explained by operation of a similar mechanism *in vivo*.

4.6 Lutheran Blood Groups

This antigen system is rarely of clinical importance. The Lu(a+b+) phenotype present in around 8% of the population and the Lu(a−b+) present in 92% of the population are the most common gene products. The Lu^a antigen, although stimulating the most common antibody, is in fact poorly immunogenic and the antibodies are usually IgM 'saline' agglutinins. Only rarely have anti-Lu^a antibodies caused transfusion reactions or haemolytic disease of the newborn. Anti-Lu^a shows dosage effects, reacting best with homozygous cells; but since these are excessively rare most examples of anti-Lu^a remain undetected. Anti-Lu^b, which can only be formed in the 0.2% of population that is Lu(b−), does appear to have greater haemolytic activity.

4.7 Lewis Blood Groups

Lewis antigens

The antigens of the Lewis blood group system along with the ABO antigens have proved fascinating subjects for the study of immunogenetics and blood group biochemistry. In clinical terms, however, the Lewis system is not of major importance, but Lewis antibodies are relatively common and do cause problems during compatibility testing. The Lewis antigens are not formed primarily on the red cell membrane but are secreted by other tissues into body fluids including plasma. Interaction between the products of a series of genes—the *Lewis, H and secretor genes*—determines the immunochemical nature of the final Lewis antigens. These plasma antigens are adsorbed from the plasma on to the red cells, but also dissociate readily from the red cell surface following transfusion to 'antigen-negative' individuals.

The two antigens Le^a and Le^b are, somewhat confusingly, not allelic products. The Le^b antigen is formed *from* Le^a by interaction of the *H and secretor genes*. There are three phenotypes:

(1) Individuals having red cells of Le(a−b+) phenotype (72% of Europeans, 55% of Blacks) have their Lewis precursor plasma substance converted by the combined action of *H and secretor genes* via Le^a to Le^b but leaving some residual unconverted Le^a. Le^b is adsorbed on to the red cells but some Le^a and larger amounts of Le^b remain in the plasma.

(2) Red cells typing as Le(a+b−) (22% of Europeans) result when secretor gene activity is absent (non-secretors). As a result H gene activity has no opportunity to affect the Lewis precursor substance, which is therefore converted by Lewis gene enzymes to Le^a substance alone. Le^a substance is adsorbed on to the red cells and is also present in the plasma.

(3) The Le(a−b−) phenotype, accounting for 6% of Europeans and 22% of Blacks, results from complete absence of the Lewis genes. Apparent Le(a−b−) phenotypes due to unexplained weakening of Lewis antigen expression are common during pregnancy and also characteristic of the red cells of newborn infants.

Lewis antibodies

These are generally found in genetically Le(a−b−) people as well as during pregnancy when Lewis antigens are weakened. Anti-Le^a is commonest and occurs usually as IgM complement-fixing antibody. In this form it cannot cause haemolytic disease, which is fortunate since it is one of the antibodies most frequently encountered during examination of antenatal sera. Anti-Le^a cannot be made by Le(a−b+) individuals since, as described above, these people have residual Le^a substance in their plasma. Although typically room temperature-acting saline agglutinins, many examples of anti-Le^a fix complement and react by the antiglobulin technique. These must be considered potentially haemolytic, and rare haemolytic transfusion reactions due to anti-Le^a have been described. In contrast, anti-Le^b seems to be clinically quite unimportant either when it occurs alone or when it is found together with anti-Le^a. It is therefore unnecessary to provide Le(b−) blood for patients with anti-Le^b or for those with both anti-Le^a and anti-Le^b. This is particularly true for patients of blood groups A and B since anti-Le^b sera frequently contain an anti-H component and hence react more strongly with group O red cells.

Following transfusion of Le(a+) red cells in the presence of anti-Le^a two-component red cell survival curves have been observed. A minority of cells are destroyed rapidly from complement-mediated intravascular haemolysis. The remaining cells are cleared more slowly as complement uptake proceeds only to the C3b binding stage and the affected red cells are picked up by reticuloendothelial macrophages.

Two other facts also diminish the importance of anti-Le^a during transfusion:

(1) Anti-Le^a can be neutralized by plasma transfusions from all but Le(a−b−) donors. This will occur to a considerable extent during whole blood

transfusions but not of course as effectively with red cell concentrate suspensions.

(2) Le(a+) red cells become Le(a−) following transfusion to Le(a−) recipients due to loss of the passively adsorbed antigen. The converse can also be seen to occur when Le(a−) red cells acquire Le^a substance by passive uptake from the plasma of Le(a+) individuals.

Most, but not all, transfusion laboratories type and supply Le(a−) blood for patients with anti-Le^a. An American survey[13] showed only 11.1% transfused blood selected by cross-match alone, while the majority (56%) required Le(a−) blood to be supplied *before* compatibility testing was undertaken. Experience, however, has clearly indicated the former practice to be perfectly safe. The selection of Lewis antigen-negative blood prior to compatibility testing is wasteful of both time and materials.[14,15]

It is interesting to note that use of the patient's serum only selects blood that is apparently Le(a−) and does not differentiate between Le(a−b+) and Le(a−b−) donations. Those Le(a−b+) cells could in fact have some residual Le^a on the red cell surface which may not easily be detectable with anti-Le^a sera. This fact appears to be of little practical importance. If, however, *both* anti-Le^a and anti-Le^b are present too few donations (6%) will be cross-match compatible. It may therefore be most practicable to provide screened Le(a−) blood (80% of available donations) and discount the clinical significance of the anti-Le^b. Even if there is reluctance to ignore the presence of anti-Le^b, patients with anti-Le^b may certainly be transfused with cross-match-compatible blood which does not require to have been previously shown to be Le(b−).

4.8 The I/i Antigens

Most adults have red cells bearing the I antigen; a very small number of people are I negative but carry i antigen. Red cells of the newborn initially express i antigen alone but later this is replaced as the red cells develop progressively stronger expression of the I antigen. Antibodies of the I/i system are relatively common and comprise:

(1) Low-titre cold autoagglutinins reacting against I, or combined HI antigens. These can be troublesome during low temperature serology tests or may lead to unwanted complement (C4) sensitization of cold-stored red cells.

(2) High-titre cold agglutinins reacting similarly to the above, but of much greater potency; cause 'cold' autoimmune haemolytic anaemias. These antibodies will react with all antibody panel cells, with the patient's own cells or with units selected for transfusion. The thermal range of these cold antibodies rarely extends to as high as 37 °C. Once their specificity and thermal range have been identified and the presence of other alloantibodies has been excluded, transfusions of apparently incompatible blood can be given safely. If the serum for compatibility testing is allowed to stand 'cold' on the cells some degree of autoabsorption of the anti-I will occur which may facilitate compatibility testing. Screening and compatibility testing must of course be performed at

37 °C. The use of monospecific anti-IgG antiglobulin reagents can unmask the simultaneous presence of alloantibodies. Cold agglutinating autoantibodies are common causes of ABO grouping difficulties. Their existence may be disclosed by:

(a) The autocontrol (patient's cells and patient's serum) reaction will be positive.

(b) The serum will agglutinate all adult group O cells.

(c) The cell group and serum group results will not agree.

(3) Auto anti-i is a cold agglutinin frequently associated with infectious mononucleosis. In contrast to anti-I it reacts well with cord blood and poorly with adult red cells.

(4) Rare I-negative adults can form a haemolytic anti-I. They must be transfused with I−, i+ blood.

4.9 Miscellaneous Antigen/Antibody Problems

(1) *Anti-Wr^a (Wright system)* is a fairly common antibody in serum, occurring with a frequency of approximately 2%. The source of the stimulation is unknown since the incidence of the Wr^a antigen is rare (below 0.01%). As a result of the rarity of Wr(a+) red cells the antibody remains undetected during most routine serological procedures but it is nevertheless of importance when it occurs as a contaminant in sera to be selected for use as reagents. Anti-Wr^a occurring as a contaminant of typing antisera (e.g. anti-D) would give occasional false positive reactions when Rh D-negative, Wr(a+) red cells are encountered. For this reason reagents are screened to exclude the presence of this and other similarly troublesome antibodies. Anti-Wr^a may be clinically haemolytic, but for the reasons mentioned above it is not likely to be detected during antibody screening although its presence may be disclosed during the cross-match. The incidence of haemolytic transfusion reactions must be very small since only 2% of patients possess the antibody and less than 0.01% of donations are Wr(a+). The determination of the specificities of antibodies of this nature requires the assistance of a reference laboratory possessing a panel of both Wr(a+) and Wr(a−) cells.

(2) Anti-Vw, -M^g and a variety of other antibodies reacting against rare antigens can present similar difficulties.

(3) Anti-Yt^a (Cartwright) is an example of an uncommon antibody reacting against the high-frequency Yt^a antigen. Cross-match compatible blood is obviously difficult to obtain but it appears that at least some examples of anti-Yt^a are relatively innocuous.

(4) Anti-Sd^a (Sid) is a fairly common antibody and the antigen Sd^a is present to a highly variable degree on around 90% of red cell samples. The antibody is a common cause of weak indeterminate reactions encountered during screening and compatibility testing but has not been found to be of any clinical importance.

(5) A variety of antibodies have been described which react with both leucocyte and red cell antigens and sometimes also with antigenic material present in

plasma. Some of these are weakly reactive but extend to high dilutions (HTLA—high-titre low-avidity antibodies). Examples of these include antibodies which are discovered as cross-matching problems but are not usually capable of causing haemolysis. Expert advice is required for their analysis and the assessment of their clinical significance.

(6) *Polyagglutinable cells*: this term is applied to pathologically altered red cells which are agglutinated by all human serum samples and so cannot be grouped by routine serological methods. Examples include:
   (a) *T activation*: all red cells carry the T antigen but this remains hidden unless exposed by the action of neuraminidase, which removes sialic acid from the red cell surface. Infection with neuraminidase-producing bacteria, e.g. *Clostridium* species, can result in exposure of the T antigen. All adult human sera (and serum-based reagents) contain anti-T and agglutinate T-activated red cells, making normal serological studies impossible. There may even be a state of autoimmune haemolysis. Donor blood (containing anti-T in the plasma) cannot be transfused to such patients and washed red cells are used instead. This condition is acquired as a result of bacterial infection and returns to normal with recovery of the patient.
   (b) Tn activation is serologically similar (see Section 2.4) but appears to result from a permanent change in red cell antigenic characteristics. The cause is unknown but appears to be related to a somatic mutation arising in the erythroid precursor cells.[16]
   (c) Red cells showing very strong expression of the Sid antigen (known as 'Cad' cells) are agglutinated by the small amounts of anti-Sd^a (Sid) which are present in most sera.

(7) *Polyagglutinating sera* are those which agglutinate virtually all examples of red cells. There are various causes:
   (a) Potent cold agglutinins of anti-I or HI specificity.
   (b) Sera found in Bombay, Rh null, Ko and similar subjects.
   (c) Sera reacting against very high-frequency antigens (e.g. anti-Kp^b, anti-Lan, both directed against antigens with gene frequencies greater than 0.9998).

5 CLINICAL SIGNIFICANCE OF RED CELL ANTIBODIES: DESTRUCTION OF INCOMPATIBLE TRANSFUSED RED CELLS[17]

5.1 Intravascular Haemolysis

Antibody-mediated destruction of red cells *within* the circulation (intravascular destruction) is the most severe complication of incompatible transfusions. *Intravascular destruction* occurs when antibody binding is followed by the complete sequence of complement action from C1 uptake to final binding of the C789 complex which then enzymically damages and penetrates the red cell membrane. Holes in the red cell membrane created in this way allow entry of sodium and water; red cells then rupture, liberating haemoglobin and leaving stromal fragments.

When antibodies bind to red cells conformational changes occur in their heavy chains so that they become reactive sites for attachment of the first (C1) complement component. In the case of IgG antibodies complement binding can only occur when two molecules (particularly those of IgG subclasses 1 and 3) are bound close enough to allow reaction with both of the two receptor sites on the $C1_q$ portion of the C1 complex molecule. In contrast, uptake of one IgM molecule alone is sufficient to initiate the complement binding sequence probably because each molecule carries 10 paired heavy chains for $C1_q$ interaction.

Intravascular haemolysis is most typically seen with ABO incompatibility. Although it might be expected with other complement fixing antibodies that can lyse red cells *in vitro* it is more usual to find a predominantly extravascular destruction possibly reflecting a slower activation of the complement cascade. Complement-binding IgG antibodies that might show intravascular haemolysis include rare examples of anti-K and anti-Fy^a as well as some anti-Jk^a sera.[9]

The clinical consequences of intravascular haemolysis are discussed in chapter 23, section 2.3.

5.2 Extravascular Haemolysis

The vast majority of alloantibodies do not cause direct lysis of red cells within the circulation. Instead antibody- and complement-coated cells are destroyed within phagocytic cells (macrophages) of the reticuloendothelial system. These macrophages have receptors for the complement component C3b and also for the Fc portions of IgG1 and IgG3 but cells with bound IgM and IgA are not entrapped.

Complement uptake on to the stage of C3b alone results in sequestration and intracellular destruction of red cells but does not cause intravascular haemolysis. Complement coated red cells are cleared from the circulation predominantly by *hepatic* macrophages. Plasma C3b inactivator cleaves C3b on uncaptured freely circulating red cells to remove a portion (C3c) and leave behind C3d. A similar process affects the C4b on circulating cells, resulting in its conversion to C4d. Agglutinating IgM antibodies which are not complement fixing or capable of complete haemolysis also cause red cells to be trapped predominantly by hepatic macrophages.

In contrast, IgG antibody binding alone, not followed by complement uptake, results in capture and phagocytosis of red cells by *splenic* macrophages during destruction of incompatible blood. There may, however, be some intravascular liberation of haemoglobin if the reticuloendothelial system is overwhelmed by the presence of large amounts of incompatible blood.

Some affected red cells may escape complete phagocytosis but nevertheless still lose those portions of their membrane carrying bound antibody or complement and as a result become irregular in size or shape. Red cell damage can show in other ways; antibody- or complement-coated cells may, for example, suffer from failure of the membrane sodium pump and in consequence become spherocytes more liable to phagocytosis. Those incompatible red cells surviving immediate destruction and still remaining in the circulation can be identified by their positive reaction in the direct antiglobulin test. This reaction will be due either to the presence of membrane-bound IgG or C3d detected by the anti-IgG and anti-C3d respectively in antiglobulin sera.

5.3 Red Cell Destruction Without Demonstrable Antibodies

Uncommon instances of destruction of transfused red cells seem to occur even though alloantibodies cannot be demonstrated.[18,19] It may be that there are very small amounts of antibody and that these are just enough to cause red cell damage *in vivo* but not enough to coat red cells with the 200–500 or so molecules required for a positive antiglobulin result. In other cases undefined cellular immunological mechanisms causing red cell destruction may exist.

5.4 Haemolytic Properties of Antibodies

Antibodies reactive below 37 °C

The highest temperature of serological reaction shown by alloantibodies is important in determining their clinical importance. It now seems agreed that only those antibodies showing *in vitro* reactions at close to 37 °C are capable of destruction of transfused cells.[20] Some antibodies can cause agglutination only below 30 °C but at higher temperatures may still cause complement fixation which could lead to haemolysis of transfused blood. Antibodies that may very occasionally show this characteristic include: anti-A_1; anti-H, anti-HI, anti-I; anti-P_1; anti-M, anti-N; anti-Le^a; anti-Lu^a; anti-Vw and anti-Wr^a.

These antibodies are *not*, however, regarded as haemolytic and dangerous *unless* they show antiglobulin reactivity during 37 °C testing.[21] There is a direct correlation between ability to cause red blood cell destruction and ability to cause complement activation at temperatures above 30 °C. Antibodies not active above 30 °C do not cause any destruction whatsoever of transfused cells.[22,23] Agglutinating or complement-binding antibodies reacting between 30 °C and 37 °C may cause some premature destruction of small volumes of incompatible cells but probably do not affect the survival of normal quantities of transfused cells. The red cell destruction rate may parallel the strength of antibody as shown by *in vitro* testing.

Red cell phenotyping for P_1, Le^a, Le^b, M and N is unnecessary when providing blood for patients with cold reactive antibodies of these specificities; an acceptable practice is to use the patient's serum to screen donations using the technique in which the antibody works best. Anti-Le^a of clinical importance is detected by the antiglobulin test (anti-complement) at 37 °C and may also agglutinate at this temperature. Anti-Le^b has never been documented as being significantly haemolytic. The very rare cases of anti-P_1 of clinical importance will also be shown by their activation of complement at 37 °C.

Cold-reactive IgM autoantibodies

These will not usually cause problems during transfusion if patients are kept warm.

Warm-reacting antibodies

It is usually assumed that antibodies reacting at 37 °C do have the capacity to cause *in vivo* haemolysis. This assumption is by no means always valid but accurate prediction cannot be made from the results of currently available *in vitro* tests. There are many factors which appear to determine the degree of red cell destruction by antibodies, some of which have already been discussed. These factors include:

(1) The number of antigen sites on the red cell membrane. Examples of this effect include the more rapid destruction of homozygous red cells (e.g. Jk(a+b−) compared with Jk(a+b+), or of A_1 cells versus A_2 cells).
(2) The quantity of blood transfused. Small volumes may be removed from the circulation more rapidly than larger volumes because sometimes the larger amounts completely neutralize the circulating antibody.
(3) Immunoglobulin class of the antibody. Haemolytic antibodies are usually IgG or IgM; they rarely include examples of IgA and are never IgD or IgE.
(4) Subclass of IgG. IgG1 and IgG3 are most important in this context.
(5) The quantity of antibody bound by red cells as determined by the equilibrium constant of the antibody and its thermal range.
(6) Complement-fixing efficiency of the antibody.
(7) The presence of neutralizing antigen in plasma (e.g. Lewis substances).
(8) The phagocytic efficiency of the patient's reticuloendothelial system.
(9) Antibodies acting by enzyme methods alone are probably low affinity, weakly bound and poorly haemolytic. Only on exceptionally rare occasions are haemolytic transfusion reactions due to 'enzyme only' antibodies believed to have occurred. Some autoimmune haemolytic anaemias appear to be associated with the presence of low-affinity antibodies detectable only by enzyme methods. On some occasions 'enzyme only' antibodies represent the early phase of an immune response and are followed by antiglobulin-reacting antibodies of more definite clinical significance.
(10) The *in vivo* haemolytic activity of antibodies may be related to their *in vitro* performance in facilitating red cell phagocytosis by mononuclear phagocytes[24] or by the antibody dependent cellular cytotoxicity (ADCC) test in which *in vitro* haemolysis, effected by cytotoxic (killer cell) lymphocytes, is measured by radiochromium release from labelled target red cells.[25–27] In general the results of these studies also confirm the greater haemolytic properties of IgG1 and IgG3 antibodies.

6 ANTIBODY DETECTION

Unfortunately, no single serological technique is capable of detecting all blood group antibodies that may be present in sera. Although the antiglobulin test detects virtually all antibodies of clinical significance it also detects many that have no haemolytic potential. There are unfortunately no readily available means of separating these two categories. Antibodies of certain *specificities* (e.g. anti-K, anti-Jk[a]) are well recognized to be associated with haemolytic destruction of transfused red cells, and others (e.g. anti-P_1, anti-Le^a) have in many instances been shown not to be. Examples of these differences have been described in the foregoing sections covering the various blood group antigen systems. The relative merits of the commonly used antibody detection methods are discussed in chapter 25, section 1.3. A clue to the possible specificity of antibodies is often provided by knowledge of:

(1) Their optimal method of reaction.
(2) The incidence of incompatible cells that are found during testing against a randomly selected panel.

Some *in vitro* characteristics of antigen–antibody reactions that may be of practical help are listed below:

(1) Antibodies enhanced by use of proteolytic enzymes:
    Anti-Rh
    Anti-P_1
    Anti-HI
    Anti-Le^a.
(2) Antigens destroyed by enzymes:
    M, N, S
    Duffy (Fy^a).
(3) Antigens that are weak or lacking on red cells of the newborn:
    Lewis system
    I
    P systems
    AB antigens are weaker than in adults.
(4) Common antibodies that are detected best with antiglobulin reagents containing anti-complement activity:
    Anti-Jk^a
    Some examples of anti-Fy^a.
    Some examples of anti-K.

Table 7 Cold antibodies: their sources and the percentage of donor units expected to be found incompatible during cross-match testing

Specificity	Genotype/phenotype of patient	Percentage random units that may be incompatible
Anti-A_1	A_2	75 (gp A)
Anti-HI	autoantibodies	100
Anti-I	autoantibodies	100
Anti-P_1	P_1 – (mostly P_2)	80
Anti-Le^a and Le^b	Le(a–b–)	25 (Le^a)
Anti-Vw and $-Wr^a$	Vw and Wr^a negative	< 1
Anti-M	NN	80
Anti-E	R^1r CDe/cde	30
	R^1R^1 CDe/CDe	
	rr cde/cde	

Table 8 Immune antibodies: their sources and the percentage of donor units expected to be found incompatible during cross-match testing

Antibody	Genotype of patient	Percentage random units that may be incompatible
Anti-D	*rr (cde/cde)*	–
Anti-C+D	*rr (cde/cde)*	–
Anti-C	*rr (cde/cde), R²r, (cDE/cde), R²R² (cDE/cDE)*	85
Anti-c	R^1R^1 *(CDe/CDe)*	80
Anti-cE	R^1R^1 *(CDe/CDe)*	80
Anti-E	R^1R^1 *(CDe/CDe)*	30
	R^1r *(CDe/cde)*	
	rr (cde/cde)	
Anti-K	*kk*	10
Anti-k	*KK*	99.8
Anti-Fy^a	*Fy^b Fy^b*	65
Anti-Jk^a	*Jk^b JK^b*	77
Anti-S	*ss*	55
Anti-s	*SS*	90
Anti-Lu^a*	*Lu^b Lu^b*	8

*Clinically significant examples are rare.

(5) Antibodies causing *in vitro* lysis in the presence of fresh complement:
   Immune anti-A, anti-B
   Anti-Le^a
(6) 'Cold' antibodies. These are usually naturally occurring saline agglutinins. Commonly found examples are listed in Table 7.
(7) Antibodies that are usually immune and may be associated with transfusion reactions and haemolytic disease of the newborn.

7   INCIDENCE OF RED CELL ALLOANTIBODIES

Table 9 lists the antibodies most frequently detected in British patients. Anti-D and to a lesser extent anti-C+D formerly comprised the majority (probably over 60%) of all antibodies. The success of the Rh antenatal prophylactic programme has now reduced the combined incidence of these to around 15% of all antibodies and this should decline still further.

The antibody frequencies recorded by any one laboratory will in practice depend on the type of serology techniques in routine use. Use of room-temperature saline tests clearly increases the incidence of the 'cold' antibodies listed above. Use of sensitive enzyme techniques (e.g. two-stage papain) will increase the proportion of Rh antibodies detected. Use of antiglobulin reagents containing anti-complement activity and of homozygous screening cells will determine the success of anti-Jk^a detection. Antenatal serum samples will provide a disproportionate number of anti-D and Lewis antibodies (up to 30% of total antibodies). Approximately 0.3%[21] of routine blood donors are found to have unexpected

Table 9 Approximate frequencies of antibodies detected during serology screening[*]

Percentage of total antibodies	Specificities
10–15	Anti-D Anti-P_1 Anti-E
5–10	Anti-K Anti-Le^a Anti-HI and anti-I Anti-C+D Anti-A_1
2–5	Anti-Fy^a Anti-M Anti-Le^b Anti-E+K Anti-Le^{a+b} Anti-c+E Anti-C+D+E
1–2	Anti-N Anti-c Anti-S Anti-Jk^a Anti-Lu^a Anti-C^W
Less than	Anti-e Anti-Jk^b Anti-Kp^a Anti-Bg^a Anti-s

[*]Approximately 8–15% of samples contain various mixtures of the antibodies listed.

alloantibodies of identifiable specificities. Not surprisingly antibodies occur more often in antenatal samples as well as those from hospital patients. Incidences from 1.7%[21] to 3.0%[28] have been reported in hospital patients, with 0.5% of patients having antibodies of two specificities and 0.03% having three antibody specificities.

REFERENCES

1 Lewis, M., Antree, G.W.G., Bird E. *et al.* (1990) Blood group terminology 1990. *Vox Sang.*, **58**: 152–169.
2 Yamamoto, F., Clausen, H., White, T., Marken, J. and Hakomori, S. (1990) Molecular genetic basis of the histo-blood group ABO system. *Nature*, **345**: 229–233.

3 Mollison, P.L., Johnson, C.A. and Prior, D.M. (1978) Dose-dependent destruction of A_1 cells by anti-A_1. *Vox Sang.*, **35**: 149–153.
4 Kulkarni, A.G., Ibazebe, R. and Fleming, A.F. (1985) High frequency of anti-A and anti-B haemolysins in certain ethnic groups of Nigeria. *Vox Sang.*, **48**: 39–41.
5 Petz, L.D. and Calhoun, L. (1992) Changing blood types and other immunohematologic surprises. *N. Engl. J. Med.*, **326**: 888–889.
6 Bracey, A.E., McGinniss, M.H., Levine, R.M. and Whang-Peng, J. (1983) Rh mosaicism and aberrant MNSs antigen expression in a patient with chronic myelogenous leukaemia. *Am. J. Clin. Pathol.*, **79**: 397–401.
7 Tippet, P. (1983) Blood group chimeras: a review. *Vox Sang.*, **44**: 333–359.
8 van Rhenen, D.J. (1990) International round table conference on the definition of the Rh-negative blood donor. *Vox Sang.*, **58**: 254–255.
9 Howell, P. and Giles, C.M. (1983) A detailed serological study of five anti-JK^a sera reacting by the antiglobulin technique. *Vox Sang.*, **45**: 129–138.
10 Cheng, M.S. (1984) Potent anti-P_1 following blood transfusions. *Transfusion*, **24**: 183.
11 Yoshida, H., Ito, K., Emi, K. *et al.* (1984) A new therapeutic removal method using antigen-positive red cells: application to a p-incompatible pregnant woman. *Vox Sang.*, **47**: 216.
12 Rock, J.A., Shirey, R.S., Braine, H.G., Ness, P.M., Kickler, T.S. and Niebyl, J.R. (1985) Plasmapheresis for the treatment of repeated early pregnancy wastage associated with anti-P. *Obstet. Gynecol.*, **66**: 57–60.
13 Waheed, A., Kennedy, M.S. and Gerhan, S. (1981) Transfusion significance of Lewis system antibodies. *Transfusion*, **21**: 542.
14 Perkins, H.A., Mallory, D., Bergren, M. and Frank, B. (1982) Lewis incompatibility. *Transfusion*, **22**: 346.
15 Waheed, A., Kennedy, M.S., Gerhan, S. and Senhauser, S. (1981) Transfusion significance of Lewis system antibodies: success in transfusion with crossmatch-compatible blood. *Am. J. Clin. Pathol.* **76**: 294–298.
16 Roxby, D.J., Pfeiffer, M.B., Morley, A.A. and Kirkland, M.A. (1992) Expression of Tn antigen in myelodysplasia, lymphoma, and leukemia. *Transfusion*, **32**: 834–838.
17 Engelfriet, C.P. (1992) The immune destruction of red cells. *Transfusion Med.*, **2**: 1–6.
18 Davey, R.J., Gustafson, M. and Holland, P.V. (1980) Accelerated immune red cell destruction in the absence of serologically detectable alloantibodies. *Transfusion*, **20**: 348.
19 Baldwin, M.L., Barrasso, C., Ness, P.M. and Garratty, G. (1983) A clinically significant erythrocyte antibody detectable only by ^{51}Cr survival studies. *Transfusion*, **23**: 40–44.
20 Aubuchon, J.P. and Anderson, H.J. (1985) Report of transfusions of M- and P_1-positive red cells to a patient with anti-M and anti-P_1. *Transfusion*, **25**: 181.
21 Giblett, E.R. (1977) Blood group alloantibodies: an assessment of some laboratory practices. *Transfusion*, **17**: 299–307.
22 Millison, P.L. (1983) *Blood Transfusion in Clinical Medicine*, 7th edn. London: Blackwell Scientific.
23 Garratty, G. (1982) Correlations between in vitro compatibility testing and in vivo red cell destruction. *Biotest Bull.* **3**: 186–195.
24 Branch, D.R., Gallagher, M.T., Mison, A.P., SySiokHian, A.L. and Petz, L.D. (1984) In vitro determination of red cell alloantibody significance using an assay of monocytemacrophage interaction with sensitized erythrocytes. *Br. J. Haematol.*, **56**: 19–29.
25 Bakacs, T., Kimber, I., Ringwald, G. and Moore, M. (1984) K cell mediated haemolysis: influence of large numbers of unsensitized cells on the antibody-dependent lysis of anti-D sensitized erythrocytes by human lymphocytes. *Br. J. Haematol.*, **57**: 447–455.
26 Urbaniak, S.J. (1979) ADCC (K-cell) lysis of human erythrocytes sensitized with rhesus alloantibodies. I. Investigation of in vitro culture variables. *Br. J. Haematol.*, **42**: 303–314.
27 Urbaniak, S.J. (1979) ADCC (K-cell) lysis of human erythrocytes sensitized with rhesus alloantibodies. II. Investigation into the mechanism of lysis. *Br. J. Haematol.*, **42**: 316–328.
28 Shulman, I.A., Nelson, J.M., Saxena, *et al.* (1982) Experience with the routine use of an abbreviated crossmatch. *Am. J. Clin. Pathol.*, **78**: 178–181.

Part C
BLOOD TRANSFUSION
MATERIALS AND THEIR USES

3
Red Cell Preparations

Historically transfusion began with the use of unmodified whole blood, and this association has remained strong in the minds of many clinicians. There has been reluctance to accept that, for many transfusions, red cell suspensions alone will suffice, and that this change in practice is necessary to allow plasma and the remaining cellular components to be used for other clinical purposes. While it must be admitted that transfusion of whole blood very effectively restores both oxygen transport capacity and blood volume it is also true that normal homeostatic mechanisms are perfectly able to cope with moderate blood loss when this is replaced by transfusion of red cell suspensions combined with other crystalloid or colloid solutions.

1 COMMONLY AVAILABLE RED CELL PREPARATIONS

These are listed and described here for completeness; their uses are described in more detail in other sections.

1.1 Unmodified Stored Whole Blood

The approximate volume of each pack is 500 ml (450 ml of blood and 63 ml of anticoagulant). Stored whole blood provides *both plasma protein and red cell* replenishment. Storage results in progressive decline of the oxygen-carrying capacity but this regenerates within 24–48 hours following transfusion. Labile coagulation factors, principally Factors V and VIII, will also be reduced.[1] Functional platelets and granulocytes are absent but their antigenic residues remain.

This product was once the major item issued from transfusion centres but increased demands for other blood components have now greatly reduced its availability. This should not cause any difficulties in transfusion practice because the alternative red cell preparations, supplemented where necessary by plasma expanders or other blood components, are perfectly adequate replacements.

1.2 Freshly Drawn Blood

Freshly drawn blood (i.e., that collected within the preceding 24 hours) provides *volume, red blood cells with normal oxygen affinity, coagulation factors and platelets*. Where normal platelet function is of paramount importance blood has to be transfused as soon after collection as is practicably possible and certainly prior to refrigeration. Fresh blood was advocated for transfusion during certain haemostatic problems and also during *massive transfusion* (see chapter 12). These indications are no longer accepted in modern transfusion practice. It is rarely possible to complete the mandatory biological tests and finalize full issue requirements for release of blood in its freshest state. The arguments for overriding clinical urgency are now less persuasive against the recognized risks of virus transmission from untested blood. Formula replacement therapy—i.e., protocols entailing predetermined mixes of fresh and stored blood during massive blood replacement have accordingly lost favour. Correct practice is to monitor coagulation tests and platelet counts in order to indicate the severity of problems and to show whether more specific blood component therapy is required.

1.3 Concentrated Red Cell Suspensions (Red Cells)

These have an approximate volume of 300 ml and a haematocrit range of 0.65–0.75. They should be used for transfusion of anaemic patients and also routinely for surgical use in conjunction with plasma expanding agents.

A major clinical objection to the use of concentrated red cells during surgery is the difficulty in obtaining rapid flow rates. This understandably causes frustration and anxiety if bleeding is brisk.

Flow rate depends on:

(1) The haematocrit and blood viscosity. Dilution of the pack contents with isotonic saline* using an appropriately designed 'two pack' administration set will help. It is best if the haematocrit of packs leaving the transfusion centre

---

*No other intravenous fluids should be used for this purpose. Hypotonic fluids cause haemolysis; the calcium in lactated Ringer's will lead to coagulation of the plasma.

does not exceed 0.75. Use of optimal additive packs (see below) will overcome this problem.

(2) The height of the blood pack above the administration site.

(3) The needle gauge. A minimum of 16 G (i.d. 1.4 mm) is desirable for rapid transfusion of adults. Use of minimum length of narrow-gauge catheter tubing is important.

(4) Ensuring blood filters have not become clogged.

(5) The pressure of infusion. This must obviously be carefully supervised as pressurized infusion is dangerous if the poor flow rate is a result of needle displacement.

(6) Ensuring correct placement of the administration set needle and absence of venous spasm. Spasm may be aggravated by undesirably cool blood.

Routine use of concentrated red cell packs is recommended for initial blood replacement during all surgical procedures (see chapter 11). These can be perfectly adequately supplemented by crystalloid solutions to restore plasma volume.

1.4 Optimal Additive Red Cell Suspensions

These are red cell concentrates to which around 100 ml of a nutrient preservative solution have been added (see section 2.3). They are used under the same circumstances as concentrated red cells. Their lower haematocrit permits faster infusion flow rates.

1.5 Leucocyte-depleted Red Cells

Leucocyte-depleted blood components, now almost entirely prepared by filtration methods,[11] are advocated for a variety of purposes (see chapters 4 and 23).

While the evidence of benefit for some situations, e.g. prevention of febrile non-haemolytic transfusion reactions in multi-transfused patients is very good, the use of leucocyte-depleted blood for some of the many other purposes for which it is advocated is far less securely justified. Despite this, filter manufacturers have shown great energy in improving filter performance and in promoting their use. Accordingly, increasingly greater proportions of red cells and platelets are now filtered before transfusion.

Techniques

A moderate degree of leucodepletion (approximately 90% leucocyte removal) can be relatively easily and economically achieved by the spin and filter technique.[2,3] For this procedure blood, preferably of 1–2 weeks storage age, is centrifuged while cold to create a distinct buffy coat layer before being administered through a conventional microaggregate filter. This approach provides a convenient means of preventing the occasional febrile reactions experienced by some transfused patients. However, for most clinical circumstances in which these products are advocated the objective is to achieve the highest possible degree of leucodepletion. For this purpose 'third-generation' filter assemblies packed with cellulose acetate or polyester in either a column or flat-bed configuration are used.[4-6]

These can be highly effective when they are used under optimal circumstances but experience has shown that the filtration process is not a purely simple mechanical procedure.[7] Cell-to-matrix adhesion, cell-to-cell adhesion as well as physical entrapment occur. The success is greatly influenced by variables which may not be easy to control. These include flow rate, temperature and filter-priming efficiency. The age of the component is also important and validation data gained from the use of one component type cannot be extrapolated to cover the use of others. Prior buffy coat removal may be of benefit in achieving good post-filtration leucocyte depletion.

Leucocyte removal targets

Complete leucocyte removal is not possible. Current 'third-generation' filters achieve about a three log reduction leaving $1-5 \times 10^6$ leucocytes per unit. These levels are too low for measurement by conventional automated blood-counting techniques. The larger volume Nageotte counting chamber[8] is commonly used for post-filtration counts at this level—even lower counts and greater precision and differential analysis can be obtained by flow cytometry counting.[9]

When and where should filtration be performed?

Red cell filtration began as a laboratory technique either within hospital blood banks or regional transfusion centres. Because the original methods breached the integrity of the closed blood pack assembly, bacterial sterility could not be guaranteed. This necessitated restriction of the shelf life, usually to 24 hours at 4 °C—a definite inconvenience when several filtered units were required for patients some distance from the preparation centre. The more recent development of filters for bedside use was therefore greatly welcomed.[10] Provision of filtered blood became more timely and convenient and perhaps, though not for the soundest of reasons, use of leucocyte-depleted blood became more widespread. There is now considerable concern that filter performance in actual use may not match their alleged capabilities. This is almost entirely due to difficulties in ensuring consistent technical proficiency outside the laboratory environment and the inability to perform regular quality control. Opinion is still somewhat divided about the value of this procedure. Bedside filtration may be adequate for less stringent control of leucocyte depletion necessary for control of leucocyte-related febrile transfusion reactions (see chapter 23).

If, however, the objective is to obtain consistent and efficient leucocyte depletion, as for example in the prevention of primary HLA alloimmunization, the better quality assurance of the laboratory procedure may be essential. Fortunately, the technology now exists to enable laboratories to perform leucocyte depletion manoeuvres without the risk of microbial contamination. Linkage between filters and plastic pack assemblies can be made in which laboratory tubing segments are joined aseptically using sterile connecting devices. Alternatively, leucocyte depletion can be carried out as a routine at the time of blood collection using a filter placed in the incoming line of the collection pack—the premise being that leucocytes have a variety of adverse effects, not only clinical, but also in terms of the preservation of other blood constituents.

Cell-bound virus transmission (e.g. CMV) appears to be reduced by efficient leucocyte removal. The risk from other viruses, e.g. HIV and HBV, remains unaffected.

2 RED CELL PRESERVATION

The discovery of the ABO groups in 1901 and of the safety of giving ABO group-matched blood provided enormous impetus to the growth of transfusion. Only direct donor-to-recipient transfusions were practicable until the discovery that citrate could prevent the process of coagulation and thereby allow limited storage of blood. A later step was the discovery that the addition of dextrose as a nutrient for the red cells could allow prolongation of the 'shelf life' of stored blood units. The first widely accepted anticoagulant preservative solution was that devised in 1943 by Loutit and Mollison, who demonstrated that an acidified citrate–dextrose combination could be safely autoclaved, thereby providing a sterile anticoagulant and nutrient preservative solution. This solution, widely known as ACD (acid–citrate–dextrose), allowed storage of blood at 1–6 °C for 21 days. Heparin solution (1.0 IU/ml of blood) can be used as a temporary anticoagulant but this does not of course provide any nutrient for the red cells. The development of sterile plastic packs for blood collection led to the rapid abandonment of the use of 'taking sets' and washed reusable glass bottles for blood collection. The sterility of donor blood collection was thereby greatly improved and the use of plastic packs with attached satellites also allowed component production (e.g. platelets, cryoprecipitate and plasma) without jeopardizing microbiological safety. As a result of these developments the formerly serious risk of transfusion of infected blood has now become an extreme rarity.

There has been considerable development in red cell preservative solutions since the introduction of ACD. The following brief discussion on red cell metabolism and the assessment of red cell products is intended to illustrate the background to this work.

2.1 Red Cell Metabolism

Mature red cells retain a portion of their original glycolytic metabolism but most of the other normal cellular metabolic and synthetic activities are lost. Red cell glycolysis begins with *glucose* entry into the cell and ends with *lactic acid* and finally *pyruvic acid* formation (Figure 1); no trace remains of the tricarboxylic citric acid cycle which forms the terminal portion of glucose breakdown in most other

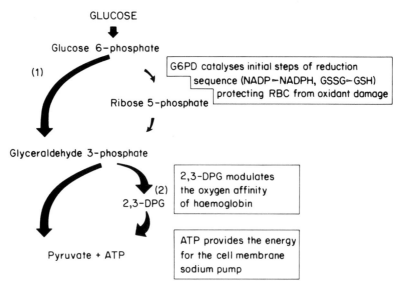

Figure 1   Red cell glycolysis. An outline showing how the three principal functional requirements of the red cells are dependent on continued glycolysis. Over 90% of the glycolytic
activity proceeds via the Embden–Meyerhof pathway.[1] The remaining 10% of glucose
6-phosphate forms a substrate for glucose 6-phosphate dehydrogenase as first step towards
GSH production and generation of reducing activity for protection against oxidant damage.
DPG is synthesized via the Rapoport–Luebering bypass[2] but this occurs at the expense
of 50% of the ATP production that can be obtained by the direct conversion of glycer-
aldehyde 3-phosphate to pyruvate

cells. Protein synthesis ceases at the reticulocyte stage with loss of the nucleus and
dissolution of the remnants of the cytoplasmic RNA.

    Red cell preservative solutions are devised to optimize performance of the resi-
dual glycolytic mechanism. Three principal energy-dependent synthetic functions
are required:

(1) *Adenosine triphosphate (ATP)* is required as energy to fuel the sodium pump of
    the cell membrane. This pump activity maintains high intracellular potassium
    concentrations and excludes extracellular sodium and water. Failure of the
    sodium pump, as a result of the run-down of glycolysis during storage, leads
    to water absorption; the red cells then lose their biconcave shape and become
    spherical. These morphological abnormalities greatly reduce the *deformability* of
    the red cells and they cannot then pass easily through the narrower areas of
    the microcirculation. It is these changes that are probably responsible for the
    progressive loss of post-transfusion viability that occurs as a result of red cell
    storage.
(2) *2,3-Diphosphoglycerate (DPG)* (see chapter 4, section 1.1) is a major determinant
    of the amount of oxygen that can be delivered to tissues by the haemoglobin
    molecule. The depletion of red cell DPG during storage leads to haemoglobin
    becoming abnormally resistant to oxygen release and this reduces the ease of
    tissue oxygenation.

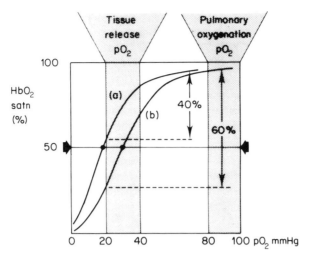

Figure 2 Oxygen dissociation curves (a) of high-affinity stored red cells (P_{50} = 18 mmHg) and (b) of freshly collected red cells (P_{50} = 27 mmHg). The deterioration in the oxygen affinity during storage results in a reduction of tissue oxygen release (from 60% to 40% in the example shown). The horizontal arrows (➤◄) show the 5% saturation scale intersecting each curve at a point (●) corresponding to the P_{50}/

(3) Reduced coenzymes, principally *NADPH* and *NADH*, are required to repair and neutralize oxidant damage to haemoglobin and other cellular or membrane proteins. While this activity has a highly important protective function *in vivo* because of the constant exposure of the circulating red cells to ingested or metabolically derived oxidant materials, it is probably of lesser importance in the sheltered environment of a blood pack.

Glucose (dextrose) in the preservative solution is the fuel for red cell glycolysis. Over 90% of glycolysis proceeds by the anaerobic Embden–Myerhof pathway: a series of enzyme–substrate stages starting with glucose and culminating in production of two molecules of ATP. DPG is produced by a shunt bypass (the Rapoport–Luebering shunt) deviating from a short portion of this enzyme–substrate sequence. The outcome of the whole glycolytic sequence is determined by the metabolic environment within the cell, which in turn is influenced by external physiological demands.

Enzyme cofactors, pH, inorganic phosphate, PO_2, PCO_2 and the concentrations of enzyme substrates or their products all interact to determine that at times ATP synthesis is favoured while under other circumstances DPG production is increased (see Figure 1). As a result of the adaptability to changing circumstances, it has proved difficult to devise red cell preservative solutions that are equally effective in maintaining physiologically desirable levels of these two organic phosphates throughout the period of refrigerated storage.

If *adenine* is added to blood it becomes converted via adenosine monophosphate (AMP) to the diphosphate (ADP) and then eventually to the triphosphate (ATP). This increase in ATP results in a substantial improvement in post-transfusion red cell viability. The extended shelf life made possible by adenine supplementation resulted in a need for increased glucose concentrations in the preservative fluids. This was particularly necessary for red cell concentrates because much of the plasma, together with preservative solution, was removed for component processing.

Plastic materials used for blood pack manufacture must also be examined for any likely effects on blood preservation. There is concern in general about untoward effects of plasticizers leaching into the blood to be transfused. Quite unexpectedly, and for unknown reasons, the plasticizer di-(2-ethylhexyl)phthalate (DEHP) used for polyvinyl chloride (PVC) bag production appears to enhance red cell deformability[12] and post-transfusion survival.

2.2 Quality Assessment of Red Cell Preparations[13]

(1) *Post-transfusion viability*: it is universally accepted that the red cell collection and preservation procedure must allow the mean recovery of at least 75% of transfused red cells in the recipient's circulation by the end of the first 24 hours following transfusion. Since the red cell life-span of normal donors varies considerably it is not surprising that post-transfusion recoveries of donor red cells, determined at any storage age, will also show considerable variability. Post-transfusion viability is measured by following the survival of radiochromium-labelled donor red cells but these studies are only performed during the evaluation stage of new preservative formulations.

(2) *Red cell ATP concentrations* appear to correlate well with post-transfusion recoveries. ATP measurements exceeding 40% of initial levels are taken to indicate that *in vivo* life-span will be acceptable. Both post-transfusion recovery figures and red cell ATP measurements show a continuous decline during storage. The rate of their fall depends on the composition of the preservation medium as discussed above.

(3) A small amount of *haemolysis* occurs during storage of red cells. This may be partly due to exhaustion of ATP in some of the cells but it is probably also caused by the action of proteolytic enzymes derived from leucocytes as well as by constituents of the preservation media. Plasma haemoglobin levels of up to 150 mg per unit are not unusual at the end of the storage period. Visibly haemolysed units have probably been infected or damaged in other ways and these should be investigated urgently. *Haemolysed units must not be transfused.*

(4) *DPG concentrations* decline rapidly after the first week and are negligible by 2 weeks of storage in most media. DPG is, however, regenerated within 24 hours following transfusion. This loss of DPG is probably of little consequence in all but massive transfusions.

(5) The *appearance* of red cell units, particularly of the supernatant plasma, may disclose certain abnormalities. These include lipaemic plasma or plasma discoloured as a result of drugs or other conditions. Donations from donors with cold agglutinins sometimes show very conspicuous red cell agglutination. The presence of *gas bubbles* or *haemolysis* is most important and may indicate bac-

terial contamination of the blood pack. Large *clots* are occasionally found, probably resulting from inadequate mixing during collection.

(6) Red cell concentrates should be subject to regular quality control to ensure that the *haematocrit* is within prescribed limits, usually between 0.65 and 0.75. This can be performed by selecting and testing on a random basis a proportion of those units that are returned unused.

(7) *Bacterial cultures* of a selected proportion of red cell packs are performed by some transfusion services as a means of verifying the efficacy of the aseptic blood collection procedures. Cultured organisms may, however, unless sufficient care is taken, represent contamination during sampling. The culture technique should permit a quantitative estimate of bacterial numbers to be made. Recovery of only a few organisms per millilitre of cultured blood is more indicative of technical problems in sampling than providing conclusive evidence for genuine contamination of the donor pack.

(8) Failure of the ATP-powered membrane cation pump results in leakage of intracellular *potassium* into the suspension medium. Unless alteration in preservation techniques is made potassium levels are not routinely measured as a quality control procedure. The known risk of high potassium levels in the plasma of stored blood[14,15] necessitates the use of relatively fresh blood for exchange transfusions of neonates although this is not a requirement for simple transfusions for anaemia[16] (see chapter 20, section 2.4).

During *routine blood banking*, where established formulations and preservation methods are in use, quality-control assessment is limited to *random bacteriological analysis, haematocrit determinations* on red cell concentrate preparations, together with common-sense *visual inspection* of packs at issue. A proportion of red cell packs are weighed as a control for accuracy of collection volumes.

2.3   Red Cell Preservative Solutions

These are generally presented as a pack containing approximately 63 ml of anti-coagulant for the collection of 450 g of blood. Blood is stored between 1 and 6 °C to slow metabolism and inhibit growth of pathogenic bacteria.

Acid–citrate–dextrose (ACD)

This contains:

trisodium citrate	1.485 g
citric acid	0.540 g
dextrose	1.687 g
in a volume of	67.5 ml

The pH of blood after collection is around 7.0, eventually falling to 6.7. A shelf life of 21 days is allowed.

Citrate–phosphate–dextrose (CPD)

This contains:

trisodium citrate	1.66 g
citric acid (monohydrate)	0.206 g
sodium dihydrogen monophosphate	0.140 g
dextrose	1.61 g
in a volume of	63 ml

The higher pH and phosphate content enhance DPG preservation but ATP levels and post-transfusion viability are not significantly improved compared with ACD.

The pH of blood collected into CPD is around 7.2, falling to 6.8 during storage.

CPDA-1

This was the first and most popularly used of the adenine-supplemented media; 0.017 g of adenine is included, resulting in a final adenine concentration of 0.25 mM in the blood pack. The dextrose content is increased by 25% over that in CPD. Addition of adenine to 0.25 mM final concentration in the blood pack improves post-transfusion viability and this correlates with improved ATP preservation. This combination of adenine and extra glucose allows satisfactory storage for at least 35 days.

At any stage of storage red cell viability is better than seen with ACD or CPD alone. The only potential toxicity of adenine, that of 2,8-dioxyadenine precipitation in renal tubules, has not been shown to be a clinical problem.[17,18] This effect is only believed to be discernible after transfusion of around one unit per kilogram of fresh whole blood. Larger amounts of older blood or of red cell concentrates could be given without risk as these contain less adenine.

Adenine does appear to be slightly detrimental to DPG preservation in a dose-dependent manner. For CPDA-1-preserved red cells DPG levels are approximately 75% of those in CPD up to around 7 days. After this time, oxygen transport functions are similar.

Adenine supplementation has not been shown to have any deleterious effects on the quality of other blood products, viz. platelets, cryoprecipitate or purified blood derivatives.

CPDA-2 and CPDA-3 (0.5 mM adenine with 75% and 100% extra glucose respectively)

These formulations have been devised as a result of concern that there may be insufficient adenine and glucose left in the plasma of hard-packed CPDA-1 red cell concentrates to guarantee 75% post-transfusion viability. In practice it seems that CPDA-1 red cell concentrates not exceeding 0.75 haematocrit have acceptable post-transfusion survival but this may not be true for units with higher haematocrits; CPDA-2 and CPDA-3 both allow storage for at least 42 days for concentrates of up to 0.85 haematocrit. The extra adenine and glucose could have metabolically undesirable effects during extensive whole blood transfusion.

Optimal additive solutions

Optimal additives are preservative solutions specially designed for the resuspension of red cell concentrates remaining after component preparation. They are presented within a separate additional pack of a multiple collection pack assembly. After plasma, platelets or buffy coats have been removed from the primary pack the optimal additive is added to the residual red cells, which are then ready for issue.

Complete removal of platelet-rich plasma and resuspension of red cells in nutrient preservative solutions offers major benefits:[19,20]

(1) Maximal procurement of plasma and other blood components.
(2) Relatively microaggregate-free red cell suspensions.
(3) Flow characteristics similar to those of unmodified whole blood.
(4) A reduced incidence of non-haemolytic febrile transfusion reactions.

It was found that addition of saline+adenine+glucose solutions could permit red blood cell preservation for up to 42 days and reduce microaggregate formation compared to that in whole blood. Haemolysis was, however, unacceptably high unless buffy coats were removed. Possibly this was due to the chymotryptic activity of leucocytes being unopposed after removal of plasma proteins. Removal of a majority of the leucocytes appears to reduce the haemolysis. It has now been clearly shown that supplementation of the medium with impermeable sugar alcohols (e.g. mannitol, 30 mmol/l, 3 mmol/pack) is also effective in reducing haemolysis.

In Europe a frequently used optimal additive is SAGM (Fenwal). This consists of 100 ml of saline–adenine–glucose medium (877 mg of sodium chloride or 150 mEq/l Na$^+$, 818 mg of dextrose, 525 mg of mannitol, 16.9 mg of adenine). The haematocrit of the final red cell suspension will generally be in the range 0.57–0.62.

In the USA, the Fenwal product ADSOL contains 900 mg of sodium chloride, 2200 mg of dextrose, 27 mg of adenine and 750 mg of mannitol. The extra glucose and mannitol allow 49 days' storage. Various other impermeable sugar alcohols such as sorbitol can be substituted for mannitol in addition to the use of other nucleotides to supplement or to replace adenine.

In view of their potential advantages both in allowing improved bank efficiency and their suitability for a large proportion of blood transfusion needs,[21] it seems likely that optimal additive supplemented red cells will become the principal red cell products to be offered by transfusion services.

Rejuvenation of red cells

Aged stored red cell products depleted of DPG and ATP can be rejuvenated by resuspension in media designed to restimulate synthesis of those essential organic phosphate compounds. A typical rejuvenation solution is the PIP cocktail,[22] which comprises pyruvate, inosine and inorganic phosphate in respective concentrations of 4, 10 and 4 μmol/ml red cells. This can produce supernormal concentrations of DPG, a right-shifted oxygen dissociation curve and recovery of ATP levels. This procedure is potentially most useful for rescuing outdated units of rare blood groups prior to freezing.

3 FROZEN PRESERVATION OF RED CELLS

Red cells are preserved excellently in the frozen state. DPG and ATP concentrations remain at the level prior to freezing and this is reflected in the satisfactory post-transfusion survival. There is, however, a disadvantage in that there may be up to 25% loss of red cells during the manipulative process.

The extensive washing necessary prior to freezing and following thawing and removal of the glycerol cryoprotectant removes all but around 0.025% of the plasma and in excess of 95% of the leucocyte and platelet antigenic material. Some viable lymphocytes do, however, persist. Free haemoglobin in the supernatant of recovered units reaches 50–100 mg/dl, which is higher than concentrations usually found in liquid stored blood. The precise product performance and specifications depend very much on the freezing and recovery technique used.

There are various advantages of frozen blood, many of which are shared with *washed red cells* or *washed and leucocyte-free* products (see section 1.5). Advantages *unique* to frozen units are:

(1) Indefinitely prolonged storage of rare blood types. A storage period of up to 10 years is normally allowed in the UK. In some circumstances such blood units may well be destined for autologous transfusion for which prolonged storage may be essential.
(2) Storage of blood units compatible with patients with complex mixtures of alloantibodies.

Disadvantages of frozen red cells include:

(1) High cost. All freezing techniques are very costly, frozen red cells being possibly three or more times more expensive than conventional red cell products.
(2) Cumbersome preparation methods. Red cells must be mixed with a *cryoprotectant* solution, usually glycerol, to prevent damage during freezing. This must be removed by an extensive washing process prior to administration.
(3) Potential wastage if blood units are no longer clinically needed when thawed.
(4) Restricted shelf life after reconstitution. Thawing and recovery of frozen blood cannot be carried out in 'closed' conditions, i.e. free from microbial exposure, and reconstituted red cells must therefore be transfused within 24 hours. This can cause problems when blood has to be transported for transfusion in outlying hospitals.
(5) Risk of errors of identification if transfer to different containers is necessary.
(6) Loss of up to 25% of *in vivo* recoverable red cells during manipulation.

The use of frozen red cells has dropped substantially over the last few years. Large numbers of units were formerly prepared for patients requiring removal of leucocytes for prevention of HLA alloimmunization. Filtration methods now have been shown to be cheaper and more effective for this purpose. Frozen storage will, however, remain the only feasible approach to the preservation of rare red cell donations.

REFERENCES

1 Nilsson, L., Hedner, U., Nilson, I.M. and Robertson, B. (1983) Shelf-life of bank blood and stored plasma with special reference to coagulation factors. *Transfusion*, **23**: 377–381.
2 Wenz, B., Gurtlinger, K.F., O'Toole, A.M. and Dugan, E.P. (1980) Preparation of granulocyte-poor red blood cells by microaggregate filtration: a simplified method to minimize febrile transfusion reactions. *Vox Sang.*, **39**: 282–287.
3 Schned, A.R. and Silver, H. (1981) The use of microaggregate filtration in the prevention of febrile transfusion reactions. *Transfusion*, **21**: 675–681.
4 Bodensteiner, D.C. (1990) Leucocyte depletion filters: a comparison of efficiency. *Am. J. Haematol.*, **35**: 184–186.
5 Pietersz, R.N.I., Steneker, I., Reesink, H.W., Dekker, W.J.A., Al, E.J.M., Huisman, J.G. and Biewenga, J. (1992) Comparison of five different filters for the removal of leucocytes from red cell concentrates. *Vox Sang.*, **62**: 76–81.
6 Koerner, K., Sahlmen, P., Zimmermann, B. and Kibanek, B. (1991) Preparation of leucocyte-poor red cell concentrates: comparison of five different filters. *Vox Sang.*, **60**: 61–62.
7 Steneker, I. and Biewenga, J. (1990) Histological and Immunohistochemical studies on the preparation of leucocyte-poor red cell concentrates by filtration: the filtration process on cellulose acetate fibres. *Vox Sang.*, **58**: 192–198.
8 Royal College of Physicians of Edinburgh (1993) Consensus Conference. Leucocyte Depletion of Blood and Blood Components.
9 Reverberi, R. and Menini, C. (1990) Clinical efficacy of five filters specific for leucocyte removal. *Vox Sang.*, **58**: 188–191.
10 MacNamara, E., Clarke, S. and McCann, S.R. (1984) Provision of leucocyte poor blood at the bedside. *J. Clin. Pathol.*, **37**: 669–672.
11 Reesink, H.W., Veldman, H., Henrichs, H.J., Prins, H.K. and Loos, J.A. (1982) Removal of leucocytes from blood by fibre filtration. *Vox Sang.*, **42**: 281–288.
12 Labow, R.S., Card, R.T. and Rock, G. (1987) The effect of the plasticizer di (2-ethylehexl) phthalate on red cell deformability. *Blood*, **70**:(1): 319–323.
13 International forum (1980) Which are the parameters to be controlled in red cell products (whole blood, red cell concentrates, washed red cells, leucocyte poor red cell concentrates, frozen red cells) in order that they may be offered to the medical profession as standardised products with specified properties? *Vox Sang.*, **39**: 229–240.
14 Latham, J.T., Jr, Bove, J.R. and Weirich, F.L. (1982) Chemical and haematologic changes in stored CPDA-1 blood. *Transfusion*, **22**: 158–159.
15 Moroff, G. and Dende, D. (1983) Characterization of biochemical changes occurring during storage of red cells: comparative studies with CPD and CPDA-1 anticoagulant-preservative solutions. *Transfusion*, **23**: 484–489.
16 Batton, D.G., Maisels, M.J. and Shulman, G. (1983) Serum potassium changes following packed red cell transfusions in newborn infants. *Transfusion*, **23**: 163–164.
17 Kreuger, A. (1976) Adenine metabolism during and after exchange transfusions in newborn infants with CPD-adenine blood. *Transfusion*, **16**: 249–252.
18 Simon, E.R. (1977) Adenine in blood banking. *Transfusion*, **17**: 317–325.
19 Hogman, C.F., Akerblom, O., Hedlund, K., Rosen, I. and Wiklund, L. (1983) Red cell suspensions in SAGM medium: further experience of in vivo survival of red cells, clinical usefulness and plasma-saving effects. 1. *Vox Sang.*, **45**: 217–223.
20 Napier, J.A.F. and Biffin, A.H. (1984) Micro-aggregate content of red cell suspensions stored in saline adenine glucose mannitol optimal additive solution. *Clin. Lab. Haematol.*, **6**: 165–169.

21 Hogman, C.F., Andreen, M., Rosen, I., Akerblom, O. and Hellsing, A. (1983) Haemotherapy with red cell concentrates and a new red cell storage medium. *Lancet* i: 269–271.
22 Valeri, C.R., Gray, A.D., Cassidy, G.P., Riordan, W. and Pivacek, L.E. (1984) The 24 hour post transfusion survival, oxygen transport function, and residual haemolysis of human outdated-rejuvenated red cell concentrates after washing and storage at 4 °C for 24 to 72 hours. *Transfusion*, **24**: 323–326.

4

Transfusion of Red Cells

1   INTRODUCTION

Red cell transfusions for anaemia should be given to *relieve symptoms* and not solely for the correction of low haemoglobin values. The expected benefit of each transfusion as regards the improvement of symptoms or the reduction of morbidity must be balanced against the particular risks to the patient concerned.

The *rate of deterioration* in the blood count is an important consideration; anaemias of rapid onset cause more severe symptoms than are found in chronic conditions in which physiological compensatory mechanisms have more time to take effect. The severity of symptoms is also dependent on the efficiency with which cardiopulmonary responses can compensate for the reduction in blood oxygen content. These compensatory reserves are lost in patients with severe *cardiac* or *pulmonary* disease in whom there is an intolerance to anaemia which becomes particularly exposed during times of crisis such as *infection, trauma* and *blood loss*. The physiological responses to acute blood loss anaemia, a state which is typically characterized by hypovolaemia, are considered in chapter 11. In contrast, the blood volume in anaemias arising from other causes is usually normal or some-times even increased. The diminished oxygen transport in chronic anaemias stems solely from the reduced blood haemoglobin concentration; unlike acute blood loss anaemia there is no problem with maintenance of blood pressure and tissue per-fusion.

1.1 Compensatory Adjustments in Anaemia

Increased cardiac output

The initial response to the onset of anaemia is an increase in ventricular stroke volume and this is followed, as anaemia becomes more severe, by an increase in heart rate. As a result the resting cardiac output shows a steady increase with declining haemoglobin until haemoglobin values of around 8.0 g/dl are reached. Below this point a sharp increase in cardiac output seems to be required in order to sustain tissue oxygen requirements. Haemoglobin values falling to around 8.0 g/dl frequently coincide with the onset of symptoms in many chronically transfused patients. Since the resting cardiac output is already increased in severe anaemia the reserve capacity normally available for exercise is lost and even mild physical exertion is liable to make the patient very short of breath, with a mark-edly increased heart rate.

Increased respiration

The hyperventilation occurring during anaemia maximizes alveolar oxygen ten-sions and blood oxygenation.

Reduced haemoglobin oxygen affinity

The haemoglobin oxygen dissociation curve is displaced to the right in anaemia; this facilitates oxygen offloading to the tissues but does not significantly reduce its uptake in the lungs. This displacement of the oxygen dissociation curve allows release of a greater amount of oxygen from haemoglobin at any given mixed venous pO_2 (see chapter 3, Figure 2). If sufficient oxygen can be released without undue reduction in venous pO_2 the oxygen tension pressure gradient from capil-lary blood to the tissues is better maintained. Without this effect tissue pO_2 would have to fall in an attempt to obtain sufficient oxygen from blood and in con-sequence the further stages of oxygen diffusion would be impeded.

The principal influence on the oxygen dissociation curve in chronic anaemia is obtained by changes in the concentration of *2, 3-diphosphoglycerate (DPG)*, an organic phosphate compound synthesized during red cell glycolysis. DPG achieves this effect by binding preferentially to haemoglobin in the deoxy con-formation and in this way DPG 'competes' with oxygen for attachment to deoxy-haemoglobin. In the presence of high DPG concentrations and low oxygen tensions the balance favours the binding of DPG to haemoglobin and release of oxygen, which is then available for tissue uptake. This mechanism also favours the requisite increase in DPG synthesis during anaemia. The tendency towards a greater degree of haemoglobin desaturation that occurs in anaemia creates an increased number of available binding sites for DPG.

The resulting uptake of free DPG by the red cell haemoglobin favours further DPG synthesis by a mass action effect in the appropriate part of the red cell glycolytic pathway (the Rapoport–Luebering shunt). The final result of these effects is an increased red cell DPG concentration, reduced haemoglobin oxygen affinity and improved release of oxygen to tissues. The degree of displacement of the oxygen dissociation curve can be expressed numerically by the P_{50} value, which specifies the partial pressure of oxygen at which 50% of the oxygen will have been released from the haemoglobin. High P_{50} values indicate that more oxygen can be released at normal mixed venous pO_2 values. P_{50} values may increase from the normal range of 27+1.0 mmHg up to 37 mmHg in anaemia. A change of this magnitude allows release of around 45% more oxygen per gram of haemoglobin at a mixed venous pO_2 of 40 mmHg.

Increased blood volume

An increase in total blood volume may occur in anaemia and this is due to plasma volume expansion. This extra volume allows capillary dilatation and an increase in the density of capillaries perfusing the tissues. Tissue oxygenation is facilitated by this increase in microvascularity because the average distance of cells from their source of oxygen supply is reduced.

1.2   Indications for Red Cell Transfusion in Anaemia

Reduction in exercise capacity

The cardiopulmonary compensations that are necessary during anaemia utilize the reserve functional capacity normally available to enable increased physical activity. Anaemia therefore limits exercise tolerance in proportion to its severity. This will be relatively less obvious in the elderly or disabled but may constitute an indication for transfusion in those whose work or life-style would otherwise be curtailed.

Coincidental medical or surgical problems

Surgery, with the attendant risks of blood loss or of other complications such as infection or adult respiratory distress syndrome, is likely to require additional cardiopulmonary performance and the effectiveness of this response would be jeopardized by the presence of anaemia. Severe infections exacerbate the severity of anaemia by placing extra demands for oxygen transport. Each case must, however, be assessed according to individual circumstances. The commonly accepted prerequisite of a minimum haemoglobin of 10 g/dl for *all* patients prior to surgery is no longer regarded as justified.

Coronary artery disease

The myocardium is highly efficient at oxygen extraction and coronary sinus oxygen-tensions are already very low. There is, therefore, little extra scope for increased oxygen extraction by the myocardium in anaemia unless coronary blood flow can be increased.

In coronary stenosis it may not be possible to match demands for increased cardiac output by an adequate increase in perfusion and oxygen delivery to cardiac muscle. Angina, therefore, may be worsened and myocardial inefficiency may result in cardiac failure. Either risk may justify transfusion to alleviate anaemia.

Pulmonary disease

This may be sufficiently severe to prevent the normal hyperventilation response that compensates for anaemia.

Anaemic symptoms

Feelings of tiredness and lethargy, which are common enough amongst the general population as well as in anaemic patients, correlate poorly with haemoglobin values. Nevertheless, some chronically anaemic patients are well aware of their progressive decline in vigour as anaemia worsens and of the converse feeling of well-being following transfusion. These patients are usually reliable witnesses of their own need for blood transfusion.

In countries where the safety of transfusions still remains problematic, a particularly rigorous approach to justifying transfusion is necessary. For example, a study of transfusion for severe anaemia in Kenyan children[1] could only confirm reduction in mortality where the haemoglobin levels were below 3.9 g/dl; or below 4.7 g/dl where respiratory distress was present. Other workers, broadly accepting the principles of this approach, emphasize the need to take into account the full clinical circumstances, e.g. age, aetiology of anaemia together with other evidence of decompensation before accepting the inevitability of transfusion.[2,3]

Rapidly deteriorating haemoglobin levels

Acute onset or deterioration of anaemia requires frequent monitoring and the ready availability of transfusion in order to avert dangerous symptoms. Despite the relatively non-controversial arguments for determining the need for red cell

Table 1 Criteria for appropriate red cell use[4]

1. Acute blood loss

   Over 25% blood volume loss *or* any of the following features present:

   General: thirst, apprehension, weakness, pallor, cool skin, Hb decrease $>2.0/\text{dl}$ in 24 hours

   Cardiovascular: chest pain, shock, orthostatic hypotension, orthostatic pulse change

   Respiratory: easy fatiguability, pulmonary oedema, adult respiratory distress syndrome, congestive heart failure, dyspnoea on exertion

   Central nervous system: syncope, restlessness, light-headedness, decline in consciousness

2. Patients without evidence of blood loss

   With chemotherapy and Hb <9 g/dl

   End-stage renal disease and Hb <8 g/dl

   Cardiovascular disease and Hb <9 g/dl

   Pre-operatively with Hb <9 g/dl

replacement in anaemia, there is evidence that a substantial proportion of transfusions do not meet agreed criteria. Criteria for red cell transfusion that could serve as a basis for audit have been published.[4,5]

Even these criteria cannot be taken as obligatory indicators for transfusion as in some cases alternative measures (e.g. erythropoietin for renal failure) would be preferred, but they do at least serve the purpose of identifying potential areas of misuse.

1.3 Relationship Between Anaemic Symptoms and Haemoglobin Level

The haemoglobin value alone is usually an unreliable guide to symptoms experienced by patients or for the need for blood transfusion. The rate of change, however, is important. A sharp fall from normal values even if only to modest degrees of anaemia (e.g. 10.0–11.0 g/dl) may cause noticeable inconvenience to otherwise fit young subjects. In contrast, chronically stable haemoglobin levels of 5 g/dl or lower can sometimes be sustained by people who may even be unaware of their relative handicap. Elderly subjects may not require normal haemoglobin levels for their usual exercise demands but may on the other hand tolerate anaemia poorly in the presence of cardiopulmonary disease. The oxygen affinity of the blood, though rarely measured in clinical practice, may also be important. Some anaemias, e.g. pyruvate kinase deficiency, are associated with such high DPG levels that these patients are less symptomatically 'anaemic' than their haemoglobin values might suggest. In other conditions such as hexokinase deficiency, in which red cell glycolysis and DPG synthesis are impaired, the converse will apply. Oxygen delivery is also reduced in anaemias with high haemoglobin F levels because oxygen dissociation from haemoglobin F is not influenced by DPG concentrations.

1.4 Transfusion Policies

Using the haemoglobin level as an indicator for transfusion

Patients requiring long-term transfusion support are best maintained with hae-moglobin levels that fluctuate as little as possible above the lowest haemoglobin level that provides acceptable relief from symptoms. These haemoglobin values will generally exceed 6–8 g/dl. The figure will very much depend on the indivi-dual patient and may well alter with time and changes in the overall clinical con-dition. Before the use of iron chelation therapy it was, for example, not unusual to see the lowest tolerable haemoglobin value rise as iron overload caused myo-cardial deterioration.

Transfusion is unlikely to be required where haemoglobin values exceed 10 g/dl. In the range between 8.0 and 10.0 g/dl the need must be considered in the context of the level of activity undertaken by the patient and the presence of car-diopulmonary or atherosclerotic disease. Below 8.0 g/dl the need for transfusion is felt by most patients, exceptions being those with renal failure or with other con-ditions such as pyruvate kinase enzyme deficiency characterized by particularly increased P_{50} values.

Quantity of blood transfused

Normal red cell production rates are of the order of 150–200 ml weekly and in those adult patients in whom endogenous red cell production is low administra-tion of two units of concentrated red cells (approximately 400 ml) every two weeks provides a convenient and acceptable transfusion regime. In many patients these amounts of blood can be administered over a 3-hour period on a day case basis. Patients managed in such a way appreciate the stability of their clinical state and predictability of transfusions. A common practice of administering four to six-unit 'top-up' transfusions only when the haemoglobin and symptoms have reached their tolerated nadir provides for a much less satisfactory state of clinical well-being, especially in the period just prior to and immediately after each indivi-dual transfusion.

Avoidance of circulatory overload

Death from congestive cardiac failure is the principal risk following transfusion of the severely anaemic. This generally follows over-enthusiastic transfusion of new patients who may be admitted already in a critical state. It can, however, also happen during the regular 'top-up' transfusions of chronically anaemic patients.

Table 2 Avoidance of circulatory overload

- Reduce the volume of blood components
- Transfuse slowly, or
- Give a partial exchange transfusion
- Give diuretics
- Transfuse patient in semi-upright position
- Observe carefully

The urgency for large increases in the red cell mass of severely anaemic patients is frequently overestimated. Simple arithmetic calculations will show that the total red cell mass of such patients may be as small as 400–500 ml. Transfusion of as little as one unit (200 ml of packed cells) will therefore increase the red cell mass by around 40%. Transfusion of two units will provide 80% extra red cells. This represents a very substantial increase in oxygen-carrying capacity and will generally be quite enough for the initial 24-hour period unless given for treatment of active blood loss. Transfusion rates of around 1–3 ml/kg per hour are usual (200 ml per hour for an average adult). For those very severely anaemic patients in cardiac failure:

(1) Red cell units no older than 5 days of age are preferred; these will have near normal oxygen affinity.
(2) Transfused blood can be given *in exchange* for simultaneous withdrawal of an equal volume of the patient's own blood.

Where straightforward transfusion without exchange is given, infusion rates not exceeding 1 ml/kg per hour may be advisable. These measures may be sufficient for immediate resuscitation and allow a more leisurely approach for future management.

Blood transfusions, except those for emergency replacement of blood loss, should always *begin slowly* and the patient must be *monitored* carefully. Body *temperature, pulse* and *blood pressure* should be recorded before each unit is given and then every 10 minutes over the first half hour and not more than every 2 hours until the transfusion is completed. No more than 1 ml/kg per hour (about 10–15 drops per minute) should be given over the first 10–20 minutes to allow time for any adverse reaction to be detected.

A permanent record should be made of these observations together with the nature and identification details of all fluids administered.

2 SPECIAL PROBLEMS OF LONG-TERM TRANSFUSION PROGRAMMES

2.1 Iron Overload

Iron overload is an invariable consequence of long-term transfusion unless steps are taken to minimize the risk. Each unit of transfused red cells provides around 200 mg of iron which cannot be eliminated from the body by normal physiological processes. Steady accumulation of unwanted iron causes structural and functional damage to the *myocardium, liver, pancreas* and other endocrine glands. Thus *cardiac* or *hepatic* failure and *diabetes* are complications that must be anticipated. Three approaches may help to minimize the risk:

(1) *Optimization of the transfusion schedule.* This entails transfusion of the minimal amount of blood required to maintain acceptable clinical status. Transfusion management of patients with thalassaemia or other anaemias with highly ineffective erythropoiesis may, however, require a slightly different approach (see section 3).

(2) *Use of iron chelation therapy.*[6,7] At present only one agent, desferrioxamine, is widely used. Desferrioxamine chelates iron and the complex is excreted via the urine. It must, unfortunately, be given parenterally. The search for a safe and effective oral iron chelation agent has so far been disappointing although one agent, deferipone (L1), is currently undergoing clinical trials.[8,9]

   Desferrioxamine is usually given in doses of around 20–60 mg/kg by slow subcutaneous infusion over periods of 8–10 hours; this is conveniently performed overnight. The optimum desferrioxamine dose appears to be related to age and the state of iron loading, the higher doses being required for adults with large amounts of accumulated iron.[10]

   Small battery-operated infusion pumps are available and the infusion needle is placed in the abdominal subcutaneous tissue. Local irritation is sometimes a problem and addition of 1 mg/ml hydrocortisone to the infusion has been claimed to be helpful in minimizing this. Oral ascorbate at a dose of 100–200 mg twice daily enhances desferrioxamine-induced iron excretion.

(3) *Use of neocytes for transfusion.* The reticulocyte-rich fraction of red cells can be harvested using apheresis machines. It has been claimed that the longer red cell life-span following transfusion reduces overall transfusion needs (and as a consequence the degree of iron overloading) by around 20%. The technique is expensive and inconvenient for widespread regular use and there is as yet no widespread agreement that a significant reduction in the rate of iron accumulation can be obtained.[11,12]

2.2   Sensitization to Leucocyte or Plasma Antigens

A high proportion of multi-transfused patients eventually develop *allergic* or even occasionally *anaphylactic reactions* to the antigenic material of donor leucocytes, platelets or plasma. These usually take the form of *pyrexias, rigors, erythematous or urticarial skin rashes* and may also include *flu-like systemic symptoms.* Sometimes *bronchospasm* or even more rarely *respiratory arrest* and *circulatory collapse* occur (see chapter 23, section 3). Minor degrees of reaction are common and can make the patient feel distinctly and unnecessarily unwell. Clinical vigilance and sympathy are required in recognizing, treating and preventing these episodes. Frequently patients come to expect this temporary malaise associated with transfusion as unavoidable when this is, in fact, not the case.

The majority of multi-transfused patients have *lymphocytotoxic antibodies* and *leucocyte agglutinins* and some component of this immunological response is almost certainly the cause of these allergic reactions (see chapter 23, section 3.1). The search for these antibodies, however, is not diagnostically of great assistance since not all patients with antibodies react clinically. Serological studies unfortunately show poor correlation with symptoms. The most definitive proof can be obtained by demonstrating that symptoms can be avoided by administration of red cell units free of leucocytes and/or plasma.

The management of acute reactions is covered in chapter 23, section 3.

Antihistamines and steroids have a place for treatment of mild or unexpected reactions, but once leucocyte sensitivity has been diagnosed an attempt should be made to avert reactions by exclusive transfusion of leucocyte-depleted blood (see chapter 3 section 1.5).

This can be prepared by filtration techniques that have now been shown to provide a product equally as good as frozen red cells, at lower cost and greater convenience.

It is important that children starting a lifelong transfusion programme are, as far as possible, prevented from developing sensitivity to leucocyte antigens. Leucocyte-depleted products should therefore be given from the start of the transfusion programme. A quality-assurance programme should govern the leucocyte depletion procedure to provide confidence that the required levels of white cell removal ($< 5.10^6$ leucocytes per pack) are consistently achieved. In practice, however, even patients receiving filtered blood develop leucocyte antibodies although this occurs more slowly and with a reduced incidence. The clinical effects of this degree of leucocyte sensitization may be greatly delayed or, in fact, may never even appear.

Indications for leucocyte depletion in transfusion

Despite the fact that leucocyte depletion is a costly process the perceived benefits of white cell removal have led to increasingly widespread use of blood filtration. This is of course not satisfactory for several reasons. There is now clear evidence that technical failures occur unless the procedure is carried out under carefully controlled conditions. Of even greater importance, much more evidence of benefit is required particularly in terms of overall morbidity and mortality in many of the situations for which filter use is proposed. The place of leucocyte depleted blood components has been reviewed in the UK and a consensus statement[13] issued. The 1993 Consensus Conference could not identify any circumstances in which controlled trials and quality of life and cost–benefit measures showed a *definite* indication for filter use. However, on the basis of published data, giving compelling evidence of clinical benefit, leucocyte depletion *could be recommended* for the following circumstances:

(1) For prevention of or delaying non-haemolytic febrile transfusion reactions in certain categories of transfusion-dependent patients.
(2) Abolition or amelioration of recurrent febrile transfusion reactions for patients receiving recurrent red cell transfusions.

(3) Newly diagnosed patients with aplasia who might be potential bone marrow graft recipients.
(4) Leucocyte depletion is also accepted as an approach to reducing CMV transmission risk if seronegative products are unavailable.

A category of *possible* indications was also identified in which a plausible rationale existed but the clinical significance of intervention remained to be proven. These included:

(1) Prevention or delay of clinically significant bleeding, due to HLA refractoriness in platelet transfusion recipients.
(2) Control of febrile transfusion reactions in platelet transfusion recipients.
(3) Prevention of adverse consequences of leucocyte-mediated immune modulation, e.g. post-operative surgical infection, tumour recurrence, progression of HIV infection and of CMV infection in CMV seropositive patients.

2.3 Formation of Red Cell Alloantibodies

With the increasing practice of blood transfusion a greater incidence of single and multiple red cell antibodies is appearing in transfusion recipients. About 0.3% of blood donors possess unexpected red cell alloantibodies, and a slightly higher incidence is observed in routine hospital admissions, the risk of possessing antibodies being greatest in those previously pregnant or transfused.

Multiply transfused patients have a much higher incidence of red cell alloantibodies and estimates ranging from 6% to over 30% have been reported.[14-17] The frequency of antibody formation appears to be much the same for patients with bone marrow failure, haemoglobinopathy,[18,19] renal failure and possibly even for those with haematological malignancy, although the evidence with regard to this latter category of patients is conflicting;[15,16] certainly alloantibody formation in patients with acute lymphoblastic leukaemia seems to be infrequent. Black patients transfused for haemoglobinopathies are more liable to form antibodies;[16] this is likely to be due to their being exposed to novel Rh and non-Rh antigens when, as is usually the case, they are transfused with random Caucasian donor blood. Because the chances of a phenotypic match are much greater, use of black donors has been advocated as a way of minimizing red cell alloimmunization.[20]

In a British series of patients with sickle cell disease a high proportion were R⁰R⁰ (*cDe/cDe*) and formed anti-C and anti-E which could have been prevented by transfusion of Rh-negative (*cde/cde*) blood.[23]

As a group of patients, delayed haemolytic transfusion reactions appeared unusually frequently, sometimes causing symptoms confusingly similar to those of sickle crises.[24]

The principal merit of the prospective matching approach is that it minimizes formation of multiple alloantibodies that would make emergency transfusion difficult.

Those patients who develop alloantibodies do so relatively early in their transfusion history, most appearing within 15 transfusions[21] or 6 months[14] of the start of the transfusion programme. For thalassaemic children in Greece, the age of starting their transfusion programme has been shown to be important.[22] Less alloimmunization was seen when transfusions were begun before 12 months of age, it being presumed that a degree of tolerance had been induced. After that age, the chances of alloimmunization could be reduced by selecting fully Rh (DcCeE) and K antigen matching, as compared to the usual ABO and Rh D selection criteria. Where it is recognized that new patients are liable to embark upon a long-term transfusion regime, the opportunity should be taken to establish the probable Rh genotype in addition to typing at least for the Kell, Ss, Kidd and Duffy system antigens. This opportunity will be lost once transfusion has begun, but the information will be helpful during analysis of the specificity of any antibodies that subsequently appear. Provision of blood matched for those blood group systems mentioned above can minimize the risk of alloantibody formation but would be costly and time consuming;[19,21] it is also wasteful of red cell typing sera and may delay the routine provision of blood. Bearing in mind that 70–80% or more patients will never develop antibodies, a more economical policy is to transfuse ABO and Rh D-compatible blood and only match more specifically when antibodies appear.[38]

3 TRANSFUSION PROBLEMS PRESENTED BY SPECIFIC ANAEMIAS

In general transfusion therapy must be reserved for those conditions that are refractory to other corrective measures. Anaemias responsive to nutritional factors or steroids should be so treated and transfusion reserved only for emergency treatment of acute problems such as congestive cardiac failure or infections.

3.1 Nutritional Anaemias

Anaemias caused by vitamin B_{12}, folate or iron deficiency rarely require transfusion. Exceptions to this policy include those iron-deficiency patients who need immediate correction of anaemia but where[4] neither oral nor parenteral iron allows sufficient bone marrow recovery to offset the rate of blood loss. Patients with *megaloblastic anaemias* presenting in severe cardiac failure may benefit from an emergency partial exchange transfusion but no more than one or two units of blood should be required. Transfusion may also be required where the diagnosis is unsure, where coincidental *infection* is present or where *inflammatory, autoimmune* or *malignant disease* makes the haematological response unreliable.

3.2 Refractory Anaemias

Anaemias due to *hypoplastic* or *ineffective erythropoiesis, sideroblastic* or *myelodysplastic* states comprise a common but heterogeneous group requiring transfusion support. Platelet therapy may additionally be required. Before a transfusion programme is instituted it is most important to ascertain whether bone marrow transplantation is a possibility as this will have an important bearing on transfusion policies (see chapter 22, section 3).

3.3   Autoimmune Haemolytic Anaemias

These anaemias, in contrast, do not commonly require transfusion. Since the auto-antibodies frequently lack any clear specificity that can be bypassed by compatibility selection, the transfused cells cannot be expected to survive better than autologous cells. In contrast, undetected alloantibodies or other less evident factors may result in an overt exacerbation of haemolysis. Serological approaches to selection of red cell units are discussed in chapter 17, section 2.4. Transfusion is, however, required occasionally. *Acute fulminating haemolysis* in which haemoglobin values may be falling rapidly requires careful monitoring and may need transfusion even in the absence of compatible blood in order to prevent circulatory failure. Transfusion may have to be continued until natural or steroid-induced remission occurs. Prophylactic folic acid is required as well as treatment of any infections that may be present. In the absence of any evident specificity the least incompatible blood units should be selected for transfusion. It is sometimes held that for *cold agglutinin haemolytic anaemia* blood units should be pre-warmed before transfusion. This may be true for rapid infusions such as may be needed during surgery but there is little evidence that pre-warming for transfusion rates of around 1 ml/min into a venous stream which may carry 50 or so times that volume is necessary.

3.4   Paroxysmal Nocturnal Haemoglobinuria

Exacerbation of *haemolysis* and also *thrombotic episodes* have been recognized to occur following transfusion in this condition. The diagnosis of paroxysmal nocturnal haemoglobinuria (PNA) must be borne in mind during investigation of haemolytic transfusion reactions, especially those that appear to defy explanation. Red cells in PNH appear to be abnormally sensitive to lysis by pathologically activated complement components. It had been believed that transfused plasma contained replacements for 'exhausted' complement components and therefore, by supplying these, blood transfusion reactivates the haemolytic process.

This supposition led to the widespread adoption of the use of *washed red cells* whenever PNH patients were to be transfused. It now seems more likely that reactions between donor antigenic material and recipient alloantibodies are the cause of complement activation and damage to the abnormally sensitive red cells. Provision of leucocyte- and platelet-depleted red cells minimizes the presentation of potentially incompatible antigens and has been found to be very effective for ensuring clinically uneventful transfusion.[25,26]

3.5   Congenital Enzyme-deficient Haemolytic Anaemias

These anaemias occasionally require transfusion. This is particularly true for those conditions presenting at birth with severe haemolysis and jaundice. These anae-

Transfusion of Red Cells   67

mias include those caused by enzyme deficiencies such as *glucose 6-phosphate dehydrogenase, hexokinase, glucose 6-phosphate isomerase* and *phosphoglycerate kinase* and also congenital *spherocytosis, elliptocytosis* and *stomatocytosis.* Transfusion management of affected babies follows the lines described for Rh haemolytic disease (see chapter 21, section 5.4). Premature infants are at greater risk of kernicterus than those with more mature hepatic function. Transfusion is generally not required on a regular long-term basis but may occasionally be needed in later life for severe acute haemolytic episodes or for exacerbations of anaemia due to aplastic crises.

3.6 Sickle Cell Disease

This generic term applies to a group of haemoglobinopathies comprising principally HbS homozygotes, HbSC heterozygotes, or some severe HbS/β-chain thalassaemia variants. In countries with developed transfusion services, blood transfusion therapy forms an important adjunct to the management of problems in these patients and the indications have been comprehensively reviewed.[27] However, where transfusion cannot be freed from a substantial risk of HIV, e.g. some Sub-Saharan African countries, use of transfusion is necessarily confined to the more clearly life-threatening occasions.[28]

The approach in blood transfusion management is to reduce HbS concentration below the levels associated with red cell sickling, but without increasing whole blood viscosity which, in its own right, is a predisposing factor for *vaso-occlusive episodes.* The following transfusion approaches are utilized:

(1) Simple additive transfusion for acute symptomatic anaemia, e.g. Hb $<$ 5.0 g/dl.
(2) Acute exchange transfusions to reduce HbS concentrations while ensuring haematocrit concentrations do not exceed the 0.35 optimum.[29]
(3) 'Super-transfusion' regimens involve sustained regular transfusions (often beginning with an exchange procedure), as a preventative measure. This strategy is often adopted following single or recurrent episodes of severe sickle cell-related symptoms and aims to maintain total haemoglobin concentration in the range 10–14.5 g/dl and HbS concentrations below 20%.

Transfusion is not required for treatment of asymptomatic patients with anaemia and is generally given only for severe anaemia, e.g. during hypoplastic episodes when marrow failure may cause a precipitate fall in haemoglobin concentration.

Transfusion may have a place for the treatment of any severe symptoms of sickle cell disease that require more energetic therapy than the usual measures such as rest, analgesia and antibiotics. These problems include *vaso-occlusive episodes,* e.g. cerebrovascular accidents, priapism, sequestration syndromes and sickle chest syndrome. Where respiratory failure exists a pO_2 of $<$ 60 mmHg is advised as an indication for exchange transfusion.[27] Symptoms due to sickling of red cells are most likely when the haemoglobin S concentration exceeds 50% of the total haemoglobin. The aim should therefore be to reduce haemoglobin S concentrations at least to below 40% and possibly below 20% for the most severe problems. This may be most rapidly accomplished by exchange transfusion. Highly dangerous events such as *cerebrovascular episodes* due to vascular stenosis and/or sickling in the cerebral vasculature may justify a regular transfusion programme.[30] Maintenance of near-normal haemoglobin values by regular transfusion suppresses endogenous erythropoiesis, and haemoglobin S concentrations below 20% may be possible. This measure substantially reduces the risk of recurrences. The role of transfusion in *pregnancy* is by no means agreed and further evaluation of pregnancies managed with or without transfusion support is needed.[31]

Those centres employing transfusion in the hope of preventing the high fetal morbidity and mortality in mothers with haemoglobin SS or SC disease usually begin this during the last 3 months of pregnancy.[32,33]

Transfusion should also be given during *severe infections* to prevent exacerbation of sickling episodes. The optimum post-transfusion haemoglobin level for these patients is not fully established. While it has been claimed from viscosity studies that haematocrits above 0.35 may be counter-productive and negate the effect of transfusion,[29] other studies have shown higher exercise capacity in patients transfused to normal haemoglobin values.[34,35]

These principles are also generally applied to the management of patients undergoing both emergency and elective *surgery*, although bearing in mind the higher rate of complications with transfusions in sickle cell disease[36] it has been argued that transfusions are over-employed and a more careful assessment of the individual patient's clinical circumstances is required.[36] Transfused patients with sickle cell disease do have a greater risk of delayed haemolytic transfusion reactions (see section 2.3).

3.7 Thalassaemia

Transfusion is most usually required for the severe anaemia of homozygous β-thalassaemia or that due to double heterozygosity for other thalassaemia disorders.

Unlike congenital enzymopathies, transfusion is not needed during the neonatal period because haemoglobin F concentrations are high. Transfusion becomes necessary later in the first year of life when β-chain production should, under normal circumstances, be fully operative.

The objectives of transfusion in these conditions are:

(1) To prevent the gross skeletal deformities that otherwise result from hyperplastic erythropoiesis.
(2) To improve the rate of growth and physical development.
(3) To prevent severe illness due to aplastic crises resulting from infections.
(4) To allow near-normal levels of physical activity.
(5) To reduce the iron overload resulting from severe anaemia and ineffective erythropoiesis.

The success with which these objectives are attained may be dependent on the average haemoglobin level achieved as a result of transfusion. Levels of around 8.0 g/dl provide conventionally acceptable results but evidence now exists that attainment of haemoglobin values of the order of 10 g/dl significantly reduces the pathological degree of iron absorption. Maintenance of higher target values (e.g. haemoglobin exceeding 12.0 g/dl) has been claimed to be even more successful in this respect.[37]

Iron overload resulting from a combination of pathologically increased gastro-intestinal iron absorption and transfusional iron leads to death, generally before adulthood, unless preventative measures are taken (see section 2.1). Desferrioxamine by regular subcutaneous infusion can be successful in preventing iron accumulation and should be instituted early in the transfusion programme. Urinary iron loss is proportional to the degree of iron loading and this is related to age and the total amount of transfusion. Daily losses of up to 200 mg can be achieved.

Alloimmunization to leucocyte and red cell antigens can become a major problem in thalassaemic children on lifelong transfusion regimens (see section 2.2).

REFERENCES

1 Lackritz, E.M., Campbell, C.C., Ruebush II, T.K. *et al.* (1992) Effect of blood transfusion on survival among children in a Kenyan hospital. *Lancet*, **340**: 524–528.
2 Newton, C.R.J.C., Marsh, K., Peshu, N. and Mwangi, I. (1992) Blood transfusions for severe anaemia in African children (letter). *Lancet*, **340**: 917–918.
3 Brewster, D.R. (1992) Blood transfusions for severe anaemia in African children (letter). *Lancet*, **340**: 917.
4 Saxena, S., Rabinowitz, A.P., Cage Johnson and Shulman, I.A. (1993) Iron-deficiency anaemia: a medically treatable chronic anaemia as a model for transfusion overuse. *Am. J. Med.*, **94**: 120–124.
5 Carmel, R. and Shulman, I.A. (1989) Blood transfusion in medically treatable chronic anaemia: pernicious anaemia as a model for transfusion overuse. *Arch. Pathol. Lab. Med.*, **113**: 995–997.
6 Leading article (1984) High-dose chelation therapy in thalassaemia. *Lancet* i: 373–374.
7 Brittenham, G.M., Griffith, P.M., Nienhuis, A.W. *et al.* (1994) Efficacy of deferoxamine in preventing complications of iron overload in patients with thalassemia major. *N. Engl. J. Med.*, **331**: 567–573.
8 Oral chelation in the treatment of thalassaemia and other disease. *Drugs Today* (1992), **26** (Suppl. A): 1–187.
9 Kontoghiorghes, G.J. (1992) Advances in oral iron chelation in man. *Int. J. Haematol.*, **55**: 27–38.
10 Pippard, M.J. and Callender, S.T. (1983) Clinical annotation. The management of iron chelation therapy. *Br. J. Haematol.*, **54**: 503–507.
11 Propper, R.D., Button, L.N. and Nathan, D.G. (1980) New approaches to the transfusion management of thalassaemia. *Blood*, **55**: 55–66.
12 Corash, L., Klein, H., Deisseroth, A. *et al.* (1981) Selective isolation of young erythrocytes for transfusion support of thalassaemia major patients. *Blood*, **57**: 599–606.
13 Royal College of Physicians of Edinburgh (1993) Consensus Conference. Leucocyte depletion of Blood and Blood Components.
14 Lasky, L.C., Rose, R.R. and Polesky, H.F. (1984) Incidence of antibody formation and positive direct antiglobulin tests in a multitransfused hemodialysis population. *Transfusion*, **24**: 198–200.
15 Blumberg, N., Peck, K., Ross, K. and Avila, E. (1983) Immune response to chronic red blood cell transfusion. *Vox Sang.*, **44**: 212–217.
16 Kim, H.C., Barnsley, W. and Sweisfurth, A.W. (1984) Incidence of alloimmunisation in multiply transfused pediatric patients. AABB Meeting Abstracts. *Transfusion*, **24**: S8, 417.
17 Sarnaik, S., Schornack, J. and Lusher, J.M. (1986) The incidence of development of irregular red cell antibodies in patients with sickle cell anemia. *Transfusion*, **26**: 249–252.

18 Sirchia, G., Zanella, A., Parravicini, A., Morelati, F., Rebulla, P. and Masera, G. (1985) Red cell alloantibodies in thalassemia major: results of an Italian cooperative study. *Transfusion*, **25**: 110–112.
19 Coles, S.M., Klein, H.G. and Holland, P.V. (1981) Alloimmunisation in two multi-transfused patient populations. *Transfusion* 21: 462–466.
20 Sosler, S.D., Jilly, B.J., Saporito, C. and Koshy, M. (1993) A simple, practical model for reducing alloimmunization in patients with sickle cell disease. *Am. J. Hematol.*, **43**: 103–106.
21 Blumberg, N., Ross, K., Avila, E. and Peck, K. (1984) Should chronic transfusions be matched for antigens other than ABO and $RH_o(D)$? *Vox Sang.*, **47**: 205–208.
22 Merianou, V.M., Panousopoulou, L.P., Lowes, L.P., Pelegrinis, E. and Karaklis, A. (1987) Alloimmunization to red cell antigens in thalassaemia: comparative study of usual versus better-match transfusion programmes. *Vox Sang.*, **52**: 95–98.
23 Davies, S.C., McWilliam, A.C., Hewitt, P.E., Devenish, A. and Brozovic, M. (1986) Red cell alloimmunisation in sickle cell disease. *Br. J. Haematol.*, **63**: 241–245.
24 Cummins, D., Webb, G., Shah, N. and Davies, S.C. (1991) Delayed haemolytic transfusion reactions in patients with sickle cell disease. *Postgrad. Med. J.*, **67**: 689–691.
25 Brecher, M.E. and Taswell, H.F. (1989) Paroxysmal nocturnal heamoglobinuria and the transfusion of washed red cells: a myth revisited. *Transfusion*, **29**: 681–685.
26 Rosse, W.F. (1989) Transfusion in paroxysmal nocturnal haemoglobinuria: to wash or not to wash? *Transfusion*, **29**: 663–664.
27 Davies, S.C. and Brozovic, M. (1989) Sickle cell anaemia: the presentation, management and prophylaxis of sickle cell disease. *Blood Rev.*, **3**: 29–44.
28 Fleming, A.F. (1989) Sickle cell anaemia: the presentation, management and prevention of crisis in sickle cell disease in Africa. *Blood Rev.*, **3**: 18–28.
29 Jan, K., Usami, S. and Smith, J.A. (1982) Effects of transfusion on rheological properties of blood in sickle cell anaemia. *Transfusion*, **22**: 17–20.
30 Russell, M.O., Goldberg, H.I., Hodson, A. *et al.* (1984) Effect of transfusion therapy on arteriographic abnormalities and on recurrence of stroke in sickle cell disease. *Blood*, **63**: 162–169.
31 Morrison, J.C. and Foster, H. (1979) Transfusion therapy in pregnant patients with sickle cell disease: a National Institutes of Health Consensus Development Conference. *Ann. Intern. Med.*, **91**: 122–123.
32 Morrison, J.C., Blake, P.G. and Reed, C.D. (1982) Therapy for the pregnant patient with sickle hemoglobinopathies: a national focus. *Am. J. Obstet. Gynecol.*, **144**: 268–269.
33 Westney, L.S., Callender, C.O., Stevens, J., Bhagwanari, S.G., George, J.P.A. and Mun, S.O.L. (1984) Pregnancy sickle cell, renal allograft: pathophysiology of sickle cell anemia. *Obstet. Gynaecol.*, **63**: 753.
34 Miller, D.M., Winslow, R.M., Klein, H.G., Wilson, K.C., Brown, F.L. and Statham, N.J. (1980) Improved exercise performance after exchange transfusion in subjects with sickle cell anemia. *Blood*, **56**: 1127–1131.
35 Charache, S., Bleecker, E.R. and Bross, D.S. (1983) Effects of blood transfusion on exercise capacity in patients with sickle-cell anemia. *Am. J. Med.*, **74**: 757–764.
36 Bischoff, R.J., Williamson, A. III, Dalali, M.J., Rice, J.C. and Kerstein, M.D. (1988) Assessment of the use of transfusion therapy perioperatively in patients with sickle cell hemoglobinopathies. *Ann. Surg.*, **207**: 435–438.
37 Masera, G., Terzoli, S., Avanzini, A. et al. (1982) Evaluation of the supertransfusion regimen in homozygous beta-thalassaemia children. *Br. J. Haematol.*, **52**: 111–113.
38 Ness, P.M. (1994) To match or not to match: the question for chronically transfused patients with sickle cell anemia. *Transfusion.*, **34**: 558–560.

5
Platelet Transfusion

The ready availability of platelet transfusion has removed thrombocytopenic haemorrhage as the major cause of death in patients with haematological malignancy.
Platelet transfusions can now be given routinely to control or prevent bleeding
due to thrombocytopenia whenever this is encountered in medical, surgical or
obstetric practice. These transfusions are usually assumed to be effective, although
in individual instances it may be difficult to obtain objective proof of benefit.
Platelet therapy is less reliably effective than red cell transfusion for various
reasons:

(1) Alloimmunization occurs much more frequently and the serological analysis is
    also more complex.
(2) Compatibility testing is not as well developed or reliable as a means of pre-
    dicting post-transfusion platelet survival.
(3) The frequency of compatible donors for alloimmunized patients is usually low.

(4) Platelets have a shorter *in vivo* life-span, they store less well *in vitro* and post-transfusion recovery is less predictable.

For these reasons and also because of the frequency of alloimmunization, it is not so certain that transfusion will confer a significant benefit analogous to the predictable rise in haemoglobin concentration following red cell transfusion.

1 INDICATIONS FOR PLATELET TRANSFUSION

Platelets are required for the treatment of *thrombocytopenic patients* who are *actively bleeding* or who are judged to be *at risk of haemorrhagic symptoms*. Where platelet function is normal the risk of haemorrhage depends on the platelet count.

Relation between platelet count and bleeding

- Below $20 \times 10^9/1$ *High risk*. Patients who are not showing thrombocytopenic symptoms may need *prophylactic therapy*.
- $20-50 \times 10^9/1$ Platelets should be transfused to patients showing *symptoms* and those *requiring surgery*.
- $50-100 \times 10^9/1$ Platelet therapy not usually required. Bleeding risks only slightly increased. Platelets may be required where bleeding would be particularly dangerous, e.g. during neurosurgery or ophthalmic surgery.

These categorizations should not be applied too literally. Other circumstances may need to be considered:

(1) The *direction of change* of the platelet count is important. The risk of bleeding is greater with falling counts than with rising counts.
(2) *Platelet kinetics* affect the bleeding tendency. At any given platelet count the risk of bleeding appears less in high turnover states, e.g. idiopathic thrombocytopenic purpura, than it is in thrombocytopenia due to aplasia.
(3) *Infections* and *febrile episodes* increase the risk of bleeding. These episodes justify the use of prophylactic platelets when counts are low. It follows that prophylactic platelets are more likely to be required when granulocyte counts are also low.
(4) The *haematocrit* appears to affect the risk of bleeding.[1] Severe anaemia, when associated with increased haemorrhagic symptoms, should be treated.
(5) Concomitant *drug therapy* may be important. Drugs such as aspirin which inhibit platelet cyclooxygenase activity should be avoided in thrombocytopenia. Cytotoxic drugs associated with mucosal ulceration may predispose to bleeding.

The value of the bleeding time for determining the need for treatment

The standardized template bleeding time has been traditionally used to provide a measurement of the bleeding tendency in both thrombocytopenia and disorders of platelet function. Prolongation of the bleeding time begins when platelet counts fall below $100 \times 10^9/l$ and it increases progressively with declining counts until around a level of $20 \times 10^9/l$, at which point indefinite lengthening occurs. A two-fold prolongation of the normal bleeding time, e.g. to around 15 minutes, is indicative of a significant risk of bleeding.

There is no point in performing bleeding times in severe thrombocytopenia associated with leukaemia or aplasia. The result is certain to be abnormal and the test will cause unnecessary discomfort and inconvenience. Bleeding times may be useful for screening patients prior to invasive procedures or for investigation of patients with bleeding symptoms not fully explained by platelet count changes.[2] The place of the bleeding time in the evaluation of platelet concentrates is considered in section 8.

2 CLINICAL CONDITIONS REQUIRING PLATELET THERAPY

Haematological malignancies

Haematological malignancies, in particular adult *acute myeloid leukaemia*, constitute by far the largest category of patients requiring regular platelet therapy. Thrombocytopenia may be due to the underlying condition or result from cytotoxic drugs or radiotherapy. As a result of the successful experience gained in use of platelets for this condition, bleeding has ceased to be the principal cause of death. The use of platelet therapy has allowed development of more intensive cytotoxic treatment regimens and as a result remission rates have improved.

Thrombocytopenia associated with bone marrow failure (aplastic, hypoplastic, sideroblastic or refractory anaemia)

Platelets can be valuable in the treatment of acute self-limiting conditions or for isolated bleeding episodes. In chronic states long-term blood transfusion or platelet therapy inevitably leads to *alloimmunization* against a broad range of HLA or platelet-specific antigens. This complication seriously diminishes the chances of providing serologically compatible and clinically effective therapy.

Massive transfusion

This is discussed more fully in chapter 12. *Dilutional thrombocytopenia* occurs less readily than commonly supposed. It is expected that platelet counts will only fall below $100 \times 10^9/l$ when at least 1.5–2.0 blood volumes have been replaced with stored blood. Platelet therapy may be considered at this point but is certainly needed at levels of $50–60 \times 10^9/l$ or less. Administration of platelets during rapid surgical bleeding is wasteful and ineffective. Therapy may be more valuable when conserved until surgical haemostasis is secured. Generalized oozing unrelated to fresh surgical incisions suggest the presence of significant thrombocytopenia or *disseminated intravascular coagulation* which should then be investigated.

Surgery in thrombocytopenia

Major surgery requires platelet counts to be above $50 \times 10^9/l$. Although not routine practice, the bleeding risk can be assessed pre-operatively by means of the template bleeding time and it can also help in confirming that pre-operative platelet transfusions have been effective. Higher platelet counts may be required during neurosurgery or ophthalmic surgery when excessive bleeding would be highly dangerous. Cardiopulmonary bypass surgery (chapter 14) can be associated with an *acquired platelet functional defect* which may necessitate more ready recourse to platelet therapy.

Splenectomy for idiopathic thrombocytopenia is considered below. Removal of the large adherent spleens typical of patients with myelofibrosis and thrombocytopenia presents unavoidable haemostatic difficulties. Platelets administered pre-operatively will be sequestered in the spleen and a clinically significant post-transfusion increment is unlikely. The most rational approach is to delay platelet administration until the splenic vessels can be clamped. High-dose platelet infusions will then be more effective. Multi-transfused patients may well be alloimmunized and this should be investigated prior to surgery.

Idiopathic thrombocytopenic purpura

Platelet therapy is not often indicated in this condition. The bleeding risk seems to be less than anticipated from the platelet count; possibly the higher proportion of young larger platelets associated with the high platelet turnover rate provides more effective haemostasis. This is fortunate because any transfused platelets will be destroyed as rapidly as autologous platelets; it is therefore highly unlikely that any effect, either in the form of a post-transfusion increment or corrected bleeding time, will be noticeable.

If platelets are to be given at all in idiopathic thrombocytopenic purpura (ITP) then high doses, of the order of 1.5–2 packs per 10 kg body weight, should be used. If the platelet count shows a post-transfusion increase the diagnosis of ITP is probably incorrect! Platelets are therefore only given for dangerous bleeding episodes, such as intracranial or ophthalmic haemorrhage.

Platelets are not now normally given to cover *splenectomy in ITP*; this operation is frequently and safely performed without platelet cover. It is probably prudent to make platelet concentrates available on standby in case bleeding becomes uncontrollable. Platelets are best administered *after* the splenic pedicle has been clamped. A high proportion of any platelets transfused before that time will be surgically removed with the spleen.

Congenital platelet dysfunctional states

The rare patients with normal platelet counts but defective platelet function present a heterogeneous group for whom generalizations regarding management may be inappropriate. Platelets may be needed for bleeding episodes or prior to surgery.

In the absence of more specific guidance, perform template bleeding times to assess the risk of bleeding. If platelet therapy is needed the template bleeding time can help in monitoring its effectiveness. The success of therapy can also be assessed by the degree of correction of the specific functional defect characteristic of the condition concerned, e.g. the ADP-induced platelet aggregation which is abnormal in Glanzmann's thrombasthenia.

Acquired platelet functional defects

Uraemia and *myeloma* are the commonest examples of these conditions and, in both, abnormalities of plasma composition impair platelet function. Platelet therapy will therefore be largely ineffective. Dialysis is required for uraemia and plasmapheresis for myeloma.

3 PROPHYLACTIC PLATELET THERAPY

The well-established relationship between severe thrombocytopenia and spontaneous haemorrhage has led to the widespread use of *prophylactic platelet therapy* to protect patients through periods of risk. While it seems highly likely that such policies must reduce chances of life-threatening haemorrhage, modern studies confirming the value of *prophylactic policies* have not been performed. Indeed, it has been shown by necessity that many patients can tolerate prolonged periods of profound thrombocytopenia without serious problems. There is also some debate about the threshold platelet counts at which prophylactic therapy should be considered. Counts of $20 \times 10^9/l$ are generally taken as a treatment trigger.[3,4] However, convincing evidence suggests that significantly hazardous counts are much lower[5] and utilization of a $5-10^9/l$ threshold has been shown to be perfectly safe in the absence of other risk factors.[6] Fever, coagulation dysfunction, heparin or anatomical bleeding lesions justify higher threshold values.

There are some disadvantages to use of prophylactic therapy; these include expense, increased number of donor exposures and possibly also enhanced risk of alloimmunization. The advantages of prophylactic therapy are also not universally accepted. Even when the value of prophylactic therapy is accepted the platelet count threshold at which this is justified is still very much a matter of debate[7-9] and it is certainly true that not all patients with severe thrombocytopenia should be considered automatic candidates for prophylactic therapy.

4 PLATELET PREPARATIONS

4.1 Random-donor Platelet Concentrates

Platelets collected from random donations are the most frequently used form of platelet product. Donations should be maintained close to $22\,°C$ during the 6–8-hour hold time permissible until platelet preparation.[10] This is usually carried out by subjecting the blood to a short-spin centrifugation phase after which platelet-rich plasma is left as the supernatant. *Platelet concentrates* are then prepared by displacing the platelet-rich plasma into a satellite pack and subjecting this to a second slower spin. This results in a supernatant consisting of platelet-poor plasma which is removed to leave 50–60 ml of plasma accompanying the platelet pellet at the bottom of the pack. The traumatic damage of centrifugation temporarily alters the platelets in CPD-anticoagulated blood in such a way that resuspension in the plasma residue is not possible until 1 or 2 hours have elapsed, during which time the packs must remain undisturbed to allow for spontaneous disaggregation. After completion of the rest period the platelets are gently resuspended from the platelet pellet and the pack is placed on a mixer for storage.

An alternative and increasingly used procedure for platelet concentrate production involves use of a hard spin (approx. 3000 g) to demarcate the buffy coat. After removal of the supernatant platelet-poor plasma, the buffy coat fraction can be decanted, pooled with others and then subjected to a further gentle spin to produce a pooled platelet concentrate which can be tailored to provide a conventional adult therapeutic dose. It is relatively easy to incorporate an in-line leucocyte removal filter into the separation system so as to obtain a leucodepleted final product. Preparation of platelets by the buffy coat procedure avoids the step of hard compaction into a pellet, such as occurs during the 'platelet-rich plasma' process. This appears to minimize the amount of trauma-related activation damage (see section 8).

Platelet concentrates are usually stored at 22–24 °C and presented in volumes of 50–60 ml containing 5.5–7×10^{10} platelets or proportionately larger volumes if platelets are pooled. This process represents around 80% recovery of platelets from the original donation. About 60% of the infused dose should be recovered in the recipient's circulation in the absence of bleeding or alloimmunization (see section 5).

4.2 Single-donor Platelets

Single-donor platelets are obtained by plateletpheresis using either continuous-flow or intermittent-flow centrifugation procedures.

The degree of contamination can be greatly reduced by careful selection of collection conditions but generally at the expense of platelet yields. The yields that are actually obtained during plateletpheresis depend on the donor platelet count, the machine and technique used for collection, the skill of the operator and the degree of purity selected. These will therefore be determined on an individual laboratory basis. Modern plateletpheresis techniques are now capable of obtaining platelet yields of the order of 3–6×10^{11}. The products can be virtually red cell free and some meet current standards for leucocyte-depleted products. ($< 1.0 \times 10^6$ leucocytes per 55×10^9 platelets).[11] This performance comfortably exceeds current agreed minimum quality specifications for platelet concentrates (see section 6.3) and makes plateletpheresis an attractive means for therapeutic platelet procurement.

Choice between single-donor and random-donor platelets

Single-donor plateletpheresis places the donor at greater inconvenience and also at slightly greater risk than normal blood collection and fully informed consent is essential. Venepuncture to both arms—one for collection and one for return of blood—is usually required for continuous-flow systems; intermittent centrifugation systems are, however, performed using only a single needle. The donation time may take up to 1.5 hours. The procedures are readily accepted and safe and are not as demanding as for granulocyte collection. No donor pre-medication is required. Adverse reactions are confined mainly to those caused by hypovolaemia or excessive rates of citrated blood return; both are uncommon but are more likely with intermittent flow systems. Donor platelet counts may fall by as much as 40% but significant thrombocytopenia will not occur if pre-donation counts were satisfactory.

Apheresis platelets are not always as readily available and require a greater commitment on the part of the donor. Nevertheless in some clinical units they are believed to be more efficacious and have become the favoured product.

Apheresis platelets are the only convenient means of providing HLA-matched doses; furthermore donor exposures and the opportunities for HLA sensitization as well as microbiological risks are reduced. A disadvantage with some machines has been greater yield variability necessitating increased quality-control vigilance to ensure that adequate therapeutic dosages have been achieved.

Care must be taken to ensure that plateletpheresis donors have taken no aspirin or other drugs affecting platelet function in the week preceding donation. This will impair platelet performance in inverse proportion to the number of days before donation that are free of aspirin ingestion. It is clearly best to exclude the collection of platelets from random donors who have taken aspirin but in practice it is unlikely that more than an occasional pack in a pool will be so affected.

4.3 Frozen Platelets[12]

Platelets collected either from random donations or from single donors can be frozen for prolonged storage. Dimethyl sulphoxide (DMSO) has proved to be the most successful cryoprotective agent. This material is toxic and must therefore be removed from the thawed platelets by thorough washing before use. Platelets are resuspended in autologous plasma before reinfusion.

Frozen platelet banking was originally considered as a means of meeting unexpected clinical demands, e.g. where requirements outstrip provision from freshly collected donations or, alternatively, facilitating continued support over prolonged public holidays. The expense of these procedures, technical inconvenience and poor yields have meant that this promise has not been fulfilled and frozen banking has remained relatively underdeveloped.

Uses of frozen platelets

(1) *Autologous platelet transfusions*: autologous platelets collected from patients with leukaemia in remission can be frozen and stored for future use. This

manoeuvre guarantees availability of compatible platelets for future use when alloimmunization may result in random donor platelets being ineffective.
(2) Frozen storage may be useful for provision of *HLA-matched platelets* or for storage of platelet antigen-'negative' (e.g. HPA-1a-negative donations) platelets which may otherwise be unavailable when required.

4.4   Leucocyte- and Red Cell-poor Platelets

Unwanted cellular contamination can be minimized by careful attention to centrifugation during preparation. Avoidance of folds in the blood pack or disturbances of the buffy coat interface and not sampling too close to the buffy coat layer, are all important technical considerations. Filtration is, however, now by far the most effective means of purifying random donor platelet suspensions. Leucocyte counts of below 10^6 per donation (>99% leucocyte loss) are possible with generally no more than 10–15% loss of platelets. Filters are available for use in transfusion laboratories and also for bedside filtration of platelet concentrates. There is evidence, however, that bedside procedures are less reliable than those in the laboratory which can be subject to more stringent control. Cell-free products may be indicated:

(1) To reduce red cell contamination and allow ABO-incompatible donations to be given.
(2) To diminish the likelihood of HLA sensitization (see section 5.1).
(3) To reduce the rate of febrile transfusion reactions that frequently accompany regular platelet transfusion. (Despite the expectation of benefit, two recent studies have failed to confirm that leucocyte depletion is effective)[13,14](see chapter 23).

4.5   Irradiated Platelets

Irradiated platelets must be used where graft-versus-host reaction is a possible risk (see chapter 23, section 3). Irradiation does not appear to reduce post transfusion recovery.[15]

4.6   Platelets for Paediatric Use

The volume of platelet concentrates can be further reduced for paediatric use[16] (see chapter 20, section 3).

5   DOSAGE OF PLATELETS

Platelets are usually administered on a basis predetermined by local custom; e.g. six random donor packs or their equivalent in apheresis donations to adult patients, proportionately less for children. The rationale for this should be supported by factors such as the following:

(1) Producers of platelets should provide data regarding the expected platelet count of their products. Normally this is of the order of $55-70 \times 10^9$ per random donor pack or $3-6 \times 10^{11}$ where apheresis donations are provided.
(2) The patient's estimated blood volume (BV). This is calculated approximately (in litres) from $2.5 \times$ body surface area (m^2) or $70 \, ml/kg$ body weight (kg).
(3) The desired platelet count increment (PI) should be decided.
(4) Because of splenic sequestration only about 0.67 of the infused dose will normally be recoverable in the circulation.
 Taking these factors into consideration the dose may be calculated from:

$$\text{Dose required} = \frac{\text{BV} \times \text{PI}}{0.67}$$

On this basis the common 'routine' of six packs (at 55×10^9 platelets per pack) will produce an increment of about $40 \times 10^9/l$ in a $70 \, kg$ (5 l BV) adult.

(5) Transfused platelets should raise the platelet count of recipients who have not been immunized or do not have non-immune factors that could shorten platelet survival (see below). A variety of ways of assessing post-transfusion response exist.[17] Conventionally it is accepted that a $5-10 \times 10^9/l$ 1-hour post-transfusion increment per pack should occur. More precise assessment of recovery is provided by a modification of the formula described above to give the *corrected count increment*.[18] This is calculated from:

$$\frac{\text{Observed increment} \times \text{surface area } (m^2)}{\text{Number of platelets given } (\times 10^{11})}$$

Values of $15-20 \times 10^9/l$ per square metre for each 10^{11} platelets administered are expected. Increments are usually measured at 1 hour and 20–24 hours following transfusion.

Failure to achieve satisfactory post-transfusion increments indicate one or more of the following circumstances:

(1) The occurrence of *alloimmunization*. In the absence of (2) and (3) below, failure to obtain an increment (e.g. two consecutive 1-hour increments of below 5×10^9 following random donor platelets) is highly suggestive.
(2) *Idiopathic thrombocytopenia, bleeding, infection and disseminated intravascular coagulation (DIC)* appear to cause increased platelet turnover and transfused platelets are also quickly consumed.
(3) *Splenomegaly*: as many as 30% of transfused platelets are sequestered in the normal spleen. Splenomegaly results in sequestration of an even higher proportion.

(4) *Adverse storage or preparation conditions*: these will damage platelets and reduce
    their post-transfusion viability.

Routine platelet transfusions for haematological patients are usually given on the
basis of clinical symptoms and platelet counts but without regular recourse to
measurement of increments. Increments should, however, be confirmed if clinical
improvement does not occur as a refractory state due to alloimmunization may
have developed.

During preparation of thrombocytopenic patients for major surgery a target of
at least $50 \times 10^9/l$ should be attained.

Lower doses, with correspondingly lower increments, may be acceptable for
prophylactic cover.

5.1 Compatibility Selections

Non-immunized patients are normally given ABO and Rh D-matched platelets;
where supplies of platelets are adequate this practice avoids confusion and is
simple to operate. Where this is not possible platelets of other groups can be used
provided appropriate explanation is given to clinical staff. Immunized and clinically refractory patients require special measures for selection of compatible platelets (see section 6.4).

ABO group

Platelets carry ABO blood group antigens but these are largely derived by passive
absorption from those present in plasma.[19] ABO-incompatible platelets can be
transfused and are effective even though post-transfusion survival and recovery
have been claimed to be slightly diminished. Provided red cell counts of the concentrates are below 0.4×10^9 per pack (not visibly pink) a standard adult dose of
six to eight packs will contain no more than 0.5 ml red cells which would not be
expected to cause haemolytic symptoms. Refractory patients should be transfused
with ABO-compatible platelets, if at all possible, as under these circumstances all
factors influencing platelet survival should be optimized.[20]

Group O plateletpheresis donations issued to non-group O recipients are
usually screened to identify those with *high-titre alloantibodies*, in particular haemolysins, which have been causes of haemolytic transfusion reactions during platelet
therapy.[21,22]

If these are avoided, group O donations to non-O recipients have been shown
to be effective and perfectly safe. Although positive direct antiglobulin tests may
be observed, clinical haemolysis seems not to occur.[23]

However, immune complex formation from transfused ABO alloantibodies and
incompatible blood group substances in recipient plasma might be responsible for
diminished survival, both of autologous and of transfused platelets through the
'innocent bystander' mechanism.[24]

Rh D group

This is expressed poorly, if at all, on platelets. Contaminating Rh D-positive red cells have been shown to be immunogenic; alloimmunization frequencies of up to 19% have been reported.[25] Increasing numbers of patients treated for malignancy are now surviving to have successful pregnancies. Prevention of Rh D immunization in women of childbearing age is therefore desirable. Intramuscular injections of anti-D are contraindicated. When intravenous preparations are not available a dose of 250 IU of the intramuscular preparation given subcutaneously should be adequate.[26]

6 PLATELET ALLOIMMUNIZATION[27,28]

Clinical unresponsiveness to platelet transfusions eventually occurs in a high proportion (up to 50%) of patients receiving multiple transfusions. In patients with normal immune function immunization to platelets occurs much more rapidly than that following red cell transfusions. The refractory state usually occurs after 4–8 weeks' therapy although in some patients it may develop after only 1–2 weeks. The problem appears to be accelerated when there is a history of *previous transfusion* or *pregnancy*.

The refractory state is most frequently due to immunization against *HLA antigens*; in around 25% of cases platelet-specific antibodies are also involved. To a lesser, although uncertain, extent it reflects immunization against other *non-HLA histocompatibility antigens* and in around 5% of cases to *platelet-specific antigens* alone.

The problem of alloimmunization to platelet-specific antigens, e.g. HPA-1a platelet antigens, is also considered in chapter 20 (section 4.2, neonatal alloimmune thrombocytopenia), chapter 23 (section 3, non-haemolytic transfusion reactions, post-transfusion purpura) and chapter 8 (section 3, intravenous immunoglobulin for thrombocytopenia).

Platelets carry HLA antigens (class I but not class II HLA antigens) and are therefore rendered ineffective when transfused to recipients possessing incompatible HLA antibodies. However, platelets alone do not appear capable of primary HLA immunization, this being a consequence of the leucocytes that usually contaminate platelet preparations. It is for this reason that regimens involving transfusion of *leucocyte-depleted* products are increasingly used in an attempt to prevent the development of alloimmunization. Alloimmunization has been claimed to develop less readily in patients with leukaemia on immunosuppressive treatment than in patients with normal immune function[29] although this conclusion has been in conflict with other observations.[30,31]

Most patients with bone marrow failure, in whom immune function is not typically impaired, rapidly become refractory. There is, however, some disagreement about the actual immunization rates in patients with leukaemia: incidences ranging upwards from 40% are reported.[32]

The incidence of alloimmunization is probably dose dependent,[30,33] although this again has been disputed.[34]

Dose dependence has been claimed to occur for the first 10–12 donor exposures; after this number of transfusions has been given, the risk of immunization appears to decline for the remaining unimmunized patients, and possibly a proportion never at any time become immunized.

6.1 Diagnosis of the Refractory State

Diagnosis of a refractory state due to alloimmunization usually requires the following circumstances:

(1) Failure to achieve the expected post-transfusion increment.
(2) Exclusion of non-immune causes of poor response (see section 5).
(3) Demonstration that lymphocytotoxic HLA antibodies are present. These antibodies occur in around 95% of refractory patients.
(4) A history of platelet transfusion, previous blood transfusions or pregnancy will always be obtained.
(5) Under ideal circumstances the diagnosis will be confirmed when serologically compatible platelets restore post-transfusion increments.

6.2 Delaying the Onset of Immunization

Attempts have been made to reduce the rate at which this occurs by the following methods:

(1) Use of filters for leucocyte depletion has been claimed in several studies virtually to prevent alloimmunization.[35–38] These filters do not appear to cause morphological or functional damage; post-transfusion viability and effectiveness are not impaired.[39,40] About 15–24% platelet loss may be expected,[38] the greatest depletion occurring in older units. Leucocyte depletion has been claimed to be the most cost-effective approach to management of alloimmunization,[41] and prevention of alloimmunization has been shown to diminish the need for blood component support, reduce infection rates, and improve the chance of relapse-free survival[42] in acute myelogenous leukaemia.
   It should be remembered that all red cell components must also be leucocyte depleted if this policy is adopted.
(2) *Reducing the number of platelet transfusions*: it has, for example, been suggested that the use of prophylactic transfusion should be curtailed because of the risk of alloimmunization. This practice does appear to delay alloimmunization but it is claimed that eventually most susceptible patients will become refractory irrespective of their transfusion regimen.[43]
(3) *Use of single-donor transfusions*: this has the aim of reducing the number of HLA antigens to which the recipient is exposed, thereby restricting the range of specificities of those antibodies that do develop. This does not always seem to be borne out in practice, probably because of the cross-reactivity between HLA antigens which ensures a multispecific antibody response. It has, however, been found that this approach can retard development of the clinical refractory state compared with use of multiple random donor platelets.[33]

Single-donor HLA-matched platelet transfusion regimens have also been used to delay alloimmunization. This approach is, of course, logistically difficult or sometimes impossible for those patients with uncommon HLA genotypes. Alloimmunization to non-HLA antigens or platelet-specific antigens is a possible consequence which may reduce the effectiveness of this approach.

The logistic difficulties of such regimens do not appear to be justified by the limited success that has been shown.

(4) *Reduction of HLA immunogenicity using ultraviolet (UV) irradiation*: UV irradiation in the wavelength region of 280–340 nm has been shown in numerous animal studies to remove the HLA immunogenicity of platelet transfusions. This appears to be the result of inactivation of mononuclear cell-mediated antigen presentation and can be achieved without impairment of platelet function.[44,45]

However, lymphocyte phytohaemagglutin responses, mixed lymphocyte culture (MLC) responses and interleukin production have not been shown to be abolished. Application to the human clinical situation has so far been limited—a difficulty has been the identification of plastic materials which combine both the gas permeability requirements for platelet storage as well as permitting adequate transmission of UV light. If this problem can be resolved the use of UV irradiation may provide a valuable advance in prophylaxis of the refractory state.

In conclusion, leucocyte depletion appears at the present time to offer the most effective means of reducing alloimmunization. This is, however, a costly procedure which has to be balanced against the expense and difficulties of dealing with the established refractory state. The data so far are not sufficiently compelling to have resulted in widespread adoption of any of these measures. Platelets, including those for prophylactic use, should therefore be transfused when judged necessary on clinical grounds using random donor platelets, when these are the most conveniently available, until the development of alloimmunization.

6.3 Management of Immunized Patients

When a refractory state develops, effective long-term platelet transfusion will be considerably more difficult to achieve.

Prior to confirmed serological diagnosis, or when non-immune factors are believed to coexist, the only recourse is to provide larger and more frequent doses of unselected donor concentrates. Under these circumstances it is important to measure post-transfusion increments. This is also particularly so where excellent serological matches have been obtained as it may help to establish the relative importance of immune and non-immune causes for the unresponsive state.

For patients expecting long-term treatment the development of the alloimmunized state should be anticipated and the following procedure is advisable:

(1) Determine the HLA A and B phenotype of the patient at the start of the treatment.
(2) Screen sera regularly for emergence of lymphocytotoxic HLA antibodies.

(3) Perform post-transfusion increments if there is clinical doubt as to efficacy of transfusions.

There are a variety of approaches to the provision of compatible platelets for refractory patients, thus testifying to the fact that there is no obvious 'best buy' in terms of compatibility procedure. Platelets can be supplied from panels as either *HLA matched* or selected according to one or more of a variety of *cross-match* procedures.

Intravenous immunoglobulin is probably not effective in blocking alloantibody-mediated donor platelet destruction but is currently under investigation (see chapter 11).

6.4 HLA-matched Platelets

(1) Some centres utilize *HLA-matched* platelets as a first approach to management of refractory patients. In practice, the high degree of HLA polymorphism sometimes makes the search for compatible donors for patients with uncommon phenotypes very difficult.

Many transfusion services now have local panels of HLA-matched donors and cooperate on a regional or national basis to meet more difficult matching requirements. Required panel sizes for platelet donors have been estimated as being between 1000 and 3000.[46]

The size will depend on the degree of matching required and also on the genetic diversity of the population concerned. In the UK many transfusion centres recruit donors for the British Bone Marrow and Platelet Panel, which in 1994 amounted to 70 000 potential donors, and also utilize their own contribution to the panel as a source of platelet donors. About 60–70% of patients with the most common phenotypes will have a reasonable expectation of securing good matches;[47] many of the remainder will not be matched well. The position can be improved if HLA antigen splits and cross-reactive antigens are utilized.

It cannot be assumed that all cross-reactive antigen combinations are equally clinically compatible, although the subject has been investigated[48,49] to provide preliminary data on the potential therapeutic value of donations selected on this basis.

HLA incompatibility cannot account for all cases of failure to respond. On occasions perfect matches are unsuccessful and in other instances the opposite is found. In these instances non-HLA antigenic systems or platelet-specific antigens must be involved.[50] Certainly the fact that unrelated but otherwise apparently perfect matches are rarely as successful as those from identical siblings is suggestive evidence for the importance of minor histocompatibility differences.

In general, however, it has been shown that post-transfusion increments in refractory patients do depend on the degree of HLA compatibility. Only matching HLA-A and HLA-B antigens is necessary; there is no evidence yet for the need to consider HLA-C compatibility, and platelets do not carry class

II antigens. Full HLA-A,B antigen matches are in general more successful than donations differing by a single antigen even when the differing antigens are cross-reactive.[51]

Family members should also be investigated as possible donors. Some may be HLA identical; failing this they may share HLA haplotypes or possess minor histocompatibility antigens in common with the patient. Siblings should certainly be investigated where antibodies to platelet specific antigens, e.g. HPA-1a, are involved.

(2) *Lymphocytotoxicity tests* are the most widely performed compatibility tests for donor selection. They have been claimed to be 70% accurate in predicting donors capable of providing a post-transfusion increment. If well-matched (HLA) donations are not available it may therefore be advantageous to use donations of HLA phenotypes that are compatible with the recipient's lymphocytotoxic HLA antibodies. This approach is likely to be most successful where patients' sera react with a relatively narrow range of antigen specificities. In such instances a wider selection of donations may be eligible for consideration than would result from confining the search to good HLA matches alone.

On about 30% of occasions lymphocytotoxicity cross-matching fails to predict the transfusion outcome. The test procedure relies on complement-fixing lymphocytotoxic antibodies—accordingly non-complement-fixing HLA antibodies will not be detected and neither will platelet-specific antibodies. On the other hand, unexpected successful transfusions in the face of a positive cross-match also occur. These might be examples of occasions in which a particular HLA antigen is not well expressed on the donor platelets.[52]

(3) *Platelet cross-match testing*: a contrasting approach is to use platelet cross-matching as the first approach to compatibility selection—this argument is supported by their increasing reliability for outcome prediction and by the great expense of maintaining HLA typed panels in the knowledge that the rarer donors are unlikely ever to be called. Up to 60–70% of donors selected for refractory patients may prove to be compatible by cross-match studies and also provide good post-transfusion increments. Rather surprisingly, not all of these are found amongst the closely HLA-matched donors. It should be noted that cross-matching is particularly indicated where it is intended to use single randomly selected apheresis donations. This precaution can disclose instances in which the available donor may be completely unsuitable and be therefore even less effective than random donor platelets of mixed antigen status.

Platelet cross-match tests will detect platelet-specific antigens but in practice these procedures are most often examining the reaction between HLA antibodies and class I antigens and possibly also minor immunocompatibility antigens carried on the platelet membrane. For these reasons, the term *platelet-reactive antibodies* may be preferred.[53] The reaction frequencies of these antibodies, not all of which can be characterized, do not usually coincide with those corresponding to the best-known platelet antigen–antibody systems. A wide variety of technical procedures are in use for platelet cross-matching. These include platelet-specific immunofluorescence tests (PSIFT),[54] platelet-reactive antiglobulin tests (PRAT),[55,56] Solid-phase red cell adherence tests[57] and enzyme-linked immunoglobulin (ELISA).[58-60]

The best of the platelet cross-matching procedures are at least as successful as HLA matching or lymphocytotoxicity cross-matching for prediction of successful transfusions.[61]

A study examining the relative merits of various approaches concluded that a 95% transfusion success rate could be achieved by a combination of all three of the above procedures.[62]

7   STORAGE OF PLATELET CONCENTRATES

Storage temperature

The optimum storage temperature for platelet concentrates is 22 °C; at this temperature post-transfusion recovery and survival are best preserved although their ability to confer immediate haemostatic benefit appears to be temporarily reduced compared to the former practice of 4 °C storage. Full recovery of function appears to take up to 24 hours following transfusion[63] but the significance of this in the management of acute haemorrhage is uncertain. Blood donations that are to be used for platelet preparation should not be allowed to cool substantially below 22 °C.

The storage environment

The qualities required of platelets for their natural function of aggregating and plugging defects in the circulation do not allow for convenient laboratory manipulation and storage. Platelets are very susceptible to damage from mechanical handling. Their function and viability are adversely influenced by chilling of blood units prior to storage but on the other hand the by-products arising from their metabolism at higher temperatures also accumulate during storage and have a self-poisoning effect.

Exhaustion of oxygen supply and carbon dioxide accumulation are well-recognized problems of platelet concentrate storage; pH measurements provide an indication of their severity (see section 8.1).

Platelets deteriorate progressively during storage; the process appears to be accompanied by appearance on the platelet surface of the α-granule membrane protein 140 (GMP140) as evidence for α-granule release and platelet activation.[64]

Acceptable function appears to be retained for at least 7 days but a conspicuously increased incidence of bacterial contamination with prolonged storage of platelet concentrates has curtailed the usable shelf life to 5 days. Leucocyte removal appears to benefit platelet viability. Leucocyte metabolism almost certainly has a deleterious effect on the platelet storage milieu and furthermore proteolytic enzymes released from degranulating leucocytes may cause direct platelet damage. Similarly, coagulation system activation which occurs spontaneously during storage may accelerate platelet activation;[65] for this and other reasons synthetic storage media are under investigation as a replacement[66,67] for the plasma currently retained within platelet concentrates.

Synthetic storage media

Attempts are in progress to develop synthetic storage media for platelet concentrates to meet the metabolic requirements of platelets more specifically. Platelets, unlike red cells, have an intact Krebs citric acid cycle and are not restricted to substrates such as glucose as an energy source. Currently, saline citrate acetate solutions have been found most promising as a resuspension medium.[68,69]

8 SPECIFICATIONS, QUALITY CONTROL AND CLINICAL EVALUATION OF PLATELET PREPARATION

Quality of platelets for transfusion can be assessed in several ways.

Incremental rise in platelet count following transfusion

Measurement of post-transfusion increments can be a valuable procedure for determining the *quality* of platelet products or the presence of an *alloimmunized* state. It can only be applied during prophylactic therapy when other conditions (e.g. sepsis, DIC, bleeding) that could lead to poor results are absent (see section 5). Normal 1-hour corrected increments are around $15-20 \times 10^9/1$ per square metre per 10^{11} platelets administered.

Post-transfusion circulation time

Platelets have been labelled with various radioactive materials (e.g. $DF^{32}P$, ^{51}Cr or ^{111}In) in order to measure their post-transfusion life-span. The interpretation of these studies is subject to the caveats mentioned above. Post-transfusion survival measurements are not routinely performed but they can be valuable for assessing the quality of platelets prepared by or stored under experimental conditions. These studies usually entail reinfusion of autologous radiolabelled platelets into volunteer donors. The behaviour of control fresh platelets can be compared with an identical sample prepared by the procedure under examination. Mean platelet survivals are of the order of 6 days.

Correction of the bleeding time

Those patients who definitely need platelet therapy will have a prolonged bleeding time. Correction of this by platelet transfusion provides convincing confirmation of the clinical benefit to be expected. Only carefully performed standardized template bleeding times are at all useful in this respect. The procedure is valuable:

- during the *evaluation* of new products; or
- where a *guarantee* of therapeutic success must be obtained such as before major surgery; or

- where there appears to be a *discrepancy* between platelet counts and the severity of clinical symptoms.

The procedure is neither necessary nor suitable for the routine evaluation of platelet transfusions.

Clinical evaluation

Ideally the *cessation of bleeding* could be used to prove the efficacy of platelet therapy. In practice the severity of symptoms and their causes vary so much in individual patients that the clinical results are not very helpful in the critical assessment of platelet quality. If the clinical outcome is to be used as an index of effectiveness a system of objective scoring of symptoms in a 'blind' randomized comparison involving a substantial number of patients is required.

Morphological assessment

During storage platelets change from a discoid to a spherical shape and micro-protrusions extend from the membrane. This deterioration probably correlates with a reduction in post-transfusion recovery and survival. Suspensions containing normal discoid platelets show a characteristic opalescent swirling appearance when disturbed. A variety of techniques involving light or ultrasound transmission have been devised to measure these shape changes as an index of expected viability.[70,71] Sudden exposure of platelets *in vitro* to hypotonic solutions causes a rapid disc-to-sphere transformation which, if the platelets are viable, is followed by slower return to their original shape. These events are accompanied by a temporary change in the optical density of the platelet suspension; the degree of functional deterioration of a platelet suspension correlates with its inability to return to its original optical density following hypotonic shock. Fresh platelets will recover to around 70% of the initial optical density values, this response will decline to below 40% for poorly viable platelets.

Other tests

Many other tests can and have been used to provide information regarding likely clinical efficacy. Platelet *aggregation tests* utilizing ADP, collagen and other agents and also platelet *factor 3 availability* may indicate their haemostatic potential. *Serotonin uptake* and *ATP content* reflect membrane function and metabolic status. Release of *lactate dehydrogenase* into the surrounding medium is indicative of the degree of membrane damage such as that incurred following manipulative manoeuvres. Liberation of *β-thromboglobulin* under the same circumstances may indicate the occurrence of platelet release reactions resulting from unwanted aggregation. Measurement of the α-granule membrane protein 140 (GMP 140) has been found to be a valuable marker for loss of function due to activation damage.

The finding of a higher proportion of platelets expressing GMP 140 appears to correlate with poor post-transfusion recovery and survival[65,72]

8.1 Routine Quality Control[73,74]

A *random sample* of platelet concentrate packs should be examined in order to ensure that the production process is supplying products of likely clinical benefit. It is convenient and economical to sample immediately outdated platelet packs for this purpose. Hard and fast rules for sampling numbers cannot easily be set; they must depend on local circumstances and the scale of the overall component production programme. As a target at least 1% of random donor platelets should be investigated in the quality-control laboratory and, of those, 75% of packs sampled at expiry should exceed the minimum criteria indicated below. Clearly, poor performance will necessitate attention to laboratory production procedures and a higher rate of sampling until the cause is ascertained.

The following measurements are useful.

pH of platelet concentrates

Anaerobic glycolysis produces lactic acid and reduces the pH of the platelet concentrate plasma. Carbon dioxide and carbonic acid will accumulate from the aerobic glycolysis of the citric acid cycle. If the pH falls to 6.0, platelet function appears to be irreversibly impaired.

The fall in pH is minimized by:

(1) Ensuring an adequate volume of plasma for the platelet suspension. Platelet concentrates require in excess of $40 \, ml/55 \times 10^9$ platelets and should not exceed a platelet concentration of $1.6 \times 10^{12}/l$; the higher volume of plasma allows dilution of H^+ ions and the extra plasma proteins provide buffering capacity.
(2) Facilitating exchange of oxygen and carbon dioxide across the plastic pack wall. This is provided by:
   (a) Packs with high surface area-to-volume ratios.
   (b) The use of gas-permeable plastics. Polyolefin has proved superior to conventional polyvinyl chloride (PVC) for this purpose. Alternatively, use of thinner-walled PVC plastic, variation in plasticizer type and concentrations have been found to be practicable solutions.[75]
   (c) Gentle mixing of the platelet suspension. All platelet concentrates should be mixed continuously throughout their storage period.

Leucocyte depletion reduces the metabolic demands on the storage environment.

Ready availability of oxygen as a result of mixing and diffusion through the pack wall reduces the amount of anaerobic glycolysis and lactic acid production. Allowing carbon dioxide to escape prevents the accumulation of carbonic acid. The permissible platelet storage time during recent years has been increased from 3 to 5 days by making use of plastic packs specially designed to facilitate the exchange of carbon dioxide and oxygen.

It is important to measure the plasma pH immediately the platelet pack has been opened. Carbon dioxide will begin to be lost from the plasma as it equilibrates with atmospheric pO_2 and the pH will show a corresponding rise.

Volume of platelet concentrates

See (1) above.

Platelet counts

It is conventionally agreed that as an attainable standard 75% of whole-blood-derived platelet packs should contain $>55 \times 10^9$ platelets. It is commonly assumed that individual packs contain $55-70 \times 10^9$ platelets per 50 ml volume. Packs containing over 80×10^9 per pack will not store well because of the increased rate of pH drop. Apheresis concentrate platelet counts should be in the range 55×10^9/ 50 ml volume provided.

Red cell and leucocyte counts

Conventional random-donor-derived packs containing below 0.4×10^9 red cells (approx. 0.04 ml) per pack will not show visible contamination. Target values of $<1.0 \times 10^9$ per pack are usually set as limits for red cell contamination. It is uncertain whether ADP release from red cells has any adverse effect on the platelets.

Leucocyte counts are usually required not to exceed 0.2×10^9 per 50 ml pack. However, low counts are desirable for several reasons:

(1) Leucocytes are the most immunogenic constituents and use of leucocyte-poor products may slow development of the refractory state.
(2) Leucocyte contamination is the principal cause of the febrile reactions commonly associated with platelet transfusions.
(3) Leucocyte metabolism probably makes a significant contribution to lactic acid and carbon dioxide production.
(4) Proteolytic enzymes released from degenerating granulocytes may be harmful to stored platelets.

Platelets offered as leucocyte-depleted products should contain below 1×10^6 leucocytes per 55×10^9 platelets. At these low levels, leucocytes cannot be counted by conventional electronic blood count analysers. Manual counting using a large-volume Nageotte haemocytometer is the method most usually employed.[76] Flow cytometry gives greater precision and enables differential analysis.[77,78]

Bacterial cultures

In view of the low incidence of significant findings and the inability of routine culturing to predict the likelihood of transfusion-transmitted infection, the value of routine sterility testing is not universally accepted. Cultures are usually performed on outdated packs to provide assurance that aseptic conditions during blood collection and component preparation have been maintained and that significant bacterial counts that might constitute a risk to patients do not occur. If recoverable microorganisms are found, it is important to perform quantitative counts and to sample in a way that enables distinction between genuine bacterial contamination and that arising from faulty culture technique.

Visual inspection

Platelet packs should be inspected to show they contain a uniform 'swirling' platelet suspension and no particles of aggregated matter.

REFERENCES

1 Anonymous (1984) The bleeding-time and the haematocrit. *Lancet*, **i**: 997–998.
2 Lind, S.E. (1991) The bleeding time does not predict surgical bleeding. *Blood*, **77**: 2547–2551.
3 Consensus Conference (1987) Platelet transfusion therapy. *JAMA*, **257**: 1777–1780.
4 British Committee for Standards in Haematology (1992) Guidelines for Platelet Transfusions. *Transfusion Med.*, **2**: 311–318.
5 Roy, A.J., Jaffe, N. and Djerassi, I. (1973) Prophylactic platelet transfusions in children with acute leukaemia: a dose response study. *Transfusion*, **13**: 283–290.
6 Gmur, J., Burger, J., Schanz, U., Fehr, J. and Schaffner, A. (1991) Safety of stringent prophylactic platelet transfusion policy for patients with acute leukaemia. *Lancet*, **338**: 1223–1226.
7 Patten, E. (1992) Controversies in transfusion medicine: prophylactic platelet transfusion revisited after 25 years: con. *Transfusion*, **32**(4): 381–385.
8 Baer, M.R. and Bloomfield, C.D. (1992) Controversies in transfusion medicine: prophylactic platelet transfusion therapy: pro. *Transfusion*, **32**(4): 377–380.
9 Schiffer, C.A. (1992) Prophylactic platelet transfusion. *Transfusion*, **32**(4): 295–297.
10 International Forum (1993) What is the optimal storage temperature for whole blood prior to preparation of blood components. *Vox Sang.*, **65**: 320–327.
11 Burgstaler, E.A., Pineda, A.A. and Brecher, M.A. (1993) Plateletpheresis: comparison of platelet yields, processing time, and white cell content with two apheresis systems. *Transfusion*, **33**: 393–398.
12 Angelini, A., Dragani, A., Berardi, A., Iacone, A., Fioritoni, G. and Torlontano, G. (1992) Evaluation of four different methods for platelet freezing: in vitro and in vivo studies. *Vox Sang.*, **62**: 146–151.
13 Williamson, L.M., Copplestone, J.A., Wimperis, J.A. and Norfolk. D.R. (1994) Bedside filtration of blood products in the prevention of HLA alloimmunization: a prospective randomized study. *Blood*, **83**: 3028–3035.
14 Goodnough, L.T., Riddell, J., Lazarus, H. *et al.* (1993) Prevalence of platelet transfusion reactions before and after implementation of leukocyte-depleted platelet concentrates by filtration. *Vox Sang.*, **65**: 103–107.
15 Duguid, J.K.M., Carr, R., Jenkins, J.A., Hutton, J.L., Lucas, G.F. and Davies, J.M. (1991) Clinical evaluation of the effects of storage time and irradiation on transfused platelets. *Vox Sang.*, **60**: 151–154.
16 Moroff, G., Friedman, A., Robkin-Kline, L., Gautier, G. and Luban, N.L.C. (1984) Reduction of the volume of stored platelet concentrates for use in neonatal patients. *Transfusion*, **24**: 144–146.

17 Bishop, J.F., Matthews, J.P., Yuen, K., McGrath, K., Wolf, M.M. and Szer, J. (1992) The definition of refractoriness to platelet transfusions. *Transfusion Med.*, **2**: 35–41.
18 Correspondence (1993) Correction of the corrected count increment units. *Transfusion*, **33**: 358–359.
19 Kelton, J.G., Hamid, C., Aker, S. and Blajchman, M.A. (1982) The amount of blood group A substance on platelets is proportional to the amount in the plasma. *Blood*, **59**: 980–985.
20 Heal, J.M., Blumberg, N. and Masel, D. (1987) An evaluation of crossmatching, HLA, and ABO matching for platelet transfusions to refractory patients. *Blood*, **70**: 23–30.
21 McLeod, B.C., Sassetti, R.J., Weens, J.H. and Vaithianathan, T. (1982) Haemolytic transfusion reaction due to ABO incompatible plasma in a platelet concentrate. *Scand. J. Haematol.*, **28**: 193–196.
22 Pierce, R.N., Reich, L.M. and Mayer, K. (1985) Hemolysis following platelet transfusion from ABO-incompatible donors. *Transfusion*, **25**: 60–62.
23 Shanwell, A., Ringden, O., Wiechel, B., Rumin, S. and Akerblom, O. (1991) A study of the effect of ABO incompatible plasma in platelet concentrates transfused to bone marrow transplant recipients. *Vox Sang.*, **60**: 23–27.
24 Heal, J.M., Masel, D., Rowe, J.M. and Blumberg, N. (1993) Circulating immune complexes involving the ABO system after platelet transfusion. *Br. J. Haematol.*, **85**: 566–572.
25 Heim, M.U., Bock, M. and Mempel, W. (1993) Dose of Anti-D immunoglobulin for the prevention of Rh D immunisation after RhD-incompatible platelet transfusions. *Vox Sang.*, **65**: 74.
26 Murphy, M.F. and Lee, D. (1993) Dose of Anti-D immunoglobulin for the prevention of RhD immunisation after RhD-incompatible platelet transfusions. *Vox Sang.*, **65**: 73.
27 Murphy, M.F. and Waters, A. H. (1985) Immunological aspects of platelet transfusions. *Br. J. Haematol.*, **60**: 409–414.
28 Godeau, B., Fromont, P., Seror, T., Duedari, N. and Bierling, P. (1992) Platelet alloimmunization after multiple transfusions: a prospective study of 50 patients. *Br. J. Haematol.*, **81**: 395–400.
29 Holohan, T.V., Terasaki, P.I. and Deisseroth, A.B. (1981) Suppression of transfusion-related alloimmunisation in intensively treated cancer patients. *Blood*, **58**: 122.
30 Howard, J.E. and Perkins, H.A. (1978) The natural history of alloimmunisation to platelets. *Transfusion*, **18**: 496–503.
31 Tosato, G., Applebaum, F.R. and Deisseroth, A.B. (1978) HLA-matched platelet transfusion therapy of severe aplastic anemia. *Blood*, **52**: 846–854.
32 Kutti, J., Zaroulis, C.G., Dinsmore, R.E., Reich, L., Clarkson, B.D. and Good, R.A. (1982) A prospective study of platelet-transfusion therapy administered to patients with acute leukemia. *Transfusion*, **22**: 44–47.
33 Sintnicolaas, K., Sizoo, W., Haije, W.G. *et al.* (1981) Delayed alloimmunisation by random single donor platelet transfusions. *Lancet*, **i**: 750–754.
34 Dutcher, J.P., Schiffer, C.A., Aisner, J. and Wiernik, P.H. (1981) Alloimmunisation following platelet transfusion: the absence of a dose–response relationship. *Blood*, **57**: 395–398.
35 Saarinen, U.M., Koskimies, S. and Myllyla, G. (1993) Systematic use of leukocyte-free blood components to prevent alloimmunization and platelet refractoriness in multitransfused children with cancer. *Vox Sang.*, **65**: 286–292.
36 Ten Haaft, M.A., Van den Berg-Loonen, P.M. and Van Rhenen, D.J. (1992) Prevention of primary HLA class 1 allo-immunization with leucocyte-poor blood components produced without the use of platelet filters. *Vox Sang.*, **63**: 257–261.
37 Murphy, M.F., Metcalfe, P., Thomas, H. *et al.* (1986) Use of leucocyte poor blood components and HLA matched platelet donors to prevent HLA alloimmunization. *Br. J. Haematol.*, **62**: 529–534.
38 Oksanen, K., Kekomaki, R., Ruutu, T., Koskimies, S. and Myllyla, G. (1991) Prevention of alloimmunization in patients with acute leukemia by use of white cell-reduced blood components: a randomized trial. *Transfusion*, **31**: 588–594.

39 Brecher, M.E., Pineda, A.A., Zylstra-Halling, V.W. *et al.* (1990) In vivo viability and functional integrity of filtered platelets. *Transfusion*, 30: 718–721.

40 Holme, S., Ross, D. and Heaton, W.A. (1989) In vitro and in vivo evaluation of platelet concentrates after cotton wool filtration. *Vox Sang.*, 57: 112–115.

41 Balducci, L., Benson, K., Lyman, G.H. *et al.* (1993) Cost-effectiveness of white cell-reduction filters in treatment of adult acute myelogenous leukemia. *Transfusion*, 33: 665–670.

42 Oksanen, K. and Elonen, E. (1993) Impact of leucocyte-depleted blood components on the haematological recovery and prognosis of patients with acute myeloid leukaemia. *Br. J. Haematol.*, 84: 639–647.

43 Murphy, S., Litwin, S., Herring, L.M. *et al.* (1982) Indications for platelet transfusion in children with acute leukaemia. *Am. J. Hematol*, 12: 347–356.

44 Andreu, G., Boccaccio, C., Lecrubier, C. *et al.* (1990) Ultraviolet irradiation of platelet concentrates: feasibility in transfusion practice. *Transfusion*, 30: 401–406.

45 Pamphilon, D.H., Potter, M., Cutts, M. *et al.* (1990) Platelet concentrates irradiated with ultraviolet light retain satisfactory in vitro storage characteristics and in vivo survival. *Br. J. Haematol.*, 75: 240–244.

46 Bolgiano, D.C., Larson, E.B. and Slichter, S.J. (1989) A model to determine required pool size for HLA-typed community donor apheresis program. *Transfusion*, 29: 306–310.

47 Schiffer, C.A., Keller, C., Dutcher, J.P. *et al.* (1983) Potential HLA matched platelet donor availability for alloimmunized patients. *Transfusion*, 23: 286–289.

48 Dahlke, M.B. and Weiss, K.L. (1984) Platelet transfusion from donors mismatched for crossreactive HLA antigens. *Transfusion*, 24: 299–302.

49 Duquesnoy, R.J., Filip, D.J., Rodey, G.E., Rimm, A.A. and Aster, R.H. (1977) Successful transfusion of platelets 'mismatched' for HLA antigens to alloimmunised thrombocytopenic patients. *Am. J. Hematol.*, 2: 219–226.

50 Tosato, G., Applebaum, F.R. and Deisseroth, A.B. (1978) HLA-matched platelet transfusion therapy of severe aplastic anemia. *Blood*, 52: 846–853.

51 Moroff, G., Garratty, G., Heal, J.M., *et al.* (1992) Selection of platelets for refractory patients by HLA matching and prospective crossmatching. *Transfusion*, 32: 633–640.

52 Szatkowski, N.S. and Aster, R. H. (1980) HLA antigens of platelets: IV. Influence of 'private' HLA B locus specificities on the expression of Bw4 and Bw6 on human platelets. *Tissue Antigens*, 15: 361–368.

53 Brubaker, D.B. and Romine, M. (1987) Relationship of HLA and platelet-reactive antibodies in alloimmunized patients refractory to platelet therapy. *Am. J. Haematol.*, 26: 341–352.

54 Pegels, J.G., Bruynes, E.C.E., Engelfriet, C.P. *et al.* (1982) Serological studies in patients on platelet and granulocyte substitution therapy. *Br. J. Haematol.*, 52: 59–68.

55 Myers, T.J., Kim, B.K., Steiner, M. *et al.* (1981) Selection of donor platelets for alloimmunized patients using a platelet-associated IgG assay. *Blood*, 58: 444–450.

56 Kickler, T.S., Braine, H. and Ness, P.M. (1985) The predictive value of crossmatching platelet transfusion for alloimmunized patients. *Transfusion*, 25: 385–389.

57 Rachel, J.M., Summers, T.C., Sinor, L.T., *et al.* (1988) Use of solid phase red blood cell adherence method for pretransfusion platelet compatibility testing. *Am. J. Clin. Pathol.*, 90: 63–68.

58 Gudino, M. and Miller, W.V. (1981) Application of the enzyme linked immunospecific assay (ELISA) for the detection of platelet antibodies. *Blood*, 57: 32–37.

59 Sintnicolaas, K., van der Steuijt, K.J.B., van Putten, W.L.J. *et al.* (1987) A microplate ELISA for the detection of platelet alloantibodies: comparison with platelet immunofluorescence test. *Br. J. Haematol.*, 66: 363–367.

60 Nordhagen, R. and Flaathen, S.T. (1983) Chloroquine stripping of HLA antigens on platelets for the platelet immunofluorescence test. Seventh Meeting, International Society of Haematology (European and African Division), Barcelona. Abstract. 618.

61 Moroff, G., Garratty, G., Heal, J.M. *et al.* (1992) Selection of platelets for refractory patients by HLA matching and prospective crossmatching. *Transfusion*, 32: 633–640.

62 Freedman, J., Garni, A., Garvey, M.B. *et al.* (1989) A cost-effectiveness evaluation of

platelet crossmatching and HLA matching in the management of alloimmunized thrombocytopenic patients. *Transfusion*, **29**: 201–207.

63 Owens, M., Holme, S., Heaton, A., Sawyer, S. and Cardinali, S. (1992) Post transfusion recovery of function of 5-day stored platelet concentrates. *Br. J. Haematol.* **80**: 539–544.

64 Rinder, H.M., Murphy, M., Mitchell, J.G., Stocks, J., Ault, K.A. and Hillman, R.S. (1991) Progressive platelet activation with storage: evidence for shortened survival of activated platelets after transfusion. *Transfusion*, **31**: 409–414.

65 Triulzi, D.J., Kickler, T.S. and Braine, H.G. (1992) Detection and significance of alpha granule membrane protein 140 expression on platelets collected by apheresis. *Transfusion*, **32**: 529–533.

66 Schiffer, C.A., Patten, E., Reilley, J. *et al.* (1987) Effective leukocyte removal from platelet preparations by centrifugation in a new pooling bag. *Transfusion*, **27**: 162–164.

67 Beutler, E. (1993) Artificial preservatives for platelets. *Transfusion*, **33**: 279–280.

68 Shimizu, T. and Murphy, S. (1993) Roles of acetate and phosphate in the successful storage of platelet concentrates prepared with acetate containing additive solution. *Transfusion*, **33**: 304–310.

69 Guilliksson, H. (1993) Storage of platelets in additive solutions: the effect of citrate and acetate in in vitro studies. *Transfusion*, **33**: 301–303.

70 Bellhouse, E.L., Inskip, M.J., Davis, J.G. and Entwistle, C.C. (1987) Pre-transfusion non-invasive quality assessment of stored platelet concentrates. *Br. J. Haematol.*, **66**: 503–508.

71 Trenchard, P.M. (1987) Ultrasound-induced light transmission change within platelet suspensions as an indirect measure of platelet morphology: preliminary correlation with stirring-induced light transmission change. *Ultrasound Med. Biol.*, **13**: 197–208.

72 Rinder, H. M., Murphy, M., Mitchell, J.G., Stocks, J., Ault, K.A. and Hillman, R.S. (1991) Progressive platelet activation with storage: evidence for shortened survival of activated platelets after transfusion. *Transfusion*, **31**: 409–414.

73 Aster, R.H. (1981) Which are the parameters to be controlled in platelet concentrates in order that they may be offered to the medical profession as a standardised product with specific properties? *Vox Sang.*, **40**: 115–126.

74 *Guidelines for the Blood Transfusion Service (UK)* (1993) London: HMSO.

75 Carmen, R. (1993) The selection of plastic materials for blood bags. *Transfusion Med. Rev.* 7(1): 1–10.

76 Masse, M., Naegelen, C., Pellegrini, N., Segier, J.M., Marpaux, N. and Beaujean, F. (1992) Validation of a simple method to count very low white cell concentrations in filtered red cells or platelets. *Transfusion*, **32**: 565–571.

77 Sheckler, V.L. and Loken, M.R. (1993) Routine quantitation of white cells as low as 0.001 per μ L in platelet components. *Transfusion*, **33**: 256–261.

78 Vachula, M., Simpson, S.J., Martinson, J.A. *et al.* (1993) A flow cytometric method for counting very low levels of white cells in blood and blood components. *Transfusion*, **33**: 262–267.

6
Granulocyte Transfusion

Prolonged *neutropenia* is a common and serious consequence of *chemotherapy* or *radiotherapy* for *haematological malignancies* and following *bone marrow transplantation*. Work in the 1970s and later seemed to suggest that intensive transfusions of *granulocytes* might help in treatment of established infection[1] and possibly also prevent infections during periods of severe neutropenia. For a decade or so, granulocytes were tried in a variety of clinical settings largely supported by some encouraging data from clinical trials. More concerted and objective studies have not, however, confirmed this initial enthusiasm.

The successful management of neutropenia-related infection is now very much dependent on recent improvements in *antibacterial chemoprophylaxis*.[2] It has also been shown that the vulnerable period of severe neutropenia can also be shortened by use of *recombinant growth factors* such as granulocyte–macrophage-stimulating factor (rHu GM-CSF) or granulocyte colony-stimulating factor (rHu G-CSF). These accelerate the maturation and differentiation of residual stem cells. Peripheral blood granulocyte counts recover more quickly although the granulocytes may be less functionally mature.[3] Because of the success of these alternative measures and the rather modest evidence supporting the value of granulocyte therapy, the use of granulocyte transfusions is now rare. When granulocyte therapy is used it is mainly in a supporting role for the treatment of severe life-threatening infections proving refractory to other measures.[8]

1 INDICATIONS FOR THERAPY

The use of *neutrophil granulocytes* for treatment should only be considered when the following circumstances are combined:

- Severe neutropenia.
- Proven bacterial infection.
- Failure to respond to appropriate antibiotic therapy.

The patients most frequently considered for granulocyte therapy are those with *marrow aplasia* or *haematological malignancy* without any immediate prospect of recovery from their episode of infection.[4,5] Granulocytopoiesis will be virtually absent and the blood will show profound neutropenia (below 0.5×10^9/l). Granulocytes are sometimes also used for treatment of *sepsis in neonates* for whom different indications and criteria apply. This is discussed in chapter 20, section 4.1. Granulocytes have also been used successfully for treatment of severe infection in chronic granulomatous disease[6,7] and for other congenital disorders of *granulopoiesis*.

Patients who have *granulocytopenia* as a result of cytotoxic therapy are more liable to sepsis than those with chronic aplasia. This is largely due to the presence of such factors as: mucosal ulceration induced by chemotherapy, cutaneous wounds following invasive procedures and generalized immunosuppression.

2 GRANULOCYTE PREPARATIONS

Granulocytes are best obtained from *single-donor leukapheresis* procedures.[8,9] These usually entail either continuous or, more usually, intermittent flow of the donor's circulation through apheresis machines which centrifuge the blood and allow collection of the requisite cell from the appropriate sedimented layer.

Apheresis enables collections of $1.5–2.0 \times 10^{10}$ granulocytes in a volume of 500 ml and these can be obtained over a donation period of 3–4 hours. Pre-medication of the donor with *corticosteroids* (e.g. dexamethasone $4\,\text{mg}/\text{m}^2$ or prednisone 60 mg orally at least 2 hours before donation) is necessary in order to maximize yields. In addition, sedimenting agents such as hydroxyethyl starch (HES) (e.g. 6% HES in saline) are added to the blood as it leaves the donor to improve leucocyte separation and reduce red cell contamination. HES can cause plasma volume expansion and as a result reduction of the donor's haemoglobin concentration. On a more experimental basis, rHu G-CSF has been used to stimulate higher yields (e.g. $>4 \times 10^{10}$ granulocytes).[8]

Therapeutic doses of granulocytes can also be obtained from the *buffy coat layers* of freshly collected random-donor blood packs. Each donation should contain around $0.5–1.0 \times 10^9$ per pack and the haematocrit will be approximately 0.3–0.5. A total of 10–20 buffy coat donations is required to obtain an adequate dose of granulocytes.

Single-donor preparations are necessary if *HLA-matched granulocytes* are required. These may be selected as compatible when HLA antibodies are already present or chosen to reduce exposure to novel HLA antigens in unsensitized patients. Donors who are relatives should probably not be used if bone marrow transplantation from a family member is likely as there appears to be a risk of sensitization to minor histocompatibility antigens also shared by the prospective donor.

3 DOSAGE OF GRANULOCYTES AND GRANULOCYTE KINETICS

Clinical and experimental evidence indicates that a dosage in excess of 1×10^{10} granulocytes and ideally approaching 5×10^{10} granulocytes is required. These amounts are still only of the order of 10–50% of the healthy *in vivo* daily production and are considerably less than the numbers available during a normal neutrophil leucocytosis.

The post-transfusion kinetics and distribution of granulocytes differ from those of red cells and platelets. After transfusion the majority of granulocytes lodge in the pulmonary vasculature and marginal pools of the bloodstream before release and reappearance as circulating cells some hours later. Normally around 50% of all granulocytes may, at any one time, be lodged in tissues or in the marginal pool.

4 STORAGE AND COMPATIBILITY TESTING

Red cell compatibility

In practice, because of their high red cell content, ABO-compatible donations are usually used. Recipients should be screened for irregular red cell antibodies before administration. If screening is negative conventional cross-match testing will not be necessary, but the ABO groups should be confirmed to be compatible at least by an immediate spin procedure before infusion. Granulocytes do not appear to carry ABH or Rh D antigens and could therefore be given in pure form without regard to these blood groups.[10,11]

HLA compatibility The degree of HLA similarity between donor and recipient appears to influence both the magnitude of post-transfusion increments and the survival of transfused cells. However, therapeutic effectiveness is not noticeably affected unless HLA or granulocyte-specific antibodies are present. Accordingly, HLA matching is not carried out for unsensitized recipients.

Granulocytes are usually administered as soon as possible after collection.[12] Only limited storage[13] (up to 6 hours at 22°C) appears possible. This situation is somewhat arbitrary since the optimal preservation conditions for granulocytes still remain to be determined.

5 COMPLICATIONS OF GRANULOCYTE TREATMENT

(1) Adverse *allergic reactions*, e.g. fevers, chills and pulmonary reactions, are quite frequent during granulocyte administration. Sometimes severe pulmonary reactions are seen. These have been ascribed to accumulation of antibody and complement-damaged granulocytes in pulmonary capillaries (see chapter 23, section 3.2). In some instances concomitant amphotericin B has been blamed.
(2) *Graft-versus-host disease* is an important risk. Granulocyte preparations contain

large numbers of lymphocytes and require irradiation if given to severely immunosuppressed patients. At conventional doses, granulocyte function does not seem to be damaged.[14]

(3) Cytomegalovirus infection (see chapter 24, section 7).
(4) HLA immunization.

Not only do granulocytes and lymphocytes carry class 1 HLA antigens, but in addition preparations contain class II antigen-presenting cells capable of facilitating the establishment of the primary immune response (see chapter 5 section 6).

REFERENCES

1　Strauss, R.G. (1983) Granulocyte transfusion therapy. *Clin. Oncol.*, **2**: 635–655.
2　Rogers, B.J.H. (1991) Prevention of infection during neutropenia (clinical annotation). *Br. J. Haematol.*, **79**: 544–549.
3　Macey, M.G., Sangster, J., Kelsey, S.M. and Newland, A.C. (1993) Pilot study: effects of G-CSF on neutrophil ex-vivo function post bone marrow transplantation. *Clin. Lab. Haematol.*, **15**: 79–85.
4　Anonymous (1980) Infection complicating severe granulocytopenia. *Lancet*, **ii**: 25–26.
5　Brown, A.E. (1984) Neutropenia, fever and infection. *Am. J. Med.*, **76**: 421–428.
6　Yomtovian, R., Abramson, J., Quie, P. and McCullough, J. (1981) Granulocyte transfusion therapy in chronic granulomatous disease. *Transfusion*, **21**: 739.
7　Dougherty, S.H., Peterson, P.K. and Simmons, R.L. (1983) Granulocyte transfusion as adjunctive therapy for qualitative granulocytopenia. *Arch. Surg.*, **118**: 873–874.
8　Huestis, D.W. and Glasser, L. (1994) The neutrophil in transfusion medicine. *Transfusion*, **34**: 630–640.
9　Strauss, R.G., Goeken, J.A., Eckermann, I., McEntegart, C.M. and Hulse, J.D. (1986) Effects of intensive granulocyte donation on donors and yields. *Transfusion*, **26**: 441–445.
10　Gaidulis, L., Branch, D.R., Lazar, G.S., Petz, L.D. and Blume, K.G. (1985) The red cell antigens A, B, D, U, Ge, Jk3 and Yt^a are not detected on human granulocytes. *Br. J. Haematol.*, **60**: 659–668.
11　Dunstan, R.A., Simpson, M.B. and Borowitz, M. (1985) Absence of ABH antigens on neutrophils. *Br. J. Haematol.*, **60**: 651–657.
12　McCullough, J., Weiblen, B.J. and Fine, D. (1983) Effects of storage of granulocytes on their fate in vivo. *Transfusion*, **23**: 20–24.
13　Miyamoto, M. and Sasakawa, S. (1987) Studies on granulocyte preservation III. Effect of agitation on granulocyte concentrates. *Transfusion*, **27**: 165–166.
14　Eastlund, D.T. and Charbonneau, T.T. (1988) Superoxide generation and cytotactic response of irradiated neutrophils. *Transfusion*, **28**: 368–370.

7
Coagulation Factor Materials for Therapeutic Use

A variety of blood components and products are available for the treatment of abnormal coagulation. These range from simple donations of fresh frozen plasma, useful principally for treatment of acquired broad-spectrum abnormalities, to more highly purified coagulation factor concentrates designed to rectify specific deficiency states. The more widely available of these are described below, followed by an outline of the principal disorders for which coagulation factor treatment is indicated.

The terms *blood products* and *blood components* are frequently rather loosely interchanged and this applies particularly to those used for treatment of haemostatic problems. It is preferable to reserve the term blood products for those materials that have been extracted and purified from crude plasma, frequently sterilized and presented in a stable concentrated form. These materials principally include coagulation factor concentrates, albumin and immunoglobulins. Blood components are best regarded as those materials relatively easily separated from the main body of the donation by means of differential separation followed by expression into satellite packs attached to the original donor blood pack. Examples of these include fresh plasma, cryoprecipitate, platelet and red cell concentrates.

1 FRESH FROZEN PLASMA

Freshly collected separated and frozen plasma contains all the clotting factors required for haemostasis and was the first transfusion material to be devised for treatment of coagulation deficiencies. It has, however, some obvious shortcomings which have led to the development of more highly purified materials designed for specific purposes. The volume of fresh frozen plasma (FFP) is, for example, too large to permit adequate correction of severe single-factor deficiency states without the risk of causing circulatory overload. The specific activity, i.e. the ratio of concentration of the desired factor to that of other proteins, is low. As a result most of the protein actually transfused is unwanted and unnecessary. Despite this, FFP is a useful, though almost certainly overused, material for treatment of a variety of conditions as described below.

1.1 Composition[1]

At the time of freezing, small numbers of platelets, red cells and leucocytes may still remain in the plasma. After freezing and thawing plasma will be largely free of intact cells (a few lymphocytes are claimed to survive) but cellular debris and antigenic material will be present. The pack volume will be around 200–240 ml. This will comprise approximately 1 part anticoagulant solution to 4 parts plasma; the pH and electrolyte composition of CPD plasma are shown in Table 1.

Table 1 Composition of fresh frozen CPD plasma and normal plasma

	FFP	Normal plasma
Sodium	167.5 mmol/l	140.0 mmol/l
Chloride	76.0 mmol/l	100.0 mmol/l
Glucose	26.0 mmol/l	6.0 mmol/l
Osmolality	320.0 mOsm/k	290.0 mOsm/kg
pH	7.07	7.4
Inorganic phosphate	3.5 mmol/l	1.1 mmol/l

Coagulation factor content of FFP

The coagulation factor content of FFP must vary since:

(1) The donors' individual coagulation factor concentrations vary. Normal Factor VIII levels, for example, can range from 50 IU/dl to 200 IU/dl.
(2) The speed of freezing, stability and duration of storage may affect the product. Labile factors, e.g. V and VIII, may fare less well than others.

In general it may be best to assume that FFP contains, on a volume-to-volume basis, around 70% of normal *in vivo* plasma coagulation factor levels.

Preparation and storage of FFP

Each pack of plasma should have been separated from the red cells, leucocytes and platelets by a fast spin and frozen. FFP should be stored below −30 °C and is customarily given a shelf life of 12 months. Frozen storage above −30 °C appears to accelerate its deterioration.

1.2 Dosage and Administration

The generally accepted dose for infusion is 12–15 ml/kg or approximately four donor packs for a 70 kg recipient. This cannot be expected to increase coagulation factor levels by more than 12–15%, but the increase may be sufficient to reduce the risk of bleeding. During active blood loss larger volumes can of course be infused as part of the plasma volume replacement. FFP is usually thawed in a 37 °C water-bath before administration. There is a danger that microbial growth in the water-bath together with undetected pin-hole leaks in the FFP packs may cause a risk of bacterial infection to the recipient. For this reason use of protective plastic bag over-wraps is advised for thawing of all plasma products. The thawed plasma should be administered with the minimum of delay (e.g. no more than 2 hours) to avoid loss of potency.

It is least confusing to clinical staff if FFP of the same ABO group as the recipient is provided. Logically, of course, group A plasma can be safely given to both group A and O recipients, and group AB plasma to any group. Group AB plasma is the single most useful group of holding stock if turnover is small. Special liaison with ward staff is required if non-identical ABO group transfusion is to be practised as this may appear to conflict with routine blood administration policies. The small amount of red cell stroma present in FFP packs is possibly capable of producing Rh immunization[2,3] and certainly appears capable of boosting anti-D titres. This latter problem has been observed in women undergoing plasma exchange for Rh haemolytic disease. It is therefore advisable to transfuse Rh D-negative donations to Rh D-negative women of childbearing age.

1.3 Clinical uses of FFP[4,5]

The clinical use of FFP has grown enormously in recent years but surveys have shown that it is mostly used for plasma volume expansion in situations in which there are little or no valid indications for coagulation factor support.[6] This is a wasteful practice; FFP should be used only for its coagulation factor content. Despite the popular use of FFP there is little proof that it is efficacious in many circumstances in which it is used. Coagulation screening tests correlate poorly with clinical bleeding and often remain unaffected by FFP therapy.[7] Recommended uses include the following:

(1) *Broad-spectrum coagulation factor replacement*: FFP can be used for treatment of the following:
   - Bleeding or surgery in liver disease.
   - Oral anticoagulant overdosage.
   - Massive transfusion coagulation problems (but only when indicated by clinical and laboratory assessment).
   - During apheresis procedures when combined plasma volume and coagulation factor replacement are required.
   - Disseminated intravascular coagulation.
   - Coagulation disorders of the newborn (e.g. disseminated intravascular coagulation, bleeding due to haemorrhagic disease; see chapter 20, section 5).
   - Thrombotic thrombocytopenic purpura (chapter 8 section 6.1).

(2) *Replacement of single-factor deficiencies*: historically FFP was used for treatment of haemophilia but the high volume required and the inadequate increments in Factor VIII recovery severely limited its usefulness. Use of FFP is still justified for those rare single-factor deficiencies where specific concentrates are unavailable. Deficiencies of Factor II and Factor X are usually managed with prothrombin complex. FFP may be the most readily available material for treatment of *Factor V, VII, XI and XIII deficiency states* although specific concentrates have been prepared. FFP should certainly not be used in many of the situations for which it is often mistakenly prescribed. These include 'formula' prophylactic replacement in massive transfusion; as a routine replacement fluid in apheresis; as a replacement fluid in hypovolaemia or routinely in cardiac surgery.

Cryosupernatant plasma—the supernatant after cryoprecipitate removal—is now very much less available as a consequence of the decline in cryoprecipitate use. There are no specific indications for its use apart from its possible superiority over FFP for the treatment of *thrombotic thrombocytopenic purpura*.[8]

1.4 Adverse Reactions from FFP

FFP carries the virus transmission risk of all labile blood products. However, efforts are now under way to virus inactivate FFP using solvent detergent treatment or photochemical viral inactivation. These materials are currently under clinical trial examination.

Special risks associated with FFP administration include the following:

(1) *Allergic and anaphylactoid reactions*: these are rare but can be extremely severe. Mild reactions consist of *urticaria* and *rigors*. Severe reactions involve profound

hypotension, bronchospasm, pulmonary oedema and even *cardiopulmonary arrest*. Their pathogenesis and treatment are described in chapter 23, section 3.

(2) Transfusions of large amounts of group O plasma to non-O recipients will cause *haemolysis, jaundice* and sometimes a positive direct antiglobulin test on recipient red cells. As donations of plasma are normally screened to exclude those with high titres of ABO haemolysins this is not usually a problem, but administration of incompatible ABO group plasma should, whenever possible, be avoided.

2 CRYOPRECIPITATE

The care of haemophilia A patients improved dramatically following the introduction of this, the first partially purified Factor VIII preparation. This advance was made possible following the demonstration that most of the Factor VIII and fibrinogen coprecipitated in the cold and could be extracted from plasma relatively easily for therapeutic purposes.

2.1 Preparation of Cryoprecipitate

Cryoprecipitate is prepared by controlled thawing of FFP to the point where the last frozen slush has almost melted and the supernatant is still around 0 °C. Factor VIII and fibrinogen remain as a diffuse cotton-wool-like precipitate which can be extracted by centrifugation and syphoning away all but around 10–20 ml of the main body of supernatant plasma. This cryoprecipitate is rapidly refrozen and then maintained below –30 °C. A storage period of 12 months is usually assigned.

Thawing for administration should be as performed for FFP (see section 1.2). Usually the desired number of packs are pooled to enable administration of the total dose in one pack alone. Saline rinsing of the 'empty' packs minimizes the waste of residual material.

2.2 Cryoprecipitate Composition

Cryoprecipitate packs are presented in volumes varying from 10 to 25 ml. Packs should contain a minimum average of 70 IU Factor VIII, which represents around 40% recovery from the original donor plasma. Actual yields depend on the local production procedures and information regarding these should be obtained to assist calculation of correct doses. Yields exceeding 150 IU per pack have been obtained when particular care is taken to minimize losses during preparation. Quality-control procedures should aim to perform Factor VIII assays on at least 1% of all cryoprecipitate packs produced. These should include packs sampled in the first month and also during the last month of their shelf life.

The typical composition of cryoprecipitate is:
Volume   10–25 ml
Factor VIII content   70–150 IU per pack
Protein   0.1–0.2 IU/mg
Fibrinogen   100–300 mg per pack
Fibronectin   100–300 U per pack

2.3 Dosage and Administration

Cryoprecipitate was formerly used in large quantities for treatment of *haemophilia A*. Because of its content of vWF multimers in addition to Factor VIII it was also particularly valuable for *von Willebrand's disease* before the advent of suitable virus-inactivated Factor VIII concentrates.

Cryoprecipitate is now largely used as a source of fibrinogen and Factor VIII for treatment of the *defibrination syndrome* as discussed in chapter 8, section 5.5.

Cryoprecipitate, by virtue of its vWF multimers, appears both to shorten the bleeding time[9] and to improve haemostasis[10] in patients with uraemia.

Initial doses of 10–15 packs (1.5–2.0/10 kg body weight) are generally used.

Selection of the blood groups of cryoprecipitate should follow the principles discussed earlier for FFP. As small volumes are involved, use of group O donations for other patients should not cause problems unless daily high-dosage infusions are to be given. Cryoprecipitate should be administered through a small dead space filter (170 μm) assembly. Thawing should be performed as for FFP. The packs should be administered without undue delay, certainly within 2 hours, to avoid deterioration. Infusion should take not more than 30 minutes.

Cryoprecipitate is also used topically as a source of fibrin 'glue' for various surgical purposes (see section 2.5).

2.4 Adverse Reactions

These are not usually serious but include those described in chapters 23 and 24 for risks of transfusion and also in section 1.5 for those especially associated with FFP. Mild reactions to cryoprecipitate, including *fever*, *urticaria* or *pruritus*, are not uncommon.

2.5 Fibrin Sealant (Fibrin Glue)[11]

Concentrates of fibrinogen clotted with thrombin under controlled conditions have been found very effective both as an adhesive material and for producing a topically applied haemostatic effect. Although commercially prepared fibrinogen concentrates (e.g Tisseel, Immuno Vienna) are used widely in some countries apparently with complete safety, there are lingering concerns as to whether adequate virological safety can be assured. The memory of earlier fibrinogen concentrates being withdrawn from use because of their high hepatitis risk remains.

Cryoprecipitate, if prepared so as to maximize fibrinogen levels, is acceptable as an adequate substitute. Alternatively, plasma fibrinogen concentrates can be prepared from cryoprecipitate using ethanol, ammonium sulphate or polyethylene glycol as precipitating agents. Use of autologous plasma as a starting material completely avoids the possibility of virus transmission. The material is usually applied to the surgical site in conjunction with thrombin in a calcium chloride solution. The thrombin concentration can be adjusted to obtain the desired coagulation rate; the concentration of fibrinogen determines the adhesive strength. Active ingredients of cryoprecipitate include, of course, fibrinogen (approx. 20–50 mg/ml if prepared with care), together with Factor XIII (fibrin stabilizing factor), conferring obvious benefits. Fibronectin is also present which is claimed to entice the ingress of fibroblasts to enhance the repair process. Commercial fibrin sealant systems are better standardized, achieve higher fibrinogen concentrations and may also include *aprotinin* as a *fibrinolytic inhibitor* to improve the durability of the repair.

The use of fibrin glue is supported in a variety of surgical specialities.[12] These include tympanoplasty, peripheral nerve repair, maxillofacial surgery, cardiovascular surgery and dental extraction in patients with coagulation deficiencies.

3 FACTOR VIII CONCENTRATES

3.1 Manufacture

These products are partially purified Factor VIII materials usually manufactured on a large scale commercially or by national plasma-processing laboratories. Factor VIII is extracted from plasma by a variety of means which may include a combination of cryoprecipitation and precipitation by ethanol, glycine or polyethylene glycol. A variety of *intermediate* to *high-purity products* are prepared by these means. Specific activities range from 0.5–10.0 IU/mg protein (intermediate concentrates) to reach over 50 IU/mg (high purity). By the use of ion exchange chromatography, gel chromatography and particularly monoclonal antibody affinity chromatography very high purification is achieved. The monoclonal antibodies (anti-Factor VIII or anti-vWF) used as affinity absorbents are murine in origin and care has to be taken to ensure no contaminant traces of murine protein remain in the final product. The *very high-purity* products approximate to 2000–3000 IU/mg but the Factor VIII requires stabilization with added human albumin. Although this reduces the actual specific activity, in biological terms the gain in purification value is preserved. Recombinant DNA-derived Factor VIII is obtained by transfecting host mammalian cells (e.g. Chinese hamster ovary cells) with cDNA for Factor VIII or for Factor VIII and vWF together. Inclusion of the vWF synthetic system provides greater stability for Factor VIII. The resultant products must be extensively purified from the host cell proteins but, as with the affinity-purified products, human albumin must be added to the final product.

Very high-purity products have proved extremely satisfactory for the management of *haemophilia A*. They produce effective Factor VIII restoration in *von Willebrand's disease*, but will probably not correct the defective vWF-related bleeding time abnormality. Intermediate/high-purity concentrates, particularly those known to have high vWF multimer content (e.g. British NHS Factor 8 Y; Hemate P, Behringwerke, Germany), are therefore the materials of choice for treatment of von Willebrand's disease.[13,14]

3.2 Administration

Reconstituted Factor VIII is usually given as a bolus dose in order to reach effective haemostatic levels rapidly. This may be repeated daily or twice daily depending on the severity of the problem. Some treatment regimens utilize a bolus loading dose followed by prolonged infusion to maintain effective levels of circulating Factor VIII.[15]

Very high-dosage regimens, such as may be required for saturation of Factor VIII inhibitors (see chapter 8, section 1.2), require high-purity concentrates.

3.3 Complications of Factor VIII Therapy

Viral infection[16]

Both Factor VIII and IX concentrates (see section 4) are prepared from the pooled plasma of around 2000 or more donations. As a result they formerly carried the highest risk of virus transmission of any blood product. This risk has changed totally as a result of improved donor screening methods and virus inactivation stages introduced into the purification process. During the 1980s enormous advances were made in the reduction of virus transmission risks. Work begun originally to reduce the non-A non-B hepatitis transmission risk provided a sound basis for preventing HIV transmission when that virus emerged as a new hazard. Coagulation factor concentrates now rely on a complementary combination of chemical-partitioning purification stages and viral inactivation steps to abolish viable virus. Some purification steps, e.g. affinity chromatography, and Factor VIII precipitation steps proved particularly effective at reducing the viral load. The virucidal treatments include the use of heat applied to products either in a wet or dry state or chemical inactivation, e.g. use of solvent detergent treatment. The end result for clinical prescribers has been an array of products from different manufacturers, differing according to source of donations, paid or voluntary, donor screening procedures, purification steps, purity levels and viral inactivation procedures. Recombinant Factor VIII, currently rather expensive, has been shown to be safe and effective and is an additional candidate for users' attention.[17]

Most authorities now agree that all licensed products now available appear to be extremely safe[18-20] with respect to HBV, HBC and HIV transmission although risk cannot be discounted entirely. Not all viruses are so efficiently destroyed. Parvovirus B19 seems to be more resistant but the clinical significance of this transfusion-transmissible virus is not very clear. Solvent detergent techniques are less effective where non-lipid envelope viruses are concerned, which may explain an apparent outbreak of HAV transmission in one solvent detergent-treated Factor VIII product although the causal link is still in dispute.

Allergic reactions

Febrile reactions, rigors, headaches, nausea and *vomiting* are very occasional problems following administration of less pure Factor VIII but these usually pass off rapidly without needing treatment.

High concentrations of anti-A or anti-B blood group alloantibodies in intermediate-purity products have sometimes been observed to cause haemolysis in group A or B recipients. Manufacturers usually monitor levels of blood group antibodies to prevent this occurrence.

3.4 Immunological Abnormalities Following Factor VIII Treatment/ Relationship of Purity to HIV Disease Progression

Factor VIII antibodies appearing as a consequence of replacement therapy are discussed in chapter 8, section 1.2.

One of the most hotly debated issues in current haemophilia management is the assertion that the now generally acknowledged immunological consequences of long-term intermediate-purity therapy hasten disease progression in HIV-infected patients. Low specific activity products lead to elevation of suppressor (CD8) lymphocyte counts and reduced helper (CD4) cells. Cellular immune function, e.g. PHA lymphocyte transformation and pokeweed mitogen responses, become reduced. The nature of the contaminating substance(s) in Factor VIII has not been determined. Some studies (but not all) appear to suggest that CD4 decline does not occur as rapidly with high-purity therapy.[21,22]

Supporters of this theory argue for the sole use of high-purity products for such patients. Others caution against the uncertain relationship between immunological function tests, and clinical consequences and the high costs of instituting such policies when all health services are faced with conflicting priorities. Even though conclusive clinical evidence is slow to materialize, the combined efforts of manufacturers (who have reduced prices) patient action groups and concerned physicians are leading to a progressive shift towards the use of high-purity products.

4 FACTOR IX CONCENTRATES

Cryosupernatant plasma from which Factor VIII has been removed is used as source material for Factor IX complex concentrate production. This product is almost exclusively used for treatment of *haemophilia B* (Christmas disease) and the even rarer congenital deficiencies of the other 'prothrombin complex' factors.[23,24]

4.1 Composition

Conventional Factor IX concentrates may contain, in addition to Factor IX, substantial amounts of Factors II and X, all of which form part of the *prothrombin complex*. Most of the preparations available are not, however, enriched for Factor VII.

Development of high-purity Factor IX has been slower than that for Factor VIII, this possibly being a reflection of the considerably smaller population of Factor IX-deficient patients. Licensed high-purity products are now available, however. These appear to have the benefit of inducing less *in vivo* coagulation activation than prothrombin complex concentrates[25,26] and may therefore be indicated when thrombogenicity of the established prothrombin complex (see section 4.3) must be avoided. The principles of product development and viral inactivation closely parallel those for Factor VIII; specific activities of up to 100 IU/mg have been attained. However, no immediate prospect of recombinant Factor IX seems likely.

4.2　Administration

The freeze-dried material is usually reconstituted to give around 20 IU of Factor IX per millilitre. Reconstituted Factor IX complex concentrates show a tendency to spontaneous activation of coagulation factors which are then dangerously thrombogenic. *Deep venous thrombosis, pulmonary embolism* or *disseminated intravascular coagulation* are reported complications. Small amounts of heparin and sometimes of antithrombin III are sometimes added to Factor IX preparations during manufacture in an attempt to reduce the amounts of coagulation factor activation. Because of the risk of spontaneous activation of reconstituted Factor IX concentrates they *must* be administered within 30 minutes after preparation. Factor IX complex concentrate is *never* given as a prolonged infusion.

4.3　Activated Factor IX Products

Activation of the coagulation factors during manufacture has always been a risk and is associated with thrombotic complications in recipients. This problem has restricted the use of conventional prothrombin complex products to patients with haemophilia B in whom the risk appears small. They cannot unfortunately be used for patients with liver disease or deficiency of vitamin K-dependent factors even though at first sight they would seem to be ideally suited.

Prothrombin complex concentrates subjected to *controlled activation* have found an unexpected use in the treatment of patients with haemophilia A who have high Factor VIII inhibitor levels.[27] There is considerable disagreement regarding their efficacy but objective clinical benefit has been claimed for haemophilia A.[28–31] They have also been used for Factor IX deficiency with inhibitors, and one report documents beneficial effects in a patient with Factor V inhibitors.[32]

Factors VII, IX and X are present partly in their active forms (e.g. Xa) and it is believed that in some way these bypass the Factor VIII-dependent coagulation steps and allow completion of the coagulation process. Conclusive information regarding their mechanism of action is so far lacking. Activated prothrombin coagulation complex products (APCC) available include Feiba (Immuno, Vienna, Austria) and Autoplex (Travenol, Glendale, California, USA). The unit of potency assigned to these products reflects the Factor VIII replacement potential based on *in vitro* testing.

5 CONCENTRATES OF OTHER COAGULATION FACTORS

Fibrinogen concentrates have been used for various forms of hypofibrinogenaemia but were associated with such a high risk of hepatitis transmission that they have been withdrawn. Cryoprecipitate is usually used instead. Plasma fibrinogen levels exceeding $0.5–1.0 \, g/l$ are regarded as necessary for normal haemostasis. Hypo-fibrinogenaemia most commonly occurs as part of *disseminated intravascular coagulation* (chapter 8, section 5) in which other haemostatic abnormalities are present. Isolated *congenital hypofibrinogenaemia* is a rare condition arising through inheritance of a dysfunctional molecule; cryoprecipitate in low doses (e.g. two to four packs) is given for this condition. Treatment every 3 days is sufficient; this time period corresponds to the fibrinogen half-life in the plasma following infusion.

Factor XIII deficiency can be treated with FFP. Relatively low concentrations of Factor XIII are sufficient to maintain normal haemostasis; only occasional doses of FFP are required because of the prolonged half-life of this factor. Although deficiency states for Factors VII and XI are very rare concentrates of these Factors have also been prepared.[33,34]

Congenital *Factor X deficiency* has been managed with FFP plasma for minor bleeding episodes, supplemented with prothrombin complex concentrate for more severe problems.[35]

Plasminogen concentrates have been used to ensure a continuous supply of substrate for plasminogen activator during fibrinolytic therapy.

Antithrombin III concentrates are discussed in chapter 8, section 6.

REFERENCES

1 Hauben, D.J., Yanai, E., Mahler, D., Neumann, L. and Kaplan, H. (1982) The constituents of fresh frozen plasma stored in citrate phosphate dextrose and their clinical implications. *Vox Sang.*, **42**: 81–86.

2 Wolfowitz, E. and Shechter, Y. (1984) More about alloimmunisation by transfusion of fresh-frozen plasma. *Transfusion*, **24**: 544.

3 McBride, J.A., O'Hoski, P., Barnes, C.C, Spiak, C. and Blajchman, M.A. (1983) Rhesus alloimmunization following intensive plasma exchange. *Transfusion*, **23**: 352–354.

4 Consensus Conference (1985) Fresh-frozen plasma: indications and risks. *JAMA*, **253**: 551–553.

5 Bove, J.R. (1985) Fresh frozen plasma: too few indications—too much use. *Anesth. Analg.*, **64**: 849–850.

6 Shaikh, B.S., Wagar, D., Lau, P.M. and Campbell, E.W. (1985) Transfusion pattern of fresh frozen plasma in a medical school hospital. *Vox Sang.*, **48**: 366–369.

7 Braunstein, A.H. and Oberman, H.A. (1984) Transfusion of plasma components. *Transfusion*, **24**: 281–286.

8 Obrador, G.T., Zeigler, Z.R., Shadduck, R.K., Rosenfeld, C.S. and Hanrahan, J.B. (1993) Effectiveness of cryosupernatant therapy in refractory and chronic relapsing thrombotic thrombocytopenic purpura. *Am. J. Hematol.*, **42**: 217–220.

9 Canavese, C., Salamone, M., Pacitti, A., Mangiarotti, G. and Calitri, V. (1985) Reduced response of uraemic bleeding time to repeated doses of desmopressin. *Lancet*, **i**: 867–868.

10 Janson, P.A. Jubelirer, S.J., Weinstein, M.J. and Deykin, D. (1980) Treatment of the bleeding tendency in uraemia with cryoprecipitate. *N. Engl. J. Med.*, **303**: 1318–1322.

11 Brennan, M. (1991) Fibrin glue. *Blood Rev.*, **5**: 240–244.
12 Gibble, J.W. and Ness, P.M. (1990) Fibrin glue: the perfect operative sealant? *Transfusion*, **30**:(8): 741–747.
13 Rodeghiero, F., Castaman, G., Meyer, D. and Mannucci, P.M. (1992) Replacement therapy with virus inactivated plasma concentrates in von Willebrand disease. *Vox Sang.*, **62**: 193–199.
14 Cumming, A.M., Fildes, S., Cumming, I.R., Wensley, R.T., Redding, O.M. and Burn, A.M. (1990) Clinical and laboratory evaluation of National Health Service Factor VIII concentrate (8Y) for the treatment of von Willebrand's disease. *Br. J. Haematol.*, **75**: 234–239.
15 Hathaway, W.E., Christian, M.J., Clarke, S.L. and Hasiba, U. (1984) Comparison of continuous and intermittent factor VIII concentrate therapy in hemophilia A. *Am. J. Hematol.*, **17**: 85–88.
16 Fricke, W.A. and Lamb, M.A. (1993) Viral safety of clotting factor concentrates. *Semin. Thromb. Hemostas.*, **19**: 54–60.
17 Lusher, J.M., Arkin, S., Arbildgaard, C.F., Schwartz, R.S. and the Kogenate Previously Untreated Patient Study Group (1993) Recombinant Factor VIII for the treatment of previously untreated patients with hemophilia A: safety, efficacy and development of inhibitors. *N. Engl. J. Med.*, **328**: 453–459.
18 Kasper, C.K., Lusher, J.M. and the Transfusion Practices Committee (1993) Recent evolution of clotting factor concentrates for hemophilia A and B. *Transfusion*, **33**: 422–434.
19 Rizza, C.R., Fletcher, M.I. and Kernoff, P.B.A. (1993) Confirmation of viral safety of dry heated Factor VIII concentrate (8Y) prepared by Bio Products Laboratory (BPL): a report on behalf of U.K. Haemophilia Centre Directors. *Br. J. Haematol.*, **84**: 269–272.
20 Fricke, W., Augustyniak, L., Brownstein, A., Kramer, A. and Evatt, B. (1992) Human immunodeficiency virus infection due to clotting factor concentrates: results of the Seroconversion Surveillance Project. *Transfusion*, **32**: 707–709.
21 Hilgartner, M.W., Buckley, J.D., Operskalski, E.A., Pike, M.C. and Mosley, J.W. (1993) Purity of Factor VIII concentrates and serial CD4 counts. *Lancet*, **34**: 1373–1374.
22 de Biasi, R., Rocino, A., Miraglia, E., Mastrullo, L. and Quirino, A.A. (1991) The impact of a very high purity Factor VIII concentrate on the immune system of human immunodeficiency virus-infected hemophiliacs: a randomized prospective, two-year comparison with an intermediate purity concentrate. *Blood*, **78**: 1919–1922.
23 Ménaché, D. and Guillin, M.C. (1975) The use of Factor IX concentrates for patients with conditions other than Factor IX deficiency. *Br. J. Haematol.*, **31**: 247–257.
24 Ragni, M.V., Lewis, J.H., Spero, J.A. and Hasiba, U. (1981) Factor VII deficiency. *Am. J. Hematol.*, **10**: 79–88.
25 Hampton, K.K., Preston, F.E., Lowe, G.D.O., Walker, I.D. and Sampson, B. (1993) Reduced coagulation activation following infusion of a highly purified factor IX concentrate compared to a prothrombin complex concentrate. *Br. J. Haematol.*, **84**: 279–284.
26 Smith, K.J. (1992) Factor IX concentrates: the new products and their properties. *Trans. Med. Rev.*, **6**: 124–136.
27 Chandra, S. and Brummelhuis, H.G.J. (1981) Prothrombin complex concentrates for clinical use. *Vox Sang.*, **41**: 257–273.
28 Aronstam, A., MeLellan, D.S., Mbatha, P.S. and Wassef, M. (1982) The use of an activated Factor IX complex (Autoplex) in the management of haemarthroses in haemophiliacs with antibodies to Factor VIII. *Clin. Lab. Haematol.*, **4**: 231–238.
29 Heisel, M.A., Gomperts, E.D., McComb, G. and Hilgartner, M. (1983) Use of activated prothrombin complex concentrate over multiple surgical episodes in a hemophilic child with an inhibitor. *J. Pediatr.*, **102**: 951–954.
30 Kasper, C.K. (1984) Prothrombin complex concentrates and inhibitors. *JAMA*, **251**: 68–69.
31 Blatt, P.M., White, G.C., McMillan, C.W. and Webster, W.P. (1984) Failure of activated prothrombin complex concentrates in a hemophiliac with an anti-factor VIII antibody. *JAMA*, **251**: 67.

32 Vickars, L.M., Coupland, R.W. and Naiman, S.C. (1985) The response of an acquired Factor V inhibitor to activated factor IX concentrate. *Transfusion*, **25**: 51–53.
33 Burnouf-Radosevich, M. and Burnouf, T. (1992) A therapeutic, highly purified Factor XI concentrate from human plasma. *Transfusion*, **32**: 861–867.
34 Stirling, D. and Ludlam, C.A. (1993) Therapeutic concentrates for the treatment of congenital deficiencies of factors VII, XI, and XIII. *Semin. Thromb. Hemostas.*, **19**: 48–52.
35 Knight, R.D., Barr, C.F. and Alving, B.M. (1985) Replacement therapy for congenital Factor X deficiency. *Transfusion*, **25**: 78–80.

8
Treatment of Coagulation Disorders

Blood transfusion component therapy may be used either to restore deficiencies in the coagulation mechanism or to curtail excessive thrombotic tendencies. Many well-recognized coagulation disorders are *congenital* and these involve hereditary deficiencies either of single procoagulant factors or of inhibitors of the coagulation mechanism. *Acquired disorders* are usually more complex and involve deficiencies of multiple factors due to reduced synthesis, increased loss or accelerated consumption. Accelerated consumption of coagulation factors usually results from release of coagulation activators or from stimulation of the fibrinolytic system. Frequently these are combined in various proportions to result in either pathological clotting or bleeding.

Acquired coagulation disorders are common secondary complications of many serious medical and surgical conditions. Sometimes, the disturbances are relatively mild and have little effect on prognosis. On other occasions fulminating haemostatic disturbances dominate the clinical picture and may dictate the final outcome.

Congenital Bleeding Disorders

1 HAEMOPHILIA A (FACTOR VIII DEFICIENCY)

Haemophilia A is an inherited bleeding disorder caused either by absence of Factor VIII or alternatively by substitution of a non-functional procoagulant Factor VIII molecule. Factor VIII normally circulates in the plasma complexed to a high molecular weight carrier protein, the *von Willebrand factor* (vWF) . The lower molecular weight protein with coagulant activity is referred to as *Factor VIII:C*. The complete complex is responsible for both Factor VIII coagulant activity and also for maintaining the ability of platelets to aggregate and adhere to damaged surfaces, thereby sealing injured capillaries. Failure of the platelet-enhancing function is indicated by prolongation of the bleeding time. These two properties, *procoagulant function* and *platelet function*, are dependent on the normal activity of the lower molecular weight and high molecular weight portions respectively. Only the procoagulant function is defective in haemophilia A; platelet enhancing function remains intact.

A small proportion of patients with haemophilia treated with Factor VIII recognize this as foreign antigen and react by producing alloantibodies (see section 1.2). This antigenic aspect of the low molecular weight Factor VIII procoagulant molecule is referred to as Factor VIII:Ag. It was, however, the high molecular weight component of the complex (von Willebrand Factor, vWF; see section 3) that was first recognized to be antigenic following its experimental injection into other species. Subsequently this antigenic activity was recognized to be associated with the bleeding time component and it became clear that this was also the portion defective in von Willebrand's disease (see section 3) in which typically both the bleeding time and Factor VIII coagulant levels are abnormal. This can be explained by the fact that the large molecular weight portion of the complex appears to be necessary as a carrier allowing normal circulation of the low molecular weight Factor VIII coagulant protein.

Haemophilia A is much the commonest of the congenital bleeding disorders and affects approximately one in 10 000 of the male population. Even at this relatively low incidence the Factor VIII requirements of haemophiliac patients present a major challenge to blood transfusion services. Factor VIII supplies in any form are, in many countries, insufficient to meet clinical needs. The necessity to meet these requirements figure prominently in the blood collection and processing plans of most transfusion services and will continue to do so until the recombinant DNA technology-derived Factor VIII becomes widely available.

Haemophilia sufferers do not usually bleed excessively from trivial cuts because vascular and platelet performance is intact. Bleeding occurs from larger *skin injuries*, and *muscle and joint bleeds* feature prominently. The latter if inadequately treated lead to much *pain, immobility* and ultimately, because of fibrosis of haematomas, to *fixed deformities* of the joints. *Urinary tract bleeding* occurs and *severe hae-morrhage accompanies dental extraction* unless prophylactic Factor VIII treatment is given. Any surgery must be carefully planned and covered by adequate Factor VIII therapy. The relative safety of modern surgery in patients with haemophilia and related disorders covered with effective Factor VIII replacement has been demonstrated by a recent large survey.[1] The complete management of the haemophilia patient goes far beyond Factor VIII replacement therapy and entails specialized medical, nursing, physiotherapy and dental care in addition to attention to educational and social needs. Apart from initial emergency treatment, patients are best managed by specialists in haemophilia centres able to coordinate these various needs.

1.1 Factor VIII Replacement Therapy

Treatment of bleeding episodes must take into account the following aspects:

- The severity of the patient's factor VIII deficiency.
- The severity of the current bleeding problem.
- Whether serious immediate complications are possible, e.g. nervous tissue or airway compression.
- The choice of Factor VIII product to be used, the duration of therapy and whether adequate supplies of Factor VIII are available.
- The possible presence of Factor VIII inhibitors.
- The target plasma Factor VIII levels that will be necessary in order to control the bleeding episode.
- Potentially risky events that may arise during the management of the patients, e.g. wound dressing, joint mobilization and physiotherapy.
- Ancillary measures that might assist in prevention or control of bleeding, e.g. desmopressin (DDAVP) or fibrinolytic inhibitors.
- The presence of HIV infection as a determinant of the choice of very high-purity Factor VIII therapy (see chapter 7, section 3.5).

Certain of these aspects must be considered in more detail.

Severity of the Factor VIII deficiency

It is advisable to collect pre-treatment Factor VIII assay samples for confirmation of the severity of the Factor VIII deficit.

Severe haemophilia is associated with Factor VIII levels below 1% (100% is defined as the Factor VIII content of fresh normal plasma and is equivalent to 100 IU/dl). Disease of this severity is associated with the full spectrum of spontaneous bleeds as described above.

In mild haemophilia patients have levels exceeding 5%. They may escape notice for years until severe blood loss occurs during trauma or surgery.

Moderately affected individuals have features intermediate between these two states.

The severity of a bleeding episode

Bleeding episodes can be classified into mild, major and very severe and the doses scheduled accordingly.

(1) *Mild bleeding episodes*, e.g. early stages of joint bleeds, haematuria, single uncomplicated dental extractions:[2] give 10 IU Factor VIII per kilogram body weight to attain blood levels of 20 IU/dl.
(2) *More severe bleeding problems*, e.g. haemarthrosis,[3] haematomas, bone fractures,[4] gastrointestinal bleeding, abdominal pain, mild head injuries without evidence of neurological damage, more extensive dental extractions: give 25 IU/kg to attain blood levels of 50 IU/dl.
(3) *Severe injuries, major surgery*: give 40 IU/kg followed by 20–30 IU/kg every 12 hours to maintain blood levels between 50–100 IU/dl.

The dose can be calculated easily since (in the absence of inhibitors) 1 IU/kg gives a 2% rise in plasma Factor VIII levels.

Duration of Factor VIII therapy

Mild bleeds may require one dose alone and no more if symptoms are alleviated. This may, for example, be sufficient for most dental extractions. For other bleeding episodes dosages are continued daily until bleeding has ceased. For severe episodes it is necessary to maintain high Factor VIII levels for at least 2 weeks. Procedures such as *wound dressing* and *mobilization* following haemarthrosis also need Factor VIII cover. Episodes of *wound infection, coughing* or *vomiting* in the *postoperative period* also require that particular attention is paid to the maintenance of adequate Factor VIII levels.

Prophylactic therapy

This is a scheme of treatment designed to treat severe haemophiliac patients, i.e. those with Factor VIII levels below 1% (who have a risk of bleeding episodes almost weekly), with sufficient Factor VIII to maintain levels of around the 5% typical of mildly affected cases. The intention is:

(1) to reduce the frequency of spontaneous bleeding episodes;
(2) to prevent joint damage, loss of work or school time;
(3) to reduce overall Factor VIII use and hospital admission; and
(4) to allow higher levels of physical activity.

Prophylactic therapy is the treatment of choice for children and is best started early. Typically, it should begin between 1 and 2 years of age and continue until 18 years of age—this covering the most vulnerable period as far as haemarthrosis and joint damage are concerned. Treatment is usually given three times weekly at doses of around 20–30 IU/kg. Good venous access is obviously a prerequisite although indwelling catheters have been successfully used.

Home therapy

Under this arrangement patients or their parents are taught to administer Factor VIII concentrate early at the first sign of haemorrhage and thus prevent development of more severe bleeding episodes. This form of management allows patients to follow a normal life-style, to prevent severe painful bleeding episodes from developing and possibly to reduce all overall requirements for Factor VIII and the need for hospital admission.

The need for Factor VIII assays

Factor VIII assays should be performed:

(1) In all patients in whom the diagnosis has not already been sufficiently documented and confirmed.
(b) Prior to and just following therapy in order to confirm the absence of inhibitor activity and that the expected increase in plasma Factor VIII levels has taken place. During emergency hours assays can be dispensed with when well-known or mildly affected patients with bleeding episodes present for treatment.
(3) For severe bleeds and following surgery regular assays are necessary in order to confirm that adequate Factor VIII levels are maintained. Assays may be required daily or even twice daily and the results used to determine Factor VIII dosage and frequency.

Factor VIII recoveries and half-life

Approximately 85% of the Factor VIII in concentrates and cryoprecipitate is recoverable in the circulation following infusion. Plasma Factor VIII levels decline rapidly following infusion. The short initial phase with a half-life of 6 hours is probably due to equilibration with extracellular fluids; it is followed by a slower rate of disappearance with a half-life of 12 hours, probably representing natural decay. For practical purposes this latter figure is assumed. Thus 50% of the infused dose will be present at 12 hours and 25% at 24 hours. The choice of products to be used, including the advantages and disadvantages of intermediate and high-purity Factor VIII concentrate, have been described above (see chapter 7, section 3). Continuous infusion programmes have been shown to permit better control of Factor VIII levels, in particular for ensuring that unacceptably low levels do not occur.[5]

Adjuncts to Factor VIII therapy in haemophilia A

Des-amino-D-arginine vasopressin (DDAVP) is a synthetic vasopressin analogue which raises Factor VIII coagulant levels in normal subjects and also to a clinically useful extent in mild haemophiliacs. It also raises vWF:Ag and ristocetin cofactor activity in mildly affected patients with von Willebrand's disease.[6] DDAVP can be helpful for increasing plasma Factor VIII levels to cover dental extractions. A dose of 0.4 μg/kg has been found, for example, to give up to a four-fold increase in Factor VIII levels. Treatment can be repeated for several days but frequently a progressively declining response occurs. The vascular effects of this synthetic analogue of vasopressin are reduced but sodium and water retention can still occur and should be anticipated. Fibrinolysis is also increased by DDAVP and this unwanted effect may require concurrent antifibrinolytic treatment. DDAVP does not carry any risk of viral transmission and should therefore be used in preference to blood products for the treatment of mild haemophilia and von Willebrand's disease.

Inhibitors of fibrinolysis (e.g. ε-aminocaproic acid, tranexamic acid). These can only be used where the formation of indissoluble clots is not hazardous. Dental extractions provide the safest example; tranexamic acid at a dose of 1 g × 3 daily for 7–10 days following extraction has now become routine practice. Epistaxis and gastrointestinal bleeding are also suitable indications but fibrinolytic inhibitors have no place in the management of haematuria.

1.2   Factor VIII Inhibitors[7]

Alloantibodies (*inhibitors*) to the Factor VIII molecule appear in around 6–16% of haemophilia A patients overall or up to 52% of those with severe disease.[8,9]

There is also some suggestive evidence that inhibitor formation is more likely in patients treated with recombinant Factor VIII; this important question is, however, not resolved and large controlled studies involving previously untreated patients are necessary. It seems likely that new knowledge regarding the individual genetic lesion in haemophilia patients and its consequential effects on the ability to synthesize the Factor VIII molecular structure will enable better prediction of those most likely to develop inhibitors. Very rarely spontaneous autoantibodies to Factor VIII arise in non-haemophiliacs and these frequently give rise to life-threatening bleeding complications.[10] The development of these antibodies severely reduces the future ability to provide effective therapy. Antibodies to Factor VIII neutralize biological activity both *in vitro* and *in vivo*. Measurement of the *in vitro* capacity of inhibitors to neutralize Factor VIII gives a guide to the most suitable choice of treatment for the patient concerned. Inhibitor activity is defined as the Factor VIII-neutralizing capacity of 1 ml of patient's plasma when allowed to react with a standardized amount of pooled normal plasma Factor VIII (Bethesda units, BU/ml) or Factor VIII concentrate (Oxford units) under laboratory conditions. The results from these two assays differ slightly; on average, Bethesda unit potency slightly exceeds estimates in terms of Oxford units.

Potency of inhibitors

Very *low levels*, around 1–2 BU, do not appear to reduce the effectiveness of therapy and may remain unchanged for long periods. *Moderate inhibitor levels* of the order of 5–10 BU may be sometimes overcome by high doses of Factor VIII; this strategy is known as saturation therapy. In some of these patients anamnestic responses (boosting of the inhibitor) does not seem to occur. In others prompt elevation of the inhibitor levels prevents future Factor VIII therapy from being effective. *High inhibitor levels* (e.g. greater than 10 BU) present major problems if bleeding episodes require Factor VIII treatment. Amongst this group are 'high responder' patients in whom prompt boosting of antibody response occurs within a few days of starting therapy. It is for these patients that alternatives to the use of human Factor VIII are considered.

Management of patients with inhibitors

It is particularly important that patients with inhibitors avoid any risk of haemorrhage. Unlike conventional patients with haemophilia, the realization that there is no certainty of providing effective treatment necessitates life-style changes and may contraindicate routine elective surgical procedures.

Knowledge of a patient's previous response to treatment should be taken into account during management of each new bleeding episode. This gives the best guide to the likely response to treatment.

Treatment options for patients with inhibitors fall into three main categories. It may be possible to overcome Factor VIII antibodies by administering high-dose *saturation treatment*, antibodies may be physically *removed* or *inhibited*, or as a final alternative the role of Factor VIII in Factor X_a activation may be bypassed by the use of *activated coagulation products*.

Any inhibitor carries some risk of being boosted by Factor VIII therapy. Some patient responses may be relatively sluggish, while in other cases a brisk rise in antibody level follows within a few days of the start of Factor VIII therapy. If the problem is not too severe, two possibilities may be available:

(1) The bleeding episode may be sufficiently mild to be managed by supportive measures (rest, immobilization and analgesia) alone and not require Factor VIII therapy.
(2) The inhibitor level may be low enough (e.g. below 5 BU) to suggest that a short high-dose Factor VIII treatment course will stop bleeding before the boosted antibody response occurs.[11]

High inhibitor levels (e.g. 10 BU or more) are very difficult to manage. The options include:

(1) *Saturation of Factor VIII inhibitor activity* with the use of exceptionally high treatment doses. This strategy may still be unsuccessful. It may require more Factor VIII than can be made available and will be enormously costly. The higher-purity Factor VIII materials are usually used for this purpose.
(2) *Porcine Factor VIII*: Factor VIII prepared from porcine plasma is less readily neutralized by antihuman Factor VIII antibodies, although in its own right it can stimulate a specific neutralizing antibody response. High doses and large quantities can now be obtained. Earlier preparations of porcine Factor VIII,

though frequently effective, caused unfavourable reactions including thrombo-cytopenia. The newer more highly purified preparations (e.g. PE Porcine Factor VIII, Speywood Laboratories) appear to be better and have been highly successful.[12] Febrile reactions still take place and very occasionally thrombocytopenia occurs. The product improvement appears to be related to removal of a platelet aggregating factor present in the older material. Although inhibitor levels are normally measured against human Factor VIII, patients who have fewer than 50 BU may be expected to benefit and doses of 50 units/kg Factor VIII are unusually employed. Above this inhibitor level post-infusion recovery and clinical benefit are less likely. Assay of specific inhibitor activity against porcine Factor VIII is possible and enables more confident expectation of success.

In most patients, but not all, repeated doses of porcine Factor VIII have been given successfully without provoking anamnestic antibody responses.

(3) *Use of Activated Factor VII$_a$*: a number of clinical studies have shown that activated Factor VII (VII$_a$) is effective[13] and formal trials may endorse its role in the management of inhibitor patients. Factor VII$_a$ and tissue factor combine to activate Factor X, thus replicating the extrinsic pathway of prothrombin activation.[14]

(4) *Factor IX preparations*, both *non-activated* and *activated* (see chapter 7, section 4.3), appear in some haemophilia centres to be a successful form of treatment. Doses of the order 50–100 Factor VIII replacement units/kg are used. There are no specific laboratory monitoring methods for control of dosage. The partial thromboplastin time and the prothrombin time may both become shortened, the latter to well below normal.

(5) *Inhibitor removal or suppression*:

    (a) *Plasmapheresis* was formerly used in attempts to reduce inhibitor levels. The more recent technique of extracorporeal immunoabsorption using immobilized staphylococcal protein A to reduce plasma IgG is an experimental approach which has been claimed to be very successful.[15]

    (b) *Immunosuppressive therapy* (e.g. cyclophosphamide) has been helpful for some patients, more particularly those with *acquired haemophilia* and *Factor VIII autoantibodies*.[16]

    (c) *Intravenous immunoglobulin* (see chapter 9) may be effective, particularly for suppression of autoantibodies.[17]

    (d) *Induction of immune tolerance*: an alternative approach that has been claimed sometimes to lead to disappearance of inhibitors is the use of continuous low-dose substitution therapy programmes.[18]

2 HAEMOPHILIA B (FACTOR IX DEFICIENCY, CHRISTMAS DISEASE)

This condition, characterized by functional deficiency of Factor IX, is clinically identical to haemophilia A. The incidence appears to be about one per 100 000— only 10% that of haemophilia A. As a result there is little difficulty in providing adequate amounts of Factor IX concentrate since this can be obtained from the same source of fresh plasma that is used for Factor VIII concentrate production. Factor IX concentrates have been described earlier (chapter 7, section 4). Dosage of Factor IX concentrate follows closely the principles established for Factor VIII but a major difference that must be considered is the lower post-transfusion recovery, this being only around 50% of that infused. The dosage scheme table shown for haemophilia A (section 1.1) may be used but double the dose of Factor IX must be given in order to obtain the same increments in plasma levels. Alternatively the size of the dose to be given can be calculated from the relation:

1 IU/kg Factor IX raises the plasma Factor IX concentration by 1%

Traditional Factor IX preparations, even those that have not been intentionally activated, are potentially *thrombogenic*. For this reason some haemophilia centres have treated mild bleeding episodes with fresh frozen plasma (FFP) infusions. Only modest increments in Factor IX levels are of course possible using FFP (see chapter 7, section 1.2). These problems appear now to be largely overcome with the development of new high-purity non-activated Factor IX concentrates.[19]

High-purity preparations are used as a priority for high-risk categories of patients; these include neonates (see chapter 20) who in any case characteristically show a thrombotic predisposition,[20] patients undergoing surgery,[21] and patients with liver disease.[22]

Use of fibrinolytic inhibitors is not advised during Factor IX therapy because of the thrombotic risk.

3   VON WILLEBRAND'S DISEASE

Von Willebrand's disease is perhaps the commonest of the congenital disorders, possibly affecting up to 1% of the population. It is, however, very heterogeneous in its clinical genetic and biochemical manifestation. Fortunately the most severe clinical disease is seen extremely rarely.

In this disorder the large molecular weight carrier protein (von Willebrand Factor, vWF) that forms the major portion of the Factor VIII molecular complex is either quantitatively reduced or functionally abnormal. As a result there may be impaired carriage of the smaller Factor VIII procoagulant protein. Laboratory investigation shows a reduction in both Factor VIII procoagulant activity and the functional performance of vWF. Deficiency of the high molecular weight protein renders platelet function defective. This is shown by reduced platelet adhesiveness to collagen, the *bleeding time is prolonged*, and a characteristic defect of von Willebrand's disease plasma is its inability to promote platelet aggregation in the presence of ristocetin. In practice diagnosis is complicated by the existence of several types of molecular defect, each of which may result in slightly different clinical and laboratory results.

The condition usually shows an autosomal dominant inheritance but a smaller number of often severely affected homozygous patients also occur. The bleeding manifestations are in the main those characteristic of a defect of primary haemostasis. These consist of *mucosal* and *oral bleeding, epistaxes, bruising* and *menorrhagia*.

The classic haemophiliac haemarthrosis and muscle haematomas are uncommon but occur in the rare cases of homozygous disease.

Treatment of von Willebrand's disease[23]

The objective of treatment in von Willebrand's disease is the correction of both low plasma VIII levels and also the abnormal bleeding time since these together cause the bleeding diathesis.

Desmopressin (des-amino-D-arginine vasopressin, DDAVP) is the first line of treatment for mild and moderate von Willebrand's disease (e.g. type 1).[24] Treatment is given as for haemophilia A (see section 1.1). DDAVP is not likely to be so clinically reliable in patients who cannot synthesize the normal vWF multimer (e.g. the various forms of type II) and may be of no value for the rare but severe type III disease in which vWF synthesis is virtually absent.

Both Factor VIII concentrate and cryoprecipitate have been traditionally used for treatment of von Willebrand's disease. The latter material has been chosen for its generally more effective, albeit transient, correction of the bleeding time. Factor VIII levels are corrected less rapidly than in classical haemophilia taking 4–24 hours to reach peak levels following infusion, although levels remain elevated for a longer period. Treatment is monitored by assay of Factor VIII coagulant levels. When major surgery or bleeding episodes occur it may be worth confirming that the bleeding time has been adequately corrected as this may also reflect the haemostatic risk. A number of intermediate-purity Factor VIII concentrates have now been shown to contain therapeutically effective levels of vWF multimers (chapter 7, section 3.1) and these materials are now the treatment of choice.[25] Stated Factor VIII dosages, however, apply only to the Factor VIII procoagulant content. No functional estimation of vWF potency is possible.

Acquired Coagulation Abnormalities

4 LIVER DISEASE

A wide variety of haemostatic abnormalities are seen in liver disease. The liver is the site of synthesis of many coagulation factors; these include fibrinogen, Factor V and antithrombin III and the vitamin K-dependent Factors II, VII, IX and X. Deranged parenchymal function leads to either true *deficiency states* or to *defective synthesis* such as incomplete post-translational modification of the coagulation factor molecules. Fibrinogen levels may either be reduced as in acute liver failure, increased as in chronically inflammatory states, or alternatively dysfunctional fibrinogen molecules may be formed. Impaired absorption of the fat-soluble vitamin K, particularly in biliary obstruction, further contributes to the reduced synthetic performance of damaged liver tissue. Low-grade *disseminated intravascular coagulation* seems to be a frequent feature of active liver damage. This may be due to reduced clearance of activated clotting factors from the circulation by the hepatic reticuloendothelial cells. The same mechanism may explain the increased frequency of thromboses that have followed attempts to use Factor IX concentrates which so frequently appear to be contaminated by activated coagulation factors. The *deficiency of antithrombin III* seen in liver disease also enhances the thrombotic predisposition.

Despite the presence of multiple *in vitro* coagulation abnormalities clinical bleeding from these causes alone is uncommon; bleeding due to oesophageal varices or gastric ulceration is much more usual. The coagulation disturbances, however, undoubtedly aggravate bleeding when it occurs and make transfusion therapy more difficult. Correction of the coagulation abnormalities is only necessary for bleeding episodes or prior to liver biopsy or surgery. Treatment is best attempted with FFP, at doses of 12–15 ml/kg. Care is particularly necessary to prevent plasma volume overload. Taking into consideration the predictably poor improvements in plasma coagulation factor concentration following FFP administration (see chapter 7, section 1.2), it can be appreciated that effective replacement is at times impossible within the tolerable volume that can be administered. Diuretics are likely to be required. Vitamin K (10–20 mg) should be administered first in case restricted supplies of this have played a significant part in causing the deficiency state. There is no certainty that laboratory tests will show significant improvement after FFP therapy for the coagulation disturbances of liver failure. Progress may be assessed by means of the prothrombin time ratio, but there is no clear agreement as to safe levels for surgery; values of 1.6–1.8 are probably realistic.

4.1 Bleeding Due to Vitamin K Deficiency and Warfarin Therapy[26]

Treatment requires vitamin K (10–20 mg) orally or intravenously if absorption is doubtful. For bleeding patients or those requiring emergency surgery, particularly when oral anticoagulation must be continued, FFP at a dose of at least 12–15 ml/kg must be given. FFP is also necessary for the emergency treatment of bleeding patients with particularly high prothrombin time ratios.

Prothrombin complex concentrates (PCC) have been advocated for anticoagulant reversal. Most PCC products do not, however, have adequate Factor VII enrichment, this can be provided separately in the form of Factor VII concentrates. However, suitable PCC with Factor VII concentrates are not generally as readily available as FFP for emergency treatment.

5 DISSEMINATED INTRAVASCULAR COAGULATION AND FIBRINOLYSIS

Disseminated intravascular coagulation (DIC) denotes pathological coagulation and thrombosis throughout the vascular system. This is often accompanied by increased *fibrinolysis*, probably reflecting a compensatory attempt to maintain vascular patency. DIC probably results from failure of the normal protective mechanism whereby the enzymatic stages of the potentially explosive coagulation cascade are restrained so as to permit clotting only where the lining of the circulation is damaged. Unwanted activation of the coagulation system is normally self-limiting. A balance probably exists between the generation of activated factors by injured surfaces and by thromboplastic materials and their destruction by natural inhibitors (e.g. antithrombin III) and fibrinolysis. These arrangements appear to break down in some patients who are severely ill and as a consequence the constraint to DIC is removed.

5.1 Causes of Disseminated Intravascular Coagulation

DIC can to a lesser or greater degree be seen in a variety of conditions, some of which are listed here:

- Shock and hypoxia.
- Heat-stroke.
- Release of coagulant materials from disseminated tumours, e.g. acute promyelocytic leukaemia.
- Trauma and burns.
- Haemolytic transfusion reactions.
- Obstetric problems, e.g. retained dead fetus, abruptio placenta, septic abortion, amniotic fluid embolism.
- Purpura fulminans and haemolytic uraemic syndrome.
- Administration of activated Factor IX preparations.

5.2 Pathological Mechanisms

The above conditions probably initiate DIC as a result of *contact activation* of the initial stages of the coagulation cascade, by release of *thromboplastic materials* from damaged tissues, or by the effects of *proteolytic enzymes* released from tissues which then activate Factors II or X. DIC ranges in severity from *low-grade chronic states* to *fulminating acute defibrination syndromes*. In the former, *thrombotic* events tend to predominate. Acute DIC, on the other hand, is usually characterized by extensive consumption of platelets and clotting factors and sometimes uncontrollable *blood loss*. Widespread vascular thrombosis results in ischaemic organ failure. Red cell destruction and fragmentation through entrapment in microthrombi produce the characteristic microangiopathic haemolytic anaemia. Deterioration of the primary condition that has led to DIC is sometimes followed by transition from a smouldering to a more explosive state. Under these circumstances the greatly accelerated coagulation activity consumes coagulation factors faster than they can be replaced. Factors V and VIII, fibrinogen and platelets show the most severe depression but levels of others may also be depleted. ATIII may also be reduced and cause heparin resistance if that form of treatment is used.

5.3 Laboratory Findings

Not surprisingly, results of laboratory tests depend to a large degree on the nature of the clinical condition, the aggressiveness of the consumptive process and the amount of fibrinolysis. Screening assays, e.g. prothrombin time and activated partial thromboplastin time tests, are liable to be prolonged if a reduction in procoagulant factor concentrations predominates. Alternatively, they can be accelerated by the presence of activated products, e.g. Factor X_a. Because of this there is no consistently diagnostic profile of test results and specialist help is needed for interpretation and diagnosis. A list of the more commonly used screening tests with their expected results is given below:

Prothrombin time	Prolonged
Thrombin time	Prolonged
Partial thromboplastin time	Prolonged
Platelet count	Reduced
Fibrinogen level	Reduced
Fibrinogen degradation products	Increased

Demonstration of reduced *antithrombin III (ATIII)*, and assays for *Fibrin D-dimer*, *plasminogen* and *plasmin* provide more specific confirmation of DIC.

5.4   Abnormal Fibrinolysis

DIC is usually accompanied by evidence of increased fibrinolytic activity. This is usually termed *secondary fibrinolysis* and occurs as a compensatory response to excess coagulation, as distinct from the *primary* form where plasminogen activators introduced into the circulation lead to plasmin formation and fibrinogen lysis. In both conditions a haemorrhagic diathesis results from a combination of fibrinogen deficiency and the anticoagulant effect of fibrinogen degradation products. Secondary fibrinolysis is characterized by the appearance of thrombin split products of fibrin, e.g. *D-dimer fragments* in addition to fibrinogen split products (FDP) which are the end results of *plasmin digestion*.

5.5   Treatment of Disseminated Intravascular Coagulation

Treatment must be tailored to match both the haemostatic disturbances and the symptoms of each individual patient. There is unfortunately no firm agreement about the safety or value of the principal therapeutic materials that are used to gain control over the disordered coagulation system.

Treatment of the primary cause

The central importance of this is not disputed. Circulatory shock and hypoperfusion, for example, must be corrected, sepsis treated or delivery expedited in obstetric defibrination. It is unlikely that the measures described below for correction of the haemostatic abnormalities will have any significant benefit until the episode precipitating the DIC is brought under control.

Heparin therapy

This is most easily justified for low-grade DIC with thrombotic rather than bleeding symptoms. Numerous case reports have shown heparin to arrest the consumption of fibrinogen and platelets, to prevent further thrombosis and allow clinical recovery. Large controlled studies of the use of heparin for DIC have been less convincing. Heparin treatment would also seem to be inappropriate for DIC complicated by acute bleeding episodes. Nevertheless, *heparin therapy* does have proponents[27,28] claiming value of a less nihilistic approach, depending on the circumstances, and expert advice should be sought.

Blood component replacement therapy

Factor V, Factor VIII fibrinogen and platelets are the principal factors reduced in DIC. These deficiencies, together with the antithrombotic effect of fibrinogen split products and excess fibrinolysis, cause the pathological bleeding. Fresh platelet concentrates (one pack per 10 kg) and cryoprecipitate (1.5 packs per 10 kg) provide a suitable combination for attempting to correct the deficiency state. It must be recalled that Factor V and ATIII are not concentrated in these preparations and will be replaced least effectively. *FFP* (12–15 ml/kg) is better, *ATIII concentrates* are sometimes also used. Repeat dosage with platelets and cryoprecipitate will be required as determined by clinical progress and laboratory findings. Critics of the use of component therapy argue that replacement therapy 'feeds the fire' by providing more haemostatic factors leading to further thrombosis and continued production of the anticoagulant fibrin split products. On balance the clinical evidence does not seem to substantiate this hypothetical risk. Replacement therapy is most clearly justified when consumptive coagulopathy and pathological bleeding predominate.

Fibrinolytic inhibitors

The role of *fibrinolytic inhibitors* is particularly uncertain. Their use could be highly dangerous in many circumstances but they may be indicated for the rare conditions involving predominantly fibrinolysis, especially where bleeding is external and where the formation of indissoluble clots would not be dangerous. *Secondary fibrinolysis* appears to abate once the process of disseminated intravascular coagulation is controlled.

Monitoring the success of treatment

Fibrinogen and platelet determinations provide the most readily available laboratory guide to the success of treatment. Where available these can be supplemented by *FDP, D-dimer, and ATIII assays.*[28]

5.6   Treatment of Bleeding due to Thrombolytic Therapy[29]

Initial treatment of bleeding usually requires interruption of thrombolytic therapy together with anticoagulation and reversal of heparin where appropriate. If these measures are unsuccessful blood components, e.g. cryoprecipitate, may be needed to restore fibrinogen and Factor VIII; FFP provides Factor V, and platelets, which also carry substantial amounts of Factor V, should be used.

6   OTHER COAGULATION DISORDERS

Neonatal coagulation problems are dealt with in chapter 21. The haemostatic disturbances found during *cardiac surgery* and *massive transfusion* are discussed in chapters 12 and 14 respectively. Coagulation abnormalities also occur in other protein-losing states, particularly in the *nephrotic syndrome*. Preferential loss of antithrombin III may account for the thrombotic tendency seen in this condition.

6.1   Thrombotic Thrombocytopenic Purpura/Haemolytic Uraemic Syndrome[30]

Central to the pathology of this spectrum of conditions is the presence of *widespread platelet activation* leading to *multiple vascular thrombosis* and associated end-organ infarction. Abnormally high molecular weight vWF multimers appearing in the blood may be the precipitating agent for platelet activation. Normal plasma appears to have an inhibitory effect on the formation of these abnormal vWF multimers. FFP infusion or, even better, plasma exchange (see chapter 19) have proved markedly effective in this extremely severe condition. It has been claimed that cryosupernatant plasma (the residue after cryoprecipitate manufacture) is even more effective; the rationale is presumably based on its depleted vWF content compared to FFP.[31]

6.2   Antithrombin III Deficiency[32]

ATIII deficiency appears to be the best understood cause of *hypercoagulable thrombotic states*. Problems such as *defective fibrinolysis* or abnormalities of *protein C*, or *protein S*, another antagonist of activated coagulation factors, may explain other cases. ATIII is the principal natural thrombin antagonist; its role can be demonstrated *in vitro* by watching the natural decay of thrombin in plasma and this is the basis of ATIII bioassays. Without ATIII, thrombin generated in the bloodstream could cause uncontrolled coagulation. ATIII also has a role in neutralizing activated Factors IX, X, XI and XII.

ATIII deficiency occurs as a rare *congenital disorder* characterized by recurrent thrombotic episodes. *Acquired deficiency states* are much more common. These include nephrotic syndrome (because of the renal protein loss), disseminated intravascular coagulation and liver cirrhosis, and ATIII deficiency is also associated with intra-abdominal sepsis. ATIII can become depleted during surgical blood loss if this is replaced by asanguineous fluids, but ATIII is stable in banked blood so routine transfusion provides some replacement. It is generally believed that at least 60% of normal ATIII levels are needed to prevent an increased thrombotic risk. This degree of intolerance to mild deficiencies is unusual amongst haemostatic proteins but may not hold true if there is a simultaneous deficiency of the opposing plasma coagulation factors.[33] Concentrates of ATIII have been used for treatment of thrombotic problems in patients with ATIII deficiency. The British National Health Service ATIII product is presented as freeze-dried vials with a nominal content of 1000 IU. Loading doses of 50 IU/kg followed by 25 IU/kg on alternate days have been found effective. The biological half-life appears to be around 3 days; thus effective replacement therapy should be feasible. Several commercial ATIII concentrates are also now available. ATIII combined with subcutaneous heparin has been used successfully during prophylactic management of pregnancy in patients with congenital ATIII deficiency.[34,35] The use of ATIII concentrates has also been explored in a variety of other clinical settings with apparently encouraging results. These include, for example, management of DIC and prophylaxis of the thrombosis following orthopaedic operations. FFP can also be used as a source of ATIII. ATIII has an important therapeutic role as a cofactor for heparin anticoagulation. Heparin acts by potentiation of ATIII and in deficiency states the anticoagulant effect of heparin is therefore reduced. Prolonged heparin therapy appears to result in complexing or consumption of ATIII leading to a deficiency state which shows itself as increasing resistance to heparin therapy. ATIII concentrates could possibly have a role in this situation.

REFERENCES

1 Kitchens, C.S. (1986) Surgery in haemophilia and related disorders: a prospective study of 100 consecutive procedures. *Medicine*, **65**: 34–35.
2 Steinberg, S.E., Levin, J. and Bell, W.R. (1984) Evidence that less replacement therapy is required for dental extractions in hemophiliacs. *Am. J. Haematol.*, **16**: 1–13.
3 Aronstam, A., Wassef, M., Hamad, Z., Cartlidge, J. and McLellan, D. (1983) A double-blind controlled trial of two dose levels of factor VIII in the treatment of high risk haemarthroses in haemophilia A. *Clin. Lab. Haematol.*, **5**: 157–163.
4 Wolff, L.J. and Lovrien, E.W. (1982) Management of fractures in hemophilia. *Paediatrics*, **70**: 431–436.
5 Martinowitz, U., Schulman, S., Gitel, S., Horozowski, H., Heim, M. and Varon, D. (1982) Adjusted dose continuous infusion of Factor VIII in patients with haemophilia A. *Br. J. Haematol.*, **82**: 729–734.
6 Mariana, G., Ciavarella, N., Mazzucconik, M.G. *et al.* (1984) Evaluation of the effectiveness of DDAVP in surgery and in bleeding episodes in haemophilia and von Willebrand's disease: a study on 43 patients. *Clin. Lab. Haematol.*, **6**: 229–238.
7 Macik, B.G. (1993) Treatment of factor VIII inhibitors: products and strategies. *Semin. Thromb. Hemostas.*, **19**: 13–20.
8 Editorial (1989) Anti-Factor VIII inhibitors in haemophilia. *Lancet*, **ii**: 363–364.
9 Ehrenforth, S., Kreuz, W., Scharrer, I. *et al.* (1992) Incidence of development of Factor VIII and Factor IX inhibitors in haemophiliacs. *Lancet*, **339**: 594–598.
10 Hultin, M.B. (1991) Acquired inhibitors in malignant and nonmalignant disease states.

Symposium: Acquired Factor VIII inhibitors in the non hemophiliac: historical perspectives, current therapy and future approaches. *Am. J. Med.*, **91**: 5A–9S.

11 Bloom, A.L. (1978) Clotting factor concentrates for resistant haemophilia. *Br. J. Haematol.*, **40**: 21–27.

12 Morrison, A.E. and Ludlam, C.A. (1991) The use of porcine Factor VIII in the treatment of patients with acquired hemophilia: the United Kingdom experience. Symposium: Acquired Factor VIII inhibitors in the non hemophiliac: historical perspectives, current therapy and future approaches. *Am. J. Med.*, **91**: 5A–23S.

13 Limentani, S.A., Roth, D.A., Furie, B.C. and Furie, B. (1993) Recombinant blood clotting proteins for hemophilia therapy. *Semin. Thromb. Hemostas.*, **19**: 62–70.

14 Schulman, S. (1992) A therapeutic alternative for haemophiliacs with inhibitors. *Acta Paediatr.*, **81**: 564–565.

15 Watt, R.M., Bunitsky, K., Faulkner, E.R. *et al.* and the Hemophilia Study Group (1992) Treatment of congenital and acquired hemophilia patients by extracorporeal removal of antibodies to coagulation factors: a review of US clinical studies 1987–1990. *Transfusion Sci.*, **13**: 233–253.

16 Green, D. (1991) Cytotoxic suppression of acquired factor VIII:C inhibitors. Symposium: Acquired Factor VIII inhibitors in the non hemophiliac: historical perspectives, current therapy and future approaches. *Am. J. Med.*, **91**: 5A–14S.

17 Sultan, Y., Kazatchkine, M.D., Nydegger, U., Rossi, F., Dietrich, G. and Algiman, M. (1991) Intravenous immunoglobulin in the treatment of spontaneously acquired Factor VIII:C inhibitors. Symposium: Acquired Factor VIII inhibitors in the non hemophiliac: historical perspectives, current therapy and future approaches. *Am. J. Med.*, **91**: 5A–53S.

18 Van Leeuwen, E.F., Mauser-Bunschoten, E.P., van Dijken, P.J., Kok, A.J., Sjamsoedin-Visser, E.J.M. and Sixma, J.J. (1986) Disappearance of Factor VIII:C antibodies in patients with haemophilia A upon frequent administration of Factor VIII in intermediate or low dose. *Br. J. Haematol.*, **64**: 291–297.

19 Shmith, K.J. (1992) Factor IX concentrates: the new products and their properties. *Transfusion Med. Rev.*, **6**: 124–136.

20 Kasper, C.K., Lusher, J.M. and the Transfusion Practices Committee (1993) Recent evolution of clotting factor concentrates for hemophilia A and B. *Transfusion*, **33**: 422–434.

21 Conlan, M.G. and Hoots, W.K. (1990) Disseminated intravascular coagulation and hemorrhage in hemophilia B following elective surgery. *Am. J. Hematol.*, **35**: 203–207.

22 Goldsmith, J.C., Kasper, C.K., Blatt, P.M. *et al.* (1992) Coagulation Factor IX: Successful surgical experience with a purified Factor IX concentrate. *Am. J. Hematol.*, **40**: 210–215.

23 Scott, J.P. and Montgomery, R.R. (1993) Therapy of von Willebrand Disease. *Semin. Thromb. Hemostas.*, **19**: 1.

24 Rodehgiero, F., Castaman, G., Meyer, D. *et al.* (1992) Replacement therapy with virus inactivated plasma concentrates in von Willebrand disease. *Vox Sang.*, **62**: 193–199.

25 Cumming, A.M. (1990) Clinical and laboratory evaluation of National Health Service Factor VIII concentrate (8Y) for the treatment of von Willebrand's Disease. *Br. J. Haematol.*, **75**: 234–239.

26 British Committee for Standards in Haematology. Working Party of the Blood Transfusion Task Force (1992) Guidelines for the use of fresh frozen plasma. *Transfusion Med.*, **2**: 57–63.

27 Baker, W.F. (1989) Clinical aspects of disseminated intravascular coagulation: a clinician's point of view. *Semin. Thromb. Hemostas.*, **15**: 1–57.

28 Bick, R.L. (1988) Clinical review of disseminated intravascular coagulation. *Semin. Thromb. Hemostas.*, **14**: 315.

29 Sane, D.C., Califf, R.M., Topol, E.J., Stump, D.E., Mark, D.B. and Greenberg, C S. (1989) Bleeding during thrombolytic therapy for acute myocardial infarction: mechanisms and management. *Ann. Intern. Med.*, **111**: 1010–1021.

30 Moake, J.L. (1990) TTP: desperation, empiricism, progress. *N. Engl. J. Med.*, **325**: 426–428.

31 Byrnes, J.J., Moake, J.L., Klug, P. and Periman, P. (1990) Effectiveness of the cryosupernatant fraction of plasma in the treatment of refractory thrombotic thrombocytopenic purpura. *Am. J. Hematol.*, **34**: 169–174.

32 Menache, D., Grossman, B.J. and Jackson, C.M. (1992) Antithrombin III: physiology, deficiency, and replacement therapy. *Transfusion*, **32**: 580–587.

33 Lundsgaard-Hansen, P., Ehrengruber, E., Frei, E., Papp, E., Senn, A. and Tschirren, B. (1983) Antithrombin III and related parameters in surgical patients receiving blood components. *Vox Sang.*, **46**: 19–28.

34 Samson, D., Stirling, Y., Woolf, L., Howarth, D., Seghatchian, M.J. and De Chazal, R. (1984) Management of planned pregnancy in a patient with congenital antithrombin III deficiency. *Br. J. Haematol.*, **56**: 243–249.

35 Hellgren, M., Tengborn, L. and Abildgaard, U. (1982) Pregnancy in women with congenital antithrombin III deficiency: experience of treatment with heparin and antithrombin. *Gynecol. Obstet. Invest.*, **14**: 127–141.

9
Therapeutic Immunoglobulins

Since the early 1980s the use of immunoglobulin therapy has expanded to become one of the most clinically important (and expensive) new areas of transfusion practice. This has been a consequence of the development of safe high-dose intravenous products primarily intended to enable better replacement therapy in immunodeficiency states. Arising from somewhat serendipitous observations has come the realization that large doses of infused IgG have a powerful modulating effect on the immune system and are capable of producing remissions in some autoimmune disorders. In addition, the recognition that many of the infective problems faced by patients with secondary forms of immunodeficiency might be combated by effective replacement therapy opens up further possibilities for use.

Immunoglobulin for therapeutic use is extracted and purified from large pools, typically comprising 5000–15 000 donations of plasma. Pooled plasma from normal people contains the full spectrum of antibodies to the microorganisms causing illnesses prevalent in the community. The range of specific antibody activities in pooled normal immunoglobulins will, therefore, vary from one geographic zone to another. *Polyspecific immunoglobulin* derived in this way can be used as an anti-infective agent for the treatment of *broad-spectrum antibody deficiency states*. In contrast, plasma collected from naturally immune 'convalescent' donors, or donors artificially hyperimmunized against microbial antigens, can provide *specific* immunoglobulin. This can be used to confer passive immunity to subjects at particular risk from the infective agent concerned.

Immunoglobulins can be used in a *prophylactic* or a *therapeutic* role. The major categories of clinical problems in which these products may be used include:

(1) Congenital antibody deficiency syndromes.
(2) Acquired antibody deficiency states.
(3) When specific antimicrobial immunoglobulin therapy is needed.
(4) Certain autoimmune disorders, e.g. idiopathic thrombocytopenia.

1 IMMUNOGLOBULIN PREPARATIONS AVAILABLE

Immunoglobulin therapy began historically with the transfusion of crude normal or hyperimmune plasma. Currently available products are partially purified IgG materials prepared from the Cohn fraction II ethanol precipitate from normal or immune plasma.

The first immunoglobulin preparations contained relatively large amounts of denatured or multimeric aggregated molecules. These caused severe, often anaphylactic reactions if infused intravenously. Their use was therefore of necessity confined to intramuscular administration and the large dose volumes required limited the effective replacement levels that could be achieved. Recently normal immunoglobulin preparations for the treatment of immunodeficiency states have become available which can be given *intravenously*. These are derived from the same basic ethanol precipitation procedure but are subject to one or more of a variety of secondary chemical and physical modifications designed to prevent formation of immunoglobulin aggregates and ensure freedom from virus transmission. Currently popular is the use of low pH in the presence of pepsin, but low ionic strength ethanol, polyethylene glycol and DEAE Sephadex chromatography have also been used to remove aggregates from products designed for intravenous use. IgG is the major component of intravenous immunoglobulin products; attention is paid to reducing the content of other immunoglobulin classes; IgA in particular can be a source of serious reactions. Unlike the traditional products for intramuscular use there have been instances of hepatitis transmission with certain batches of intravenous immunoglobulin (IVIg) prepared by procedures which otherwise have exemplary safety records. This seems to indicate a very small margin of tolerance in the manufacturing process of some IVIg products. Current efforts are being directed to provide assured virucidal steps during production. In general, however, the IVIg products are very popular for the treatment of immunodeficiency syndromes and steps are even being taken to promote home treatment programmes for suitable patients.

Ideally preparations should:

(1) Contain mostly IgG.
(2) Represent all natural IgG subclasses.
(3) Contain no IgG polymers.
(4) Preserve antibody binding, complement fixing and opsonic functions.

The broad-spectrum immunoglobulins will contain a variety of antibacterial and antiviral antibodies as well as neutralizing activity against bacterial lipopolysaccharide endotoxin. It is particularly important that antibodies are present against the pathogens which commonly affect antibody-deficient patients (see section 2.1).

It is also important to bear in mind that all immunoglobulin preparations, even those for specific purposes, may contain other antibodies. Anti-D immunoglobulin may, for example, contain rubella antibodies; the finding of these in the serum following passive prophylaxis would not therefore indicate a state of active immunity to rubella.

The position with regard to immunoglobulin procurement is unlikely to remain static. There is a possibility that monoclonal cell lines may, in the future, be used for the production of certain specific immunoglobulins for therapy.

1.1 Choice of Intravenous Products

IVIg preparations are available from several of the major blood product manufacturers. These differ according to method of manufacture, product presentation and also show minor differences in IgG subclass content as well as IgA contamination. Immunoglobulin batches are analysed for titres of antibodies against a range of microbial antigens, for example measles, *Haemophilus influenzae*, group B streptoccoci, *Escherichia coli*, cytomegalovirus and hepatitis A. Unfortunately, differences in assay methodology, problems with standardization and poor correlation between *in vitro* results and *in vivo* antimicrobial potency make it very difficult to make valid conclusions as to the potential efficacy of the various products in any given clinical situation. It seems, therefore, generally agreed that for the established categories of use there is little evidence of differences in efficacy. Some products are available as ready-to-use solutions; others are freeze dried and require reconstitution. As a general rule patients with a life-long dependency are best not changed unnecessarily from one product to another. Patients become confident and accustomed to their regular form of therapy and may experience transient reactions if changed. If a change of product is necessary, the first doses are administered slowly, as is usual at the start of an IVIg therapeutic programme.

1.2 Route of Administration: Intramuscular and Intravenous Immunoglobulins

Intravenous products have become the standard choice for replacement therapy in immunodeficiency states and for immune modulation in autoimmune conditions. However most *specific* immunoglobulin products are presented for intramuscular use.

(1) The large regular intramuscular doses of immunoglobulin necessary in antibody deficiency syndromes were painful and generally greatly disliked by the recipients.
(2) The recovery of IgG in the plasma is probably about equal for either route. Absorption from subcutaneous fat is inefficient; for this reason small doses of

specific immunoglobulin are best given via the deltoid area rather than via the thigh or buttock.

Peak blood levels following intramuscular injections are reached between 2 and 5 days. Intravenous doses produce instant high plasma levels, falling by approximately 50% over a few hours as extravascular distribution occurs. Thereafter the plasma half-life of both materials appear to approximate to the 2–3 weeks characteristic of endogenous IgG.

(3) Intravenous immunoglobulin can be given in much higher doses than can intramuscular materials. This is clinically important in the treatment of antibody deficiency syndromes. In these conditions normal levels of IgG can be maintained by intravenous therapy.

2 ANTIBODY DEFICIENCY STATES

These may be either primary disorders or appear as secondary (acquired) deficiencies arising as a result of other disease or treatment. The indication to initiate treatment with immunoglobulin is based on clinical evidence of *predisposition to infection* together with *incapacity to mount an appropriate antibody response.*

2.1 Primary Antibody Deficiency Syndromes[1,2]

These clinical conditions include *transient hypogammaglobulinaemia of infancy, common variable immunodeficiency, sex-linked hypogammaglobulinaemia, late-onset hypogammaglobulinaemia,* and *hypogammaglobulinaemia with thymoma.* The humoral antibody deficiency found as a component of *severe combined immunodeficiency* will also merit immunoglobulin therapy although for these patients bone marrow transplantation is advantageous. Some patients, for example boys with Wiskott–Aldrich syndrome and patients with ataxia telangiectasia, have near-normal immunoglobulin levels but still show severely impaired antibody responses to certain microbial pathogens. Immunoglobulin levels in congenital antibody deficiency conditions are severely reduced; serum IgG concentrations, for example, are typically below 2.0 g/l compared with the normal range of 8–18 g/l. Not all such patients will be symptomatic and require treatment, but patients with congenital antibody deficiency syndrome and late-onset (common variable) hypogammaglobulinaemia generally experience a variety of infective problems. These include:

(1) Recurrent pyogenic infections, e.g. pyodema, sinusitis, otitis, pneumonia and bronchitis, arthritis, urinary tract infections, septicaemia. The organisms include *Staphylococcus* spp, *Streptococcus* spp, *Haemophilus influenzae*, *Neisseria meningitidis, Pseudomonas aeruginosa, Klebsiella spp* and *Escherichia coli.*
(2) *Mycoplasma* infections in lungs, urinary tract (ureoplasmas) and joints.
(3) Gastrointestinal infection due to *Giardia lamblia, Campylobacter* and cryptosporidia.
(4) Herpes simplex, herpes zoster and CMV.

The total body content of IgG is around 1.0 g/kg; assuming a 3-week half-life, the daily replacement needs would amount to 25 mg/kg. In practice, dosage levels of 200–400 mg/kg per month are usual.

Minimum trough levels of IgG of 5.0 g/l are usually sought on intravenous therapy. It appears that in some patients between 6 months to 1 year of continuous treatment may be required before clinical improvement is clearly evident.

Infections have occurred in infants born to mothers with hypogammaglobulinaemia even when this has, in the mother, been asymptomatic. Treatment of the mother may be needed to provide IgG for transplacental passage, the infant's immunoglobulin levels should be monitored and may need replenishment after delivery.[3]

There is some dispute over whether exogenous IgG crosses the placenta in effective amounts. It appears likely that this may take some days to occur and may also depend on the qualitative aspects of individual preparations, e.g. preservation of a high proportion of the IgG Fc receptors.

Intravenous therapy appears to make patients feel fitter, with less frequent episodes of infection, and normal plasma IgG levels can be maintained. Initial treatment, especially that given during infective episodes, characteristically appears to result in *pyrexial* symptoms. Patients also occasionally experience various other unpleasant symptoms during intravenous IgG infusion. These include backache, muscle aches, flushing feelings, nausea and sometimes vomiting. Pyrexial reactions have been attributed to reactions between microbial antigenic material and the sudden influx of immunoglobulin. Prolonged symptoms do not usually occur; slowing of the infusion rate is usually effective; antipyretics may also help. The inclusion of maltose in intravenous immunoglobulin preparations appears to reduce the incidence of unpleasant reactions. Allergic reactions may be due to IgA antibodies in those in whom this immunoglobulin is congenitally deficient.

Intravenous immunoglobulin is usually given as about a 3–6% solution at a rate of 1–3 ml/h. Higher concentrations in a smaller volume could be given via constant infusion pumps.

2.2   Secondary Immunodeficiency States[4]

Immunoglobulin deficiency is a secondary complication of a variety of acute or chronic illnesses. In many of these infection has a large influence on overall morbidity and mortality.

(1) Patients with *hypogammaglobulinaemia* associated with B cell malignancies (e.g. chronic lymphocytic leukaemia, (CLL) and non-Hodgkin's lymphoma (NHL)) have a well-recognized increase in infection rates. Intravenous immunoglobulin has been confirmed to reduce the incidence of bacterial infections but the frequency of fungal and viral infections remains unchanged. The beneficial value of either broad-spectrum or specific immunoglobulin therapy as a general policy has yet to be determined in many of these situations. Infection rates can certainly be reduced in patients with chronic lymphocytic leukaemia[5,6] but not to the extent that would justify the general use of IVIg in this

Table 1 Possible uses for IVIg in secondary immune deficiency

Haematological malignancies	Chronic lymphocytic leukaemia
	Non-Hodgkin's lymphoma
	Myeloma
	Following bone marrow transplantation
Post-trauma immunodeficiency	Burns
	Septic shock
	High sepsis risk surgery
HIV infection	
Premature neonates	

condition.[7] A decision to institute regular treatment should be based on a substantial reduction in illness and hospitalization in order to justify the very considerable inconvenience and expense.

(2) *Myeloma*: infection is particularly likely during the early phase of chemotherapy. Intravenous immunoglobulin has been found to confer some protection, but as with CLL it has not been possible to identify circumstances in which the use of IVIg can be unequivocally justified.

(3) *Bone marrow transplantation* (see chapter 22, section 3): it is now accepted that prophylactic IVIg does not produce a significant reduction in the morbidity and mortality from bacterial infections to which post-bone marrow transplant patients are particularly prone. Marginal reductions in some infection rates, e.g. from candida, staphylococal infections and Gram-negative sepsis, have been reported, but these have not been enough to justify routine prophylaxis. CMV infection (see chapter 24, section 7), in particular for seropositive recipients, is a well-recognized hazard. CMV-specific immunoglobulin was formerly used for prophylaxis and therapy. Currently it is considered that human normal IVIg is just as effective; indeed there is some contention over the value of either agent for prophylaxis. The mechanism of action is presumably not linked to specific anti-CMV titres. IVIg combined with the antiviral agent acyclovir or ganciclovir may be helpful for treatment of CMV pneumonitis.[8,9] The most convincing benefit of the use of IVIg for management of post-bone marrow transplant patients (non-T cell-depleted allogeneic grafts) seems to be a reduction of the severity of graft-versus-host disease.[10]

(4) *Septic shock, post-surgical infections, burns injury*: studies have indicated the potential benefit of IVIg for patients with these conditions.[11-13] Satisfactory studies have, however, proved difficult to perform since evenly matched treatment and controlled groups are not easily obtained. For this reason the role of IVIg for these not uncommon problems remains under investigation and cannot be supported for routine use. The pathological events in severe septic shock (synonymous with systemic inflammatory response syndrome) seem to be mediated by endotoxins or by cytokines such as tumour necrosis factor (TNF) or interleukin 1 (IL-1) and the possible beneficial effect of monoclonal antibodies against these moieties is under study[14,15] (see chapter 13, section 2).

(5) IVIg therapy has been examined for control of secondary infection in children with AIDS.[16] Even though overall immunoglobulin levels are not reduced, specific antibody responses are usually impaired. Early studies suggested significant benefit particularly for those children with severe recurrent antibiotic-resistant infections and moderately reduced CD4 counts ($>0.2 \times 10^9$/l). However, immunoglobulin therapy has not so far been shown to affect the mortality rate for this group of patients. HIV-related thrombocytopenia frequently responds, albeit temporarily, to IVIg. IVIg is therefore justified as first-choice emergency therapy for acutely symptomatic patients.[17]

(6) *Premature neonates*: intravenous immunoglobulin has been used with apparently beneficial effect in preterm very low birth weight neonates (<1500 g) as prophylaxis against infection[18,19] and for treatment of established sepsis in the newborn.[20] In both instances further studies are required before the proper role for IVIg can be defined.[21]

3   INTRAVENOUS IMMUNOGLOBULIN THERAPY FOR IDIOPATHIC THROMBOCYTOPENIA[22-24]

The unexpected observation that plasma administration appeared to improve the platelet count of patients with idiopathic thrombocytopenic purpura (ITP) led to the initial investigations into the possible role played by passively administered normal immunoglobulin in producing this effect. It is now well established that large doses of IVIg can indeed induce remission in many cases of ITP.

Acute idiopathic thrombocytopenia

IVIg is not indicated for the routine treatment of acute idiopathic thrombocytopenia since, particularly in the case of children, spontaneous remissions usually occur. Very rapid and dramatic responses have, however, been reported in severe acute ITP.[25] IVIg appears to increase the platelet count more rapidly than corticosteroids[26] (in the majority of cases studied counts reach at least 50×10/l by 2 days, with peak values at an average of 9 days) and possibly to reduce the number of patients becoming chronically thrombocytopenic. The most feared consequence of ITP, *intracranial haemorrhage*, occurs with such low frequency (below 0.25%) that it seems unlikely that any lessening of this risk could ever be shown in a trial of IVIg. The possible marginal benefits of IVIg over corticosteroids for treatment of acute ITP do not therefore justify the substantial expense of this material as the first choice of therapy. Its use has been proposed for those children with counts below 10×10^9/l judged to be at highest risk of intracranial haemorrhage,[27] particularly if response to corticosteroids is disappointing. IVIg may be most clearly justified for patients presenting with active bleeding, for emergency treatment where there has been no response to steroids, or to provide cover for essential surgery.[28]

One further possible use of IVIg is likely to be the opportunity it affords to avoid splenectomy in persistent childhood ITP.[29]

Chronic idiopathic thrombocytopenia[30]

This therapy has been most extensively examined in children. IVIg has been found to induce sustained normal platelet counts in a proportion, possibly around 20%, of cases. A similar number show no response or only transient improvement, while in the remainder a partial response occurs. These latter patients require either less steroid therapy or are able to cease steroids completely. The majority (about 70–80%) of patients do therefore show some improvement. As with acute ITP the outcome appears more favourable in children; responses reported in adults have lasted only a few weeks or have required repeated doses to maintain tolerable platelet counts. In view of its scarcity and expense, immunoglobulin should be restricted to patients not responding well to steroids and with bleeding complications, e.g. current epistaxes, mucosal bleeding, menorrhagia; when acute neurological symptoms occur or to cover trauma or surgery.[28]

IVIg has been used for the treatment of maternal ITP prior to delivery.[31–33] This should probably be given during the 2 weeks before the expected date of delivery to reduce the risk of Caesarean section and fetal haemorrhage (see chapter 20, section 3.2). Although rarely necessary, direct treatment to the affected infant has also been beneficial.[34]

Doses of IVIg for idiopathic thrombocytopenia

Most studies have used 400 mg IVIg per kilogram for 5 days followed by repeat courses if platelet counts relapse. Significant side-effects are unusual but headaches, nausea, vomiting and fever following infusions are seen in some patients.

3.1 Role of IVIg in Other Autoimmune Conditions[35–37]

No conclusive proof of the value of IVIg therapy has yet been shown in most of the many other autoimmune conditions for which it has been tried. However, a large number of uncontrolled trials and case reports provide evidence that certain patients do indeed experience benefit. *Kawasaki's syndrome* has, however, emerged as a clear indication for IVIg therapy.[38] Children should be given IVIg in conjunction with aspirin during the first 10 days in order to prevent the development of coronary aneurysms. There is evidence for improvement in thrombocytopenia associated with *systemic lupus erythematosus*, in *autoimmune neutropenia* and, possibly, also the bleeding disorder due to *autoimmune Factor VIII antibodies*.[39]

Reports have suggested improvement in dermatomyositis,[51] in severe refractory cases of myasthenia gravis treated with IVIg and in chronic inflammatory demyelinating polyneuropathy.

3.2 IVIg and Alloimmune Antibodies

IVIg therapy does not, in general, appear to be effective in alloantibody-mediated pathological processes. The most conspicuous example of benefit has been from its use in *neonatal alloimmune thrombocytopenia* (see chapter 20, section 3.1). An additional use is in the treatment of *post-transfusion purpura*.[40-42] although even in this condition the occurrence of autologous as well as transfused platelet destruction suggests a more complex mechanism is operating (see chapter 20, section 4.3). IVIg has also been evaluated in severe Rh haemolytic disease.[43] In view of the established efficacy of current protocols (see chapter 21, section 5) its use is best deserved for mothers for whom conventional management is not possible. Preliminary reports of trials of IVIg in alloimmunized *platelet transfusion* recipients have not been encouraging.[44,45]

Recently IVIg has been reported as being beneficial for children with severe steroid-dependent asthma, although the mechanism for this effect remains a matter for conjecture.

3.3 Mechanism of Action

This remains uncertain although several possible modes of action have been proposed. Some of these possibilities include:

(1) The transfused immunoglobulin may contain natural *anti-idiotypic antibodies* which by substituting for deficiencies in the patient's own immunoregulatory mechanism could suppress autoantibody formation.
(2) IVIg is prepared from large pools of plasma. It is likely that some donations will have been obtained from donors who have recovered from autoimmune diseases and these may contain anti-idiotypic antibodies with specific neutralizing capacity against the combining site of pathological autoantibodies, e.g. glycoprotein (GP) $GPII_b/III_a$ antibodies in ITP or Factor VIII autoantibodies.
(3) The high levels of circulating IgG may *saturate Fc receptors of macrophages,* creating a blockade of reticuloendothelial cell function.
(4) *Blockade of Fc receptors on B and/or T cells* may inhibit autoantibody synthesis.
(5) IVIg appears to dampen down release of inflammatory mediators (e.g. TNF, IL-1) from macrophages (see chapter 13, section 1).

4   IMMUNOGLOBULIN PREPARATIONS FOR SPECIFIC PROBLEMS

These are prepared from the plasma of donors who become immune during convalescence or who have been vaccinated to a hyperimmunized state. Most are presented as 10–20% protein solutions in 2–5 ml vials for *intramuscular use.*

(1) *Anti-D immunoglobulin*: this is presented as 3–17% solutions. Small amounts of anti-C, -E, -A and -B activity may also be present in addition to anti-D. The use of this is described in chapter 21, section 6.2.
(2) *Anti-HBs immunoglobulin* (see chapter 23, section 3.4).
(3) *Anti-tetanus toxin immunoglobulin*[46] (250 IU doses). This should be given to those with potentially contaminated injuries who have never been vaccinated or who have been vaccinated more than 10 years previously. This dose is

regarded as providing adequate protection for 1 month. Adsorbed tetanus toxoid vaccine should also be given at a different site. Efficient wound cleaning is most important.

Established tetanus requires massive doses of immunoglobulin. These should probably be of the order of 10 000 IU, part of which should be infiltrated around the wound margin. Intravenous tetanus immunoglobulin is also available in the UK for this purpose.

(4) *Anti-varicella (chickenpox)/zoster (shingles)*: This is mainly required for immunocompromised patients and neonates exposed to chickenpox or shingles. Treatment should take place as soon as possible (e.g. within 72 hours) before the virus enters cells and becomes protected. Doses of 125 IU (or 125 mg depending on the product) per 10 kg are suggested. If specific immunoglobulin is unavailable or the intramuscular route is unsuitable, as in thrombocytopenia, normal IVIg in doses of 200–300 mg/kg can be given instead.

(5) *Anti-rabies immunoglobulin* (500 IU) is also available in Britain. This is given as soon as possible after exposure; 20 IU/kg are given intramuscularly and by infiltration around the wound. Active immunization should be started at the same time.

(6) *Cytomegalovirus immunoglobulin*:[47,48] specific cytomegalovirus immunoglobulin as well as intravenous normal immunoglobulin have been used prophylactically for prevention of CMV infection following both renal and bone marrow transplantation and also in combination with acyclovir for established infection. The evidence that either agent can reduce the incidence of cytomegalovirus infection and pneumonia is now regarded as highly inconclusive. CMV antibody titres are lower in the normal IVIg preparation but this may be offset by the fact that substantially higher doses are possible. Despite promising expectations, specific CMV immunoglobulin has not proved to be a valuable product. Use of seronegative blood products and, when necessary, antiviral prophylaxis are far more effective.

(7) *Human normal immunoglobulin* is also used for:

(a) Prophylaxis for those travelling to areas where *hepatitis A* is endemic; 750 mg is assumed to provide 4–6 months' protection. Active immunization is now available and is preferred.

(b) Prevention of *non-immune pregnant women exposed to rubella* in the first trimester (dose 1.5 g). This does not, however, provide a high level of protection to the fetus and therapeutic abortion is usually advised.

(c) Prevention of *measles* in immunocompromised children.[49] Immunoglobulin with a titre of at least 80 IU/mg, at a dose of 750 mg is used for children aged over 3 years. This should be followed by 500 mg of immunoglobulin every 3 weeks until the period of risk is ended. Children with *acute lymphoblastic leukaemia* form the largest potential recipient group.

(d) Treatment of infective complications for which specific immunoglobulins are not readily available.

Gram-negative bacteraemia and *endotoxic shock*, particularly due to *Escherichia coli*, *Klebsiella pneumoniae* and *Pseudomonas aeruginosa*, are complications which carry a high mortality in hospital patients despite advances in antibiotic treatment and intensive care. The state of shock seems to be due to the liberation of bacterial lipopolysaccharides. Evidence that plasma containing high levels of neutralizing antibodies could reduce mortality led to development of a monoclonal anti-endo-toxin antibody against the lipid A endotoxin core (HA-1A) specifically to combat the high mortality associated with septic shock.[50] A major problem, however, is that of targeting this highly expensive therapy solely towards the subgroup of patients with Gram-negative infection and not those shocked from other septic causes.

Pseudomonas infections are a serious problem in severely burned patients and attempts have been made to develop specific protective immunoglobulin preparations.

REFERENCES

1 Cunningham-Rundles, C., Siegal, F.P., Smithwick, E.M. *et al.* (1984) Efficacy of intravenous immunoglobulin in primary humoral immunodeficiency disease. *Ann. Intern. Med.,* **101**: 435–439.
2 So, A., Brenner, M.K., Hill, I.D., Asherson, G.L. and Webster, A.D.B. (1984) Intravenous gammaglobulin treatment in patients with hypogammaglobulinaemia. *Br. Med. J.,* **289**: 1177–1178.
3 Hausser, C. and Buriot, D. (1982) Gamma globulin therapy during pregnancy in mother with hypogammaglobulinaemia. *Am. J. Obstet. Gynecol.,* **144**: 112.
4 Yap, P.L. (1990) Intravenous immunoglobulin for secondary immunodeficiency. *Blut,* **60**: 8–14.
5 Co-operative Group for the study of Immunoglobulin in chronic Lymphocytic Leukaemia (1988) Intravenous immunoglobulin for the prevention of infection in chronic lymphocytic leukaemia: a randomized clinical trial. *N. Engl. J. Med.,* **319**: 902–907.
6 Chapel, H.M. and Bunch, C. (1987) Mechanisms of infection in chronic lymphocytic leukaemia. *Semin. Hematol.,* **24**: 291–296.
7 Weeks, J.C., Tierney, M.R. and Weinstein, M.C. (1991) Cost effectiveness of prophylactic intravenous immune globulin in chronic lymphocytic leukaemia. *N. Engl. J. Med.,* **325**: 81–86.
8 Meyers, J.D., Reed, E.C., Shepp, D.H. *et al.* (1988) Acyclovir for prevention of cytomegalovirus infection and disease after allogeneic marrow transplantation. *N. Engl. J. Med.,* **318**: 70–75.
9 Einsele, H., Vallbracht, A., Friese, M. *et al.* (1988) Significant reduction of cytomegalovirus (CMV) disease by prophylaxis with CMV hyperimmune globulin plus oral acyclovir. *Bone Marrow Transplant.,* **3**: 607–617.
10 Guglielmo, B.J., Wong-Beringer, A. and Linker, C.A. (1994) Immune globulin therapy in allogeneic bone marrow transplant: a critical review. *Bone Marrow Transplant.,* **13**: 499–510.
11 Cafiero, F., Gipponi, M., Bonalumi, U., Piccardo, A., Sguotti, C. and Corbetta, G. (1992) Prophylaxis of infection with intravenous immunoglobulins plus antibiotic for patients at risk for sepsis undergoing surgery for colorectal cancer: results of a randomized, multicenter clinical trial. *Surgery,* **112**: 24–31.
12 Dominioni, L., Dionigi, R., Zanello, M. *et al.* (1991) Effects of high-dose IgG on survival of surgical patients with sepsis scores of 20 or greater. *Arch. Surg.,* **126**: 236–240.
13 Schedel, I., Dreikhausen, U., Nentwig, B. *et al.* (1991) Treatment of Gram-negative septic shock with an immunoglobulin preparation: a prospective, randomized clinical trial. *Crit. Care Med.,* **19**: 1104–1113.
14 Editorial (1992) Clinical trials of immunotherapy for sepsis. *Crit. Care Med.,* **20**: 721–723.

15 Editorial (1992) Monoclonal antibodies in sepsis and septic shock: recent progress, vast potential. *Br. Med. J.*, **304**: 132–133.
16 National Institute for Health and Human Development Intravenous Immunoglobulin Study Group (1991) Intravenous immunoglobulin for the prevention of bacterial infections in children with symptomatic human immunodeficiency virus infection. *N. Engl. J. Med.*, **325**: 73–80.
17 Rarick, M.U., Montgomery, T., Groshen, S. *et al.* (1991) Intravenous immunoglobulin in the treatment of human immunodeficiency virus-related thrombocytopenia. *Am. J. Haematol.*, **38**: 261–266.
18 Conway, S.P., Ng, P.C., Howel, D., Maclain, B. and Gool, H.C. (1990) Prophylactic intravenous immunoglobulin in pre-term infants: a controlled trial. *Vox Sang.*, **59**: 6–11.
19 Gonzalez, L.A. and Hill, H.R. (1989) The current status of intravenous gammaglobulin use in neonates. *Paediatr. Infect. Dis. J.*, **8**: 315–322.
20 Haque, K.N., Zaidi, M.H. and Bahakim, H. (1988) IgM enriched intravenous immunoglobulin therapy in neonatal sepsis. *Am. J. Dis. Child.*, **142**: 1293–1296.
21 Duc, G. (ed.) (1990) RSM Symposium. Prevention of infections and the role of immunoglobulin within the neonatal period. Royal Society Medicine Services International Congress & Symposium Series No. 163. London: Royal Society of Medicine Services.
22 Bussel, J.B., Kimberly, R.P., Inman, R.D. *et al.* (1983) Intravenous gammaglobulin treatment of chronic idiopathic thrombocytopenic purpura. *Blood*, **62**: 480–486.
23 Bussel, J.B. and Hilgartner, M.W. (1984) The use and mechanism of action of intravenous immunoglobulin in the treatment of immune haematologic disease. *Br. J. Haematol.*, **56**: 1–7.
24 Imbach, P., D'Apuzzo, V., Hirt, A. *et al.* (1981) High-dose intravenous gammaglobulin for idiopathic thrombocytopenic purpura in childhood. *Lancet*, **i**: 1228–1231.
25 Seeler, R.A. (1984) Overnight remission of idiopathic thrombocytopenia with intravenous immunoglobulin. *Lancet,* **i**: 961.
26 Imbach, P., Berchtold, W., Hirt, A. *et al.* (1985) Intravenous immunoglobulin versus oral corticosteroids in acute immune thrombocytopenic purpura in childhood. *Lancet*, **ii**: 464–468.
27 Blanchett, V.S. and Turner, C. (1986) Treatment of acute idiopathic thrombocytopoenic purpura (letter). *J. Pediatr.*, **108**: 326–327.
28 Eden, O.B. and Lilleyman, J.S., on behalf of the British Paediatric Haematology Group (1992) Guidelines for management of idiopathic thrombocytopenic purpura. *Arch. Dis. Child.*, **67**: 1056–1058.
29 Bussel, J.B., Schulman, I., Hilgartner, M.W. and Barundun, S. (1983) Intravenous use of gammaglobulin in the treatment of chronic immune thrombocytopenia purpura as a means to defer splenectomy. *J. Pediatr.*, **103**: 651–655.
30 Vos, J.J.E., van Aken, W.G., Engelfriet, C.P. and Kr. von dem Borne, A.E.G. (1985) Intravenous gammaglobulin therapy in idiopathic thrombocytopenic purpura. *Vox Sang.*, **49**: 92–100.
31 Mizunuma, H., Takahashi, Y., Taguchi, H. *et al.* (1984) A new approach to idiopathic thrombocytopenic purpura during pregnancy by high-dose immunoglobulin G infusion. *Am. J. Obstet. Gynecol.*, **148**: 218–219.
32 Morgenstern, G.R., Measday, B. and Hegde, U.M. (1983) Autoimmune thrombocytopenia in pregnancy: a new approach to management. *Br. Med. J.*, **287**: 584.
33 Tchernia, G., Dreyfus, M., Laurian, Y., Derycke, M., Mercia, C. and Kerbrat, G. (1984) Management of immune thrombocytopenia in pregnancy: response to infusions of immunoglobulins. *Am. J. Obstet. Gynecol.*, **148**: 225–226.
34 Chirico, G., Duse, M., Ugazio, A.G. and Rondini, G. (1983) High-dose intravenous gammaglobulin therapy for passive immune thrombocytopenia in the neonate. *J. Pediatr.*, **103**: 654–655.
35 Dwyer, J.M. (1992) Manipulating the immune system with immune globulin. *N. Engl. J. Med.*, **326**: 107–114.
36 Nydegger, U.E. (1992) Intravenous immunoglobulin in combination with other prophylactic and therapeutic measures. *Transfusion*, **32**: 72–82.

37 Ronda, N., Hurez, V. and Kazathckine, M.D. (1993) Intravenous immunoglobulin therapy of autoimmune and systemic inflammatory diseases. *Vox Sang.*, **64**: 65–72.
38 Shulman, S.T. and Rowley, A.H. (1992) Kawasaki disease and IVIg treatment. *Transfusion Sci.*, **13**: 309–315.
39 Sultan, Y., Maisonneuve, P., Kazatchkine, M.D. and Nydegger, U.E. (1984) Anti-idiotypic suppression of autoantibodies to factor VIII (antihaemophilic factor) by high dose intravenous gammaglobulin. *Lancet*, **ii**: 765–768.
40 Glud, T.K., Rosthoj, S., Jensen, M.K., Laursen, B., Grunnet, N. and Jersild, C. (1983) High-dose intravenous immunoglobulin for post-transfusion purpura. *Scand. J. Haematol.*, **31**: 495–500.
41 Mueller-Eckhardt, C., Kuenzlen, E., Thilo-Korner, D. and Pralle, H. (1983) High-dose intravenous immunoglobulin for post-transfusion purpura. *N. Engl. J. Med.*, **308**: 287.
42 Hamblin, T.J., Naorose Abidi, S.M., Nee, P.A., Copplestone, A., Mufti, G. J. and Oscier, D. G. (1985) Successful treatment of post-transfusion purpura with high dose immunoglobulins after lack of response to plasma exchange. *Vox Sang.*, **49**: 164–167.
43 Margulies, M., Voto, L.S., Mather, E. and Margulies, M. (1991) High-dose intravenous IgG for the treatment of severe Rh alloimmunization. *Vox Sang.*, **61**: 181–189.
44 Schiffer, C.A., Hogge, D.E., Aisner, J., Dutcher, J.P., Lee, E.J. and Papenberg, D. (1984) High-dose intravenous gammaglobulin in alloimmunized platelet transfusion recipients. *Blood*, **64**: 937–940.
45 Bierling, P., Cordonnier, C., Rodet, M. *et al.* (1984) High dose intravenous gammaglobulin and platelet transfusions in leukaemic HLA-immunized patients. *Scand. J. Hematol.*, **33**: 215–220.
46 Leading article (1974) Human antitoxin for tetanus prophylaxis. *Lancet*, **i**: 51.
47 Meyers, J.D., Leszczynski, J., Zaia, J.A. *et al.* (1983) Prevention of cytomegalovirus infection by cytomegalovirus immune globulin after marrow transplantation. *Ann. Intern. Med.*, **98**: 442–446.
48 Winston, D.J., Ho, W.G., Lin, C.H. *et al.* (1987) Intravenous immune globulin for prevention of cytomegalovirus infection and interstitial pneumonia after bone marrow transplantation. *Ann. Intern. Med.*, **106**: 12–18.
49 Kay, H.E.M. and Rankin, A. (1984) Immunoglobulin prophylaxis of measles in acute lymphoblastic leukaemia. *Lancet*, **i**: 901–902.
50 Ziegler, E.J., Fisher, C.J., Sprung, C.L. *et al.* (1991) Treatment of Gram-negative bacteraemia and septic shock with HA-1A human monoclonal antibody against endotoxin: a randomized, double-blind, placebo-controlled trial. *N. Engl. J. Med.*, **324**: 429–436.
51 Dalakas, M.C., Illa, I., Dambrosia, J.M., Soueidan, S.A., Stein, D.P., Otero, C., Dinsmore, S.T. and McCrosky, S. (1993) A controlled trial of high-dose intravenous immune globulin infusions as treatment for dermatomysitis. *N. Engl. J. Med.*, **329**: 1993–2000.

10
Materials for Plasma Volume Expansion

The materials available for plasma volume expansion include *crystalloid solutions, synthetic colloids* and human *albumin* or plasma. They are primarily used for restoration of volume after blood loss, and treatment of hypotensive episodes from other causes, although the various products differ in their physiological effects.[1,2]

As a group their properties include:

(1) *Plasma volume expansion*: crystalloids and isotonic materials achieve this by simple volume replenishment. Agents that raise plasma oncotic pressure (e.g. hyperoncotic synthetic colloids and albumin concentrates) obtain plasma volume expansion by absorption of water from the extracellular fluid space. This can have the beneficial effect of reducing cerebral or pulmonary oedema as well as promoting reabsorption of generalized oedema fluid.

(2) *Replenishment of extracellular salts and water* (e.g. crystalloids).
(3) *Promotion of osmotic diuresis* (e.g. gelatins and lower molecular weight dextrans).
(4) Improvement in *blood flow* as a result of *haemodilution*, reduced viscosity and reduced red cell sludging (e.g. dextrans, gelatins).

Specific properties of some products also include:

(5) *Antithrombotic* effects (e.g. dextrans).
(6) *Oxygen transport* (stroma-free haemoglobin, fluorocarbons).

1   CRYSTALLOIDS

1.1   Isotonic Solutions

Isotonic saline, sodium lactate and *Ringer's lactate (Hartmann's solution)* all have a place in blood volume restoration. They can be perfectly satisfactory as the *sole* replacement fluid for small losses *(up to 20% blood volume replacement) in fit adults*, as a supplement to red cell concentrate transfusion *during surgery or trauma* or as initial therapy for resuscitation after major haemorrhage. In this latter situation 2 : 1 combinations of crystalloid and colloid, for example sodium lactate and gelatin solution (see below), have proved perfectly satisfactory for first-line resuscitation therapy.[3]

After untreated blood loss, crystalloids are particularly indicated to replace the salt and water loss from the extracellular fluid space that accompanies prolonged haemorrhage. It may be prudent to limit their use whenever severe head injuries are suspected (there is a risk of aggravating cerebral oedema) or where particular risks of adult respiratory distress syndrome seem likely (e.g. septic shock, left ventricular failure, hypoproteinaemia).

Crystalloid solutions have the advantages of economy, ready availability and freedom from adverse reactions. They have the disadvantage that relatively large volumes must be administered (usually in excess of three times the volume lost) since most of the fluid (around 70%) will rapidly enter the extracellular space. Haemodilution, including dilution of plasma proteins, will occur. Tissue oedema and possibly pulmonary oedema (though this is controversial—see chapter 13) will occur if large volumes are given. There is evidence that interstitial fluid accumulation will not become excessive provided plasma oncotic pressure is maintained above 20 mmHg (approximately equivalent to a plasma protein concentration of 50 g/l) and positive fluid balance does not exceed 5 l.[4]

Fluid accumulation will in any case be temporary if renal function is adequate. Despite their different formulations, for most practical purposes the clinical effects of the various crystalloid electrolyte solutions are broadly similar.

Care should be taken not to infuse calcium-containing solutions (i.e. Ringer's lactate) through the administration line simultaneously with blood or coagulation will occur. The lactate in this solution is metabolized to bicarbonate and may be of value in counteracting acidosis; potassium is also included in order to counteract the tendency towards hypokalaemia.

Table 1 Crystalloids for resuscitation

Advantages
    Essential for restoration of extracellular fluid
    Cheap and readily available in unlimited amounts
    No demonstrable increase in morbidity or mortality compared to colloids
    Effective in preventing acute renal failure

Disadvantages
    Lowers colloid osmotic pressure
    Large volumes needed
    Weight gain, tissue oedema and extracellular fluid space expansion

The argument as to whether crystalloids or colloid solutions (usually albumin) are to be preferred for resuscitation purposes is still vigorously debated.[5-9]

To those on the sidelines it seems reasonable to conclude that both groups are very effective and that the pharmacological differences between them do not exert such a profound influence that the clinical benefits are clearly obvious. It seems reasonable to combine the use of crystalloids, synthetic colloids and albumin in a structured approach according to the scale of the resuscitation problem. In that way the advantages of each can be maximized and the likelihood of unwanted problems reduced.

1.2 Hypertonic Solutions[10-12]

The use of *hypertonic saline* (e.g. 7.5% NaCl or 7.5% NaCl in 6% dextran 70) is currently attracting interest as a convenient, safe and effective resuscitation agent. Given as bolus infusions rapid restoration of plasma volume is possible, water being drawn from the large reserve of extracellular fluid. Resuscitation can be achieved without the extracellular fluid overloading characteristic from use of isotonic crystalloids alone. This approach is still considered largely investigational and caution has been expressed over the potentially harmful effects of hyperosmolality and hypernatraemia.[13]

Table 2 Composition of some frequently used crystalloid solutions

	Isotonic saline	Sodium lactate	Ringer's lactate
Sodium chloride	155 mEq/l	–	102 mEq/l
Sodium lactate	–	167 mEq/l[a]	28 mEq/l[a]
Potassium chloride	–	–	4 mEq/l
Calcium chloride	–	–	4 mEq/l
pH	6.1	–	6.5

[a]Metabolically equivalent to an equal amount of bicarbonate.

2 COLLOID VOLUME EXPANDERS

2.1 Desirable Properties

Ideally colloid volume expanders should have the following characteristics:

- Stability at ambient temperature.
- Cheap to manufacture.
- Chemically inert.
- Sterilizable.
- Non-antigenic.
- Not be retained indefinitely within the body.
- Not be metabolized to toxic compounds.
- Not interfere with haemostasis or compatibility testing.
- Be retained within the plasma volume even when capillary permeability is increased.

3 SYNTHETIC COLLOIDS[1]

As a group, *synthetic colloids* are usually seen as a therapeutic alternative to albumin solutions (see section 4). Individually they are characterized in terms of their chemical composition, e.g. dextran, gelatin or hydroxethyl starch, and also by their molecular weight. Unlike human albumin, which is almost entirely a solution of albumin monomers of molecular weight 69 000, most synthetic colloids are described as polydisperse and contain a spectrum of molecular weight molecules, both smaller and larger than the nominal molecular weight. Thus the lower molecular weight population, below the 'renal threshold' will be readily excreted and encourage an osmotic diuresis. The larger molecules will have a longer intravascular retention time. The molecular weight of synthetic colloids is usually defined in terms of molecular weight average (MW_w)—the larger this number, the greater the intravascular retention and plasma viscosity—and the molecular weight number (MW_n)—the smaller numbers reflect greater oncotic activity. As a further complication the MW_w cannot be taken as the sole indicator of effective size and intravascular retention as this will also depend on the physical shape of the molecule. This could vary from that of a relatively compact globular form to a more open branched structure which might permeate less well through a capillary endothelial membrane than its molecular weight would suggest.

3.1 Dextrans

These are the longest established of the synthetic colloids. Dextrans are glucose polymers produced from starch by the action of the bacterium *Leuconostoc mesenteroides*. Fractionation is performed to produce colloid solutions of either 40 000 or 70 000 MW_w, although each product contains a considerable proportion of both higher and lower molecular sizes. Dextran solutions of nominally 110 000 or 150 000 molecular weight have also been produced but are now less frequently

	Plasma half-life	Plasma volume increase	Osmotic diuretic effect	ECF restoration	Improved capillary flow	Anti-thrombotic effect	Haemostatic failure risk	Allergic or other reactions	Dose limit	Relative cost (scale 1–10)
Crystalloids	○/●	○	○	●●	○	○	○	○	—	1
Albumin (4.5%)	●●●	●●	○	○	●	○	○	●	—	10
Albumin (20%)	●●●	●●●	○	○	●	○	○	●	—	2
Gelatin solutions	●	●●	●●	○	●●	○	○	●●	—	2
Dextran 40 (10%)	●	●●●	●●	○	●●	●●	●●●	●●	1.5 l	2
Dextran 70 (6%)	●●	●●●	●●	○	●	●●	●●●	●●	1.5 l	2
HES 450 (6%)	●●	●●	●●	○	●	?	●●	● ?	1.5 l	5
HES 200–300 (10%)	●	●●	●●	○	?	?	●	● ?	1.5 l	5

Figure 1 Comparison of the principal features of crystalloid and colloid solutions for plasma volume expansion (○, little or no effect; ● → ●●●, small to greatest effect)

used. Dextrans carry strong negative charges which can coat and accentuate the mutually repulsive negative charges on red cells and platelets. Platelet aggregation is, therefore, inhibited and this forms the basis of the *antithrombotic effect* of dextrans. Doses should not exceed 1.5 l in adults, otherwise undesirable interference with haemostasis may occur. If, on the other hand, post-operative prophylaxis against thrombosis is required, a dose of 250 ml per day 6% dextran 70 will suffice.

Dextran 40 (e.g. 10% solution in isotonic saline or dextrose) preparations are hyperoncotic solutions and cause rapid plasma volume expansion (up to twice that of the volume infused). This occurs as a result of osmotic withdrawal of fluid from the extracellular compartment. Rapid renal excretion of the smaller molecules produces an osmotic diuresis but, if renal vasoconstriction has greatly reduced urine flow rate, there is a risk that renal tubular damage will occur. For this reason it is suggested that doses should not exceed 1 l per day, and dextran 40 should not be given when the urine flow rate is below 20 ml/kg per day, the urine specific gravity is over 1045, or when the blood urea is greater than 10 mmol/l.[14]

The half disappearance time of dextran 40 from the plasma $(T_{1/2})$ is around 1 hour. Advantages of dextran 40 include:

- Haemodilution.
- Reduced blood viscosity.
- Improved blood flow.
- Anti-red cell sludging effects.

Dextran 70 (6% solution in saline or dextrose) is only slightly more hypertonic than plasma and thus causes modest plasma expansion (of the order of 120% of the infused volume). The $T_{1/2}$ plasma retention time is around 4–6 hours. Volumes of up to 1.5 l can be used to replace blood losses of the same magnitude. A similar product, dextran 60, as a 3% solution, in combination with red cell concentrates has been shown to be perfectly satisfactory for replacement of up to 50% blood volume losses.[15,16]

Dextran 70 has also been used for preoperative haemodilution, particularly in conjunction with phlebotomy for polycythaemic patients. As dextrans inhibit platelet function they are contraindicated for patients with thrombocytopenia, von Willebrand's disease and those receiving other drugs affecting platelet function. *Severe allergic reactions* to dextran are a well-recognized though infrequent problem, and appear to be due to the pre-existence of dextran-reactive antibodies. These reactions can now be largely prevented by giving a small intravenous dose of dextran–hapten prior to dextran infusion which effectively inhibits such antibodies.[17]

3.2   Gelatin Solutions (3–5% in saline)[18,19]

Gelatins are widely used colloids and have been used extensively during routine surgery combined with red cell concentrates. Gelatin solutions also appear satisfactory as the sole replacement fluid during plasma exchange[18] and have been shown to be as effective as albumin for volume replacement of the critically ill.[20]

They are prepared from hydrolysed collagen, and a colloidal solution containing an MW_w of 35 000 is obtained. The higher proportion of lower molecular weight gelatin molecules have a powerful osmotic diuretic effect. Gelatin solutions are liable to gel at low temperatures, hence various modifications, e.g. succinylation or urea linking, are applied and these are the main differences between the commercially available preparations. The physiological properties of gelatin as a plasma expander are most similar to those of dextran 40; the plasma expansion effect is around 3–4 hours. There are no haemostatic problems to restrict dosage, but it should be noted that some of the urea-linked products contain calcium in sufficient amounts to cause coagulation if directly mixed with citrated blood. Sodium lactate–gelatin combinations in the ratio 2:1 have proved satisfactory during initial resuscitation of battle casualties.[3]

3.3 Hydroxyethyl Starch[21]

These materials consist of macromolecular polymers of starch (MW_w of products range from 200 000 to 450 000) which are protected against the action of plasma amylase by hydroxyethylation. Hydroxyethyl starch preparations are very polydisperse, with individual colloid molecules small enough to pass the renal threshold as well as those of over one million molecular weight.

The popularity of these materials as plasma-expanding agents seems to be deservedly increasing. Their principal characteristics include the following:

(1) Early experience suggests they are as clinically effective as 5% albumin for resuscitation of multisystem trauma victims.[22]
(2) Oncotic properties of a 6% solution are similar to those of 5% albumin.
(3) The plasma half-life is prolonged ($T_{1/2}$ about 15 hours) compared to that of other synthetic materials.
(4) Very large volumes (up to 15 l) have been given without adverse effects. Anaphylactoid reactions are rare (incidences about 0.085%) and usually mild.[23]
(5) The cost, though greater than that of crystalloids or the other synthetic colloids, is considerably less than that of albumin.

Areas of concern include:

(1) Minor disturbance of coagulation test results (e.g. prothrombin time, partial thromboplastin time, reduction of Factor VIII, von Willebrand Factor (vWF) and prolonged bleeding time.[24] In general these have not been regarded as clinically significant,[25] although occasionally haemostatic failure has occurred.[26]
(2) Hydroxyethyl starch is cleared from the circulation and metabolized by the reticuloendothelial system. There is therefore a hypothetical risk of reticuloendothelial system impairment because of the large amounts which could be involved. Elimination of hydroxyethyl starch is prolonged, the more highly substituted preparations being retained for some weeks.

Hydroxyethyl starch has also been used as a red cell sedimenting agent during leukapheresis procedures (see chapter 6, section 2.1).

3.4 Adverse Reactions to Synthetic Colloids

These are possible with any of the colloid solutions but are generally less frequent than reactions to whole blood transfusion.[27,28] Serious reactions are very rare; surveys show incidences of less than around one in 1000 infusions,[29] although more mild side-effects may be seen in around 1% of infusions. At such low incidence rates there appears little to distinguish conclusively between the three main categories of synthetic colloids.

The *symptoms* resemble those of *anaphylactic reactions involving histamine release* and may appear after infusion of only a small volume. For this reason *infusions should, where possible, always begin slowly* while the patient is observed carefully. This anticipation is particularly important for those patients with a history of allergic illness. When reactions occur there will generally be no knowledge of pre-exposure to the particular antigen; cross-reactivity to related antigens is a possible mechanism. Sometimes, however, antibodies such as anti-dextran and anti-collagen antibodies are present. Alternative pathway complement activation by foreign materials or by macromolecular aggregates has also been shown to result in release of vasoactive amines and this may be the causative mechanism for some adverse reactions.

Hyperoncotic colloid solutions can cause excessive plasma volume expansion leading to cardiac failure in those who are susceptible.

The introduction of any new colloid into the circulation appears, possibly through its oncotic effect, eventually to cause some displacement of native proteins from the intravascular space into the surrounding extracellular fluid. Synthetic colloids may thus reduce levels of albumin and coagulation factors and elevate those in the interstitium. Changes in the plasma and extracellular fluid oncotic ratio will then not be as great as might have been expected. The reduction in coagulant factor level has been associated with increased blood transfusion requirements in resuscitated patients.[30]

Treatment of adverse reactions

(1) Stop the infusion and replace with crystalloids or a different form of colloid.
(2) Give antihistamines for mild reactions (e.g. chlorpheniramine 10 mg i.v.).
(3) For more severe reactions, give hydrocortisone 200 mg i.v. If bronchospasm is present give intravenous aminophylline.
(4) Alternatively subcutaneous adrenaline 0.2–1 ml of 1 : 1000 solution can be used for serious reactions, particularly those in which bronchospasm and angioneurotic oedema threaten the airway.

3.5 Blood Transfusion Compatibility Problems[31]

Various synthetic colloids, particularly the now rarely used very high molecular weight dextrans (molecular weight 100 000–150 000), predisposed to rouleaux formation during red cell serology studies. The rouleaux are most pronounced at

37 °C and are dispelled by saline admixture—a procedure that assists differentiation from true agglutination. These problems are probably now an over-emphasized concern with the use of modern preparations but ideally compatibility samples should be collected prior to colloid infusion. If this is not possible the laboratory should be told which products have been given.

4   HUMAN ALBUMIN PRODUCTS

4.1   Plasma Protein Fraction and Albumin Solutions

These products have replaced dried pooled plasma as the standard stable ready-to-use derivative of human plasma for restoration of blood volume. The bottled protein solutions are heated at 60 °C for 10 hours and are, as a result, bacteriologically sterile and free from transmission of viral infection.

Human albumin solutions (HAS), by definition, consist of greater than 95% albumin and are presented as 4–5% solutions or 20–25% solutions in saline. They have now superseded less pure products variously known as plasma protein fraction (PPF) or plasma protein solution (PPS) which generally comprised 4–5% protein solutions, consisting of around 83% or greater amounts of albumin in isotonic saline, the remainder being α- and β-globulins. *Plasma protein fraction and 5% albumin* have physiologically very similar effects. Their oncotic activity is similar to that of native plasma. The plasma volume expands initially by an amount equal to the volume infused but, as a result of albumin equilibration with the extracellular space, the sustained volume increase amounts to only about 60% of that originally administered. Although the fractional catabolic rate of albumin (the percentage catabolized each day) amounts to no more than 10%, the plasma $T_{1/2}$ of infused albumin is only around 15 hours, which probably reflects the extent of this equilibration process.

Albumin has a theoretical pathophysiological advantage over synthetic colloids in that its function extends beyond that of physically maintaining colloid osmotic pressure and plasma volume. Albumin acts as a reversible binding agent for

Table 3   Albumin for plasma volume expansion

Advantages
   Believed (not unanimously) to prevent pulmonary oedema and ARDS (adult respiratory
      distress syndrome)
   Smaller volumes of resuscitation fluid required as compared with crystalloids
   Tissue oedema avoided
   Binding and transport of drugs and metabolites

Disadvantages
   Expensive
   Must be derived from donor plasma
   May actually predispose to ARDS in some patients
   Some evidence of impaired myocardial performance and more frequent renal problems

anions, cations and many drugs and metabolites; it probably fulfils a transport function for these materials.

Albumin concentrates

Albumin as a 20–25% solution is presented in smaller volumes (generally 100 ml) of isotonic saline. These solutions have about four to five times the plasma oncotic potential and therefore effect *plasma volume restoration* at the *expense of the extra-cellular fluid*. In this respect they are similar to dextran 40 or gelatin solutions but volume for volume are more potent and have a more prolonged effect. Since albumin is not normally lost through the glomerulus, concentrated albumin infusion does not produce an osmotic diuresis although *improved urine output may follow the plasma volume expansion*. In hypoalbuminaemic states concentrated albumin solutions can be used to increase plasma albumin levels and, correspondingly, the plasma oncotic pressure. In this way *mobilization of oedema fluid* or improvement in shock lung syndrome may be attempted. This approach is only justified on a short-term basis; prolonged use of albumin for this purpose is ineffective and wasteful of an expensive material. Simultaneous use of diuretics is required. When increased capillary leakage of albumin, rather than external loss or synthetic failure, is the cause of the oedema, any benefit from albumin therapy alone will, of course, be short-lived. Unfortunately this is a common situation.

4.2 Clinical Uses of Albumin Solutions

The clinical indications for albumin have not proved easy to define. Perhaps for this reason and the generally favourable perception of the beneficial effects of albumin, usage has increased to such an extent that it has featured as the single most costly item of the pharmacy budget of some hospitals in the USA. This usage pattern does not bear critical scrutiny, however, and studies have shown that most albumin usage cannot be justified on sound pathological or physiological principles. Indications for transfusion of protein solutions fall into two broad categories:

(1) *Isoncotic solutions* (4–5% HAS) are used to provide volume replacement under circumstances in which significant hypoproteinaemia (total protein <50 g/l; albumin <30 g/l) has occurred or is likely to develop.
(2) *Hyperoncotic albumin concentrates* (20–25% HAS) can also be used for volume replacement but are particularly indicated when hypoproteinaemia and the resulting fall in plasma oncotic activity has already led to loss of fluid into the interstitium, e.g. pulmonary or systemic oedema, or into serous cavities in the form of ascites and pleural effusions.

However, even under these circumstances synthetic colloids should be considered first if the period of colloid oncotic support is likely to be self-limited.[28]
   Albumin is probably best justified when natural restoration of endogenous

albumin levels and plasma oncotic activity is less certain. It is generally agreed that albumin concentrates should only be used to gain control over relatively acute protein and fluid disturbances. *There is no case for continued administration in chronic disorders* when no lasting benefit can be obtained. The hypoalbuminaemia of the severely ill is a recognized marker for metabolic stress. It probably reflects a summation of abnormalities in albumin synthesis, degradation and distribution between intravascular and extravascular compartments as well as changes in total volume of distribution.[32] Albumin concentration in such patients can be improved by total parenteral nutrition[33] and this is the appropriate treatment.

Clinical circumstances justifying the use of albumin use have been proposed,[34] recommendations agreed by means of consensus conference[35] and examined in the light of clinical audit.[36,37] These include the following:

(1) As supplement to crystalloids and synthetic colloids during volume replacement of blood loss. Their use is not justified for the initial stages of resuscitation of young previously fit subjects who are not at risk of pulmonary oedema. They may be of value during extensive blood replacement (e.g. exceeding 60% blood loss) and particularly for patients who are *elderly, malnourished, hypoproteinaemic* or at risk from *congestive cardiac failure*. Unfortunately recovery of plasma albumin in such patients may be less than predicted. Increased capillary permeability allows diffusion into the larger interstitial fluid space, thereby reducing the plasma/interstitial fluid oncotic gradient.

(2) It has been suggested that albumin is preferable as plasma volume expansion agent if plasma oncotic pressures are below 20 mmHg (approximating to plasma albumin of 30 g/l). Synthetic colloids are more appropriate where the plasma oncotic pressure is not as low.

(3) *Albumin solutions* are firmly held by some to play an essential part in prophylaxis and management of adult respiratory distress syndrome occurring in surgical patients and trauma victims. An alternative view is that the pathologically increased capillary permeability so often present allows albumin to diffuse freely into the pulmonary interstitial fluid, thus making the problem worse. This is a highly controversial issue and is discussed more fully in chapter 13.

(4) *Volume and plasma protein replacement* for patients with *severe burns*, e.g. those in which more than 10% of the body's surface area is involved with second or third-degree damage (chapter 16).

(5) *Retroperitoneal surgery* where large amounts of tissue dissection are entailed. Also in surgery generally when hypoproteinaemic oedema exists which could impair tissue oxygenation and delay wound healing.

(6) Removal of substantial amounts (e.g. >1.5 l) of ascitic fluids.[38,39]

(7) *Nephrotic syndrome* (to initiate diuresis and control oedema).[40]

(8) Albumin has been used in the treatment of pre-eclamptic toxaemia and for cases of intrauterine growth retardation.[41,42] In both conditions there is maternal hypovolaemia due to a reduced plasma volume. This leads to hyperviscosity, reduced intrauterine blood flow rates and eventually to placental hypoxia.

4.3 Dosage

The total albumin deficit can be calculated on the basis of a 60:40 distribution of albumin between plasma and extravascular fluid, and dosage may be calculated accordingly. As an approximate guide one 20% or 25% 100 ml container will raise plasma levels by around 5 g/l. It must be stressed that low serum protein levels are not, by any means, invariably associated with oedema. The symptom is not, for example, shown by people with congenital deficiency of albumin. However, when *both hypoproteinaemia and oedema* are present an attempt should be made to raise albumin levels to over 30 g/l, or total serum protein to over 50 g/l and plasma oncotic pressure to over 20 mmHg.[43]

4.4 Adverse Effects of Albumin and Plasma Protein Fraction

Cardiac failure

Cardiac failure can occur after administration of concentrated albumin solutions. They are best given during the day time when nursing care and clinical observations are most easily carried out.

Hypotensive episodes

These have generally occurred with plasma protein fraction rather than albumin and appear to be due to high levels of prekallikrein activator (Hageman factor fragment, PKA). PKA initiates conversion of kallikrein to bradykinin, a peptide with powerful vasodilator activity. Bradykinin is normally destroyed rapidly in the lungs; it is therefore not surprising that hypotensive effects have been found to be more severe following direct introduction of plasma protein fraction into the arterial circulation, for example during cardiac bypass procedures. These reactions are uncommon with modern preparations in which PKA activator levels are monitored following the manufacturing process.

Allergic or anaphylactic symptoms

These may occur in a similar way to those described above for synthetic colloid materials. On rare occasions these reactions may be caused by antibodies to allotypic variants of albumin.

Residual sodium acetate

This has been associated with vasodilatation and hypotension. Aluminium as a contaminant of albumin solutions has been reported as causing bone disease in patients with poor renal function.[44]

5 FRESH FROZEN PLASMA

Fresh frozen plasma is sometimes inappropriately used for treatment of plasma volume deficits usually in conjunction with albumin or synthetic agents. However, fresh frozen plasma should *only* be used where the additional benefits of *coagulation factor replacement* are required (see chapter 7, section 1).

6 RED CELL SUBSTITUTES

The prospect of a successful artificial blood substitute simultaneously combining plasma volume expansion properties with the capacity to transport significant amounts of oxygen has enormous attractions. Although red cells represent an evolutionarily perfect vehicle for oxygen transport, they have serious drawbacks as routine transfusion materials. These disadvantages include their expense, limited shelf life, the potential for disease transmission and the need for compatibility testing and special storage as well as the dependence on a steady supply of donors. An ideal synthetic substitute would not only have to match the physiological performance of red cells but must also be safe, stable, cheap and without supply limitations and the need for pre-transfusion matching. The physiological and safety requirements are daunting and despite years of effort none of the materials so far prepared are yet suitable for introduction into routine clinical practice. In order to match the performance of a conventional blood transfusion, candidate replacement materials require the following properties:[45]

- Transport and tissue release capacity for at least 5 ml/dl oxygen.
- Transport of 4 ml CO_2/dl without significant blood pH change.
- Perfusion characteristics of normal blood.
- Prolonged intravascular retention.
- Freedom from toxicity.
- Normal oncotic pressure.

Research towards these objectives has centred around two classes of material: the haemoglobin-based solutions and the synthetic perfluorocarbon chemical emulsions.

6.1 Haemoglobin-based Oxygen Carriers[46]

Haemoglobin solutions that are free from red cell stroma appear to be non-antigenic and do not damage renal function or possess thromboplastic effects. These can be presented as 3.5–5.5% solutions, in which form they possess comparable oncotic properties to plasma and also transport oxygen. Unfortunately the P_{50} is low (13–15 mmHg) and the plasma $T_{1/2}$ is of the order of 1.5–3.5 hours. Polymerization and pyridoxylation of the haemoglobin appear to improve the P_{50}, allow use of greater haemoglobin concentrations without increasing colloid osmotic pressure and also prolong retention in the circulation. Bovine haemoglobin, in contrast to that of human origin, has no supply limitations and apart from its antigenicity would have attractions as a basis for development of an oxygen transport material. The problem of antigenicity has partly been overcome by encapsulation in a synthetic biocompatible membrane to form microspheres and these can be reinfused to provide oxygen transport throughout all parts of the circulation.

Alternative approaches under examination include use of recombinant DNA technology to engineer normal human haemoglobin production in microorganisms or to go even further introducing mutations so placed as to ensure physiologically effective oxygen delivery.

6.2   Fluorocarbons and Perfluorocarbons

These entirely synthetic substances are usually emulsified with albumin, dextrans or hydroxyethyl starch solutions to provide acceptable oncotic properties. They have the ability to transport substantial amounts of oxygen but require high inspired oxygen tensions for maximum saturation. In experimental animals they have been shown to be capable of sustaining life for short periods after complete replacement of the blood volume. One such material, marketed as Fluosol DA, has received limited clinical use in Jehovah's Witnesses who refuse blood transfusions. A variety of toxicity problems have limited its use for large-scale transfusions but applications are being found where restricted local perfusion with oxygen-carrying fluid is required, e.g. as a coronary perfusion fluid during angioplasty or for isolated organ perfusion.[47,48]

REFERENCES

1 Salmon, J.B. and Mythen, M.G. (1993) Pharmacology and physiology of colloids. *Blood Rev.*, 7: 114–120.
2 Huskisson, L. (1992) Intravenous volume replacement: which fluid and why? *Arch. Dis. Child.*, 67: 649–653.
3 Williams, J.G., Riley, T.R.D. and Moody, R.A. (1983) Resuscitation experience in the Falkland Islands campaign. *Br. Med. J.*, 286: 775–777.
4 Nielsen, O.M. and Engell, H.C. (1986) The importance of plasma colloid osmotic pressure for interstitial fluid volume and fluid balance after elective abdominal vascular surgery. *Ann. Surg.*, 203: 25–29.
5 Smith, J.A.R. and Norman, J.N. (1982) The fluid of choice for resuscitation of severe shock. *Br. J. Surg.*, 69: 702–705.
6 Metildi, L.A., Shackford, S.R., Virgilio, R.W. and Peters, R.M. (1984) Crystalloid versus colloid in fluid resuscitation of patients with severe pulmonary insufficiency. *Surg. Gynaecol. Obstet.*, 158: 207–212.
7 Haljame, H. (1985) Rationale for the use of colloids in the treatment of shock and hypovolaemia. *Acta Anaesthesiol. Scand.*, 29: 48–54.
8 Ramsay, G. (1988) Intravenous volume replacement: indications and choices. *Br. Med. J.*, 296: 1422–1423.
9 Puri, V.K. (1990) Colloid versus crystalloid war: a time for truce. *Crit. Care Med.*, 18(4): 457–458.
10 Cone, J.B., Bonny, H.W., Caldwell, F.T., Smith, S.D. and Searcey, R. (1987) Beneficial effects of a hypertonic solution for resuscitation in the presence of acute haemorrhage. *Am. J. Surg.*, 154: 585–588.

11 Younes, R.D., Aun, F., Accioly, C.Q. *et al.* (1992) Hypertonic solutions in the treatment of hypoleamic shock: a prospective, randomized study in patients admitted to the emergency room. *Surgery*, **111**: 380–385.

12 Shackford, S.R. (1992) Hypertonic saline and dextran for intraoperative fluid therapy: more for less. *Crit. Care Med.*, **20**: 160–161.

13 Dawidson, I. (1990) Hypertonic saline for resuscitation: a word of caution. *Crit. Care Med.*, **18**: 245.

14 Feest, T.G. (1974) Low molecular weight dextran: a continuing cause of acute renal failure. *Br. Med. J.*, **4**: 1300.

15 Schott, U., Sjostrand, U., Thoren, T. and Berseus, O. (1985) Three per cent dextran-60 as a plasma substitute in blood component therapy. I. An alternative in surgical blood loss replacement. *Acta Anaesthesiol. Scand.* **29**: 767–774.

16 Schott, U., Sjostrand, U., Thoren, T. and Berseus, O. (1985) Three per cent dextran-60 as a plasma substitute in blood component therapy. II. Comparative studies on pre- and postoperative blood volume. *Acta Anaesthesiol. Scand.*, **29**: 775–781.

17 Renck, H., Ljungström, K., Hedin, H. and Richter, W. (1983) Prevention of dextran-induced allergic reaction by hapten inhibition. III. Scandinavian multi-center study on the effect of 20 ml dextran I 15% administered before dextran 70 or 40. *Acta Chir. Scand.*, **149**: 355–360.

18 Stellon, A.J. and Moorhead, P.J. (1981) Polygeline compared with plasma protein fraction as the sole replacement fluid in plasma exchanged. *Br. Med. J.*, **282**: 696–697.

19 Davies, M.J. Cronin, K.D. and Domaingue, C. (1982) Haemodilution for major vascular surgery: using 3.5% polygeline (Haemaccel). *Anaesth. Intens. Care*, **10**: 265–270.

20 Stockwell, M.A., Soni, N. and Riley, B. (1992) Colloid solutions in the critically ill: a randomized comparison of albumin and polygeline. 1. Outcome and duration of stay in the intensive care unit. *Anaesthesia*, **47**: 3–6.

21 Vincent, J.L. (1991) Plugging the leaks? New insights into synthetic colloids. *Crit. Care Med.*, **19**: 316–317.

22 Shatney, C.H., Deepika, K., Milltello, P.R., Majerus, T.C. and Dawson, R.B. (1983) Efficacy of hetastarch in the resuscitation of patients with multisystem trauma and shock. *Arch. Surg.*, **118**: 804–809.

23 Ring, J., Seifert, J., Messmer, K. and Brendel, W. (1976) Anaphylactoid reactions due to hydroxyethyl starch infusion. *Eur. Surg. Res.*, **8**: 389–399.

24 Strauss, R.G., Stansfield, C., Henriksen, R.A. and Villhauer, P.J. (1988) Pentastarch may cause fewer effects on coagulation than hetastarch. *Transfusion*, **28**: 257–260.

25 Claes, Y., Hemelrijck, J.V., Gerven, M.V. *et al.* (1992) Influence of hydroxyethyl starch on coagulation in patients during the perioperative period. *Anesth. Anal.*, **75**: 24–30.

26 Lockwood, D.N.J., Bullen, C. and Machin, S.J. (1988) A severe coagulopathy following volume replacement with hydroxyethyl starch in a Jehovah's Witness. *Anaesthesia*, **43**: 391–393.

27 Isbister, J.P. and Fisher, M. McD. (1980) Adverse effects of plasma volume expanders. *Anaesth. Intens. Care*, **8**: 145–151.

28 Messmer, K.F.W. (1987) The use of plasma substitutes with special attention to their side effects. *World J. Surg.*, **69**: 69–74.

29 Ring, J. and Messmer, K. (1977) Incidence and severity of anaphylactoid reactions to colloid volume substitutes. *Lancet*, i: 466–469.

30 Lucas, C.E., Denis, R., Ledgerwood, A.M. and Grabow, D. (1988) The effects of Hespan on serum and lymphatic albumin, globulin and coagulant protein. *Ann. Surg.*, **207**: 416–420.

31 Kox, W.J. and Kox, S.N. (1988) The influence of plasma substitutes on blood typing and crossmatching in fluid resuscitation. In: Kox, W.J. and Gamble, J. (eds), *Clinics in Anaesthesiology*, Vol. 2 (No. 3), pp. 679–690. London: Baillière Tindall.

32 Klein, S. (1990) The myth of serum albumin as a measure of nutritional status. *Gastroenterology*, **99**: 1845–1846.

33 Hardin, T.C., Page, C.P. and Schwesinger, W.H. (1986) Rapid replacement of serum albumin in patients receiving total parenteral nutrition. *Surg. Gynecol. Obstet.*, **163**: 359–362.

34 Tullis, J.L. (1977) Albumin: 2. Guidelines for clinical use. *JAMA*, **237**: 460–463.
35 Durand-Zaleski, I., Bonnet, F., Rochant, H., Bierling, P. and Lemaire, F. (1992) Usefulness of consensus conferences: the case of albumin. *Lancet*, **340**: 1388–1390.
36 Alexander, M.R., Ambre, J.J., Liskow, B.I. and Trost, D.C. (1979) Therapeutic use of albumin. *JAMA*, **241**: 2527–2529.
37 Alexander, M.R., Alexander, B., Mustiion, A.L., Spector, R. and Wright, C.B. (1982) Therapeutic use of albumin: 2. *JAMA*, **247**: 831–833.
38 Bruno, S., Borzio, M., Romagnoni, M. *et al.* (1992) Comparison of spontaneous ascites filtration and reinfusion with total paracentesis with intravenous albumin infusion in cirrhotic patients with tense ascites. *Br. Med. J.*, **304**: 1655–1658.
39 Gines, P., Arroyo, V., Vargas, V. *et al.* (1991) Paracentesis with intravenous infusion of albumin as compared with peritoneovenous shunting in cirrhosis with refractory ascites. *N. Engl. J. Med.*, **325**: 829–835.
40 Davison, A.M., Lambie, A.T., Verth, A.H. and Cash, J.D. (1974) Salt-poor human albumin in management of nephrotic syndrome. *Br. Med. J.*, **i**: 481–484.
41 Buchan, P.C. (1984) Fetal intrauterine growth retardation and hyperviscosity. In: Heilmann, L. and Bucha, P.C. (eds), *Hemorheological Disorders in Obstetrics and Neonatology*. Stuttgart: F.K. Schattauer-Verlag.
42 Siekmann, U., Heilmann, L. and Ludwig, H. (1984) The therapeutic value of plasma volume expansion in pregnancies with disturbed microcirculation. In: Heilmann, L. and Buchan, P.C. (eds), *Hemorheological Disorders in Obstetrics and Neonatology*. Stuttgart: F.K. Schattauer-Verlag.
43 Grundmann, R. and Heistermann, S. (1985) Postoperative Albumin infusion therapy based on colloid osmotic pressure. *Arch. Surg.*, **120**: 911–915.
44 Maharaj, D., Fell, G.S., Boyce, B.F. *et al.* (1987) Aluminium bone disease in patients receiving plasma exchange with contaminated albumin. *Br. Med. J.*, **295**: 693–696.
45 Denison, D.N. (1988) Artificial oxygen carriers in fluid resuscitation. In Kox, W.J. and Gamble, J. (eds), *Clinics in Anaesthesiology*, Vol. 2 (No. 3), pp. 605–623. London: Baillière Tindall.
46 Bunn, H.F. (1993) The use of hemoglobin as a blood substitute. *Am. J. Hematol.*, **42**: 112–117.
47 Riess, J.G. (1991) Fluorocarbon-based in vivo oxygen transport and delivery systems. *Vox Sang.*, **61**: 225–239.
48 Biro, G.P. (1993) Perfluorocarbon-based red blood cell substitutes. *Transfusion Med. Rev.*, **7**: 84–95.

Part D
MEDICAL AND SURGICAL TRANSFUSION PROBLEMS

11

Acute Blood Loss

1 MECHANISMS OF CIRCULATORY FAILURE

Acute blood loss must have been one of the commonest life-threatening events experienced during evolutionary history. As a consequence, an elaborate but effective series of physiological responses has been developed to maintain blood flow and tissue oxygenation and these ensure recovery from all but the most serious injuries. Massive and continued haemorrhage will, however, eventually exceed the compensating capacity of all the physiological rescue mechanisms and, if left to take its natural course, is incompatible with survival. Modern resuscitation measures, including the administration of intravenous transfusion fluids, have dramatically improved the chances of recovery from severe blood loss, but it is critical that the duration of *shock* and *tissue hypoxia* is minimized. Alleviation of these latter problems is therefore the goal of transfusion therapy; failure to institute prompt and effective resuscitation leads to a series of events terminating in circulatory arrest and death. These are summarized in Figure 1.

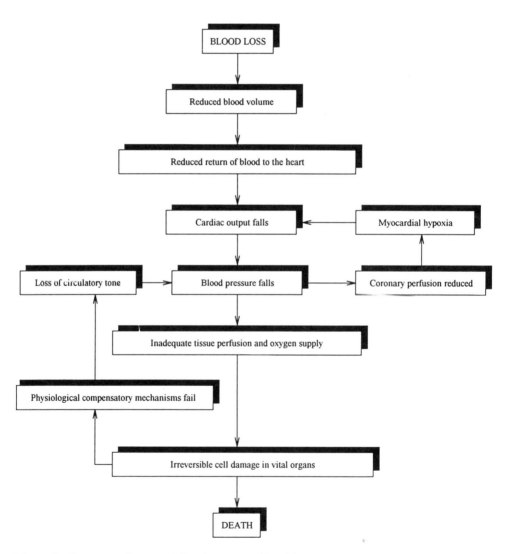

Figure 1   Sequence of events following severe blood loss

2 PHYSIOLOGICAL RESPONSES FOLLOWING BLOOD LOSS

Normal blood pressure is essential for the maintenance and control of tissue perfusion and oxygenation. Tissue perfusion is not maintained at a constant level; the normal variations in metabolic activity that occur within tissues and organs require corresponding alterations in blood flow. Tissue perfusion increases with metabolic activity; the extra demands for oxygen increase the production of *carbon dioxide* and *lactic acid*, and lead to local vasodilatation. These routine circulatory readjustments cannot take place if perfusion pressures are inadequate; tissue hypoxia therefore results.

Blood loss is followed by a series of autonomic neurological responses designed to maintain the circulation and to avert the changes shown in Figure 1. When blood volume is lost, compensating mechanisms ensure that blood *pressure* and *flow* are maintained as long as possible. The most rapid and efficient response to small blood volume losses is contraction of the size of the major veins. This reduces the volume of blood held on the venous side of the circulation and makes more available for tissue perfusion.

Continued blood volume loss inevitably threatens the maintenance of circulatory pressure. Blood pressure is a product of *cardiac output* and *peripheral resistance*; if the cardiac output is reduced as a result of the diminished venous return, the peripheral resistance must increase in order to maintain an acceptable pressure in the circulation.

2.1 Maintenance of Cardiac Output

The heart responds to blood loss by increasing:

• Rate of contraction.
• Force of myocardial contraction.
• Ventricular stroke volume.

These changes are facilitated by an increase in the excitability and conductivity of cardiac muscle. There is, therefore, an attempt to maintain cardiac output, despite a fall in right atrial filling pressures caused by the reduced return of venous blood.

These effects are mediated by a balance between the opposing *sympathetic* (sti-

Table 1 Physiological responses following blood loss

Heart rate and force of contraction increased to maintain cardiac output even though
  venous return is reduced
Vascular capacity reduced as a result of vasoconstriction
Blood supply diverted to vital organs at expense of other tissues
Pulmonary hyperventilation maintains arterial oxygenation despite increased pulmonary
  perfusion
Blood volume replenished from extracellular fluid
Kidneys conserve sodium and water to restore blood volume

---

mulatory) and *parasympathetic* (restraining) systems of the autonomic neurological control over cardiac function. The responses are triggered by signals received from two principal monitoring systems. These are:

(1) *Volume assessment*: *Stretch receptors* in the great veins and the right atrium which convey information about venous return and right atrial pressure.
(2) *Pressure assessment*: on the arterial side, *baroreceptors* in the carotid sinus or aortic arch responding to alterations in blood pressure. These mechanisms are responsible for normal homeostatic control and also bring in rapid responses to blood loss when reduced venous return and arterial hypotension both signal the need for greater sympathetic and less parasympathetic influence on cardiac function.

Although these mechanisms are autonomic and controlled by cardioregulatory centres in the medulla oblongata, cardiovascular function can also be influenced by hypothalamic and cerebral cortical activity. As a result, *anxiety* and *anaesthesia* can also modify these cardiovascular responses, sometimes exaggerating them and making them less reliable as indicators of the degree of blood loss that has taken place. For example, an anxious person who has suffered only minor blood loss can, as a result of psychogenic shock, give every outward appearance of a far more serious injury. As a further complication tissue injury also appears to exaggerate the blood pressure response and tachycardia associated with blood loss.

If haemorrhage continues these compensatory responses cease and the symptoms of bradycardia and circulatory hypotension supervene. These appear to be responses mediated by afferent vagal signals arising from the left ventricle as a consequence of impaired ventricular filling.

2.2 Adustments in the Peripheral Circulation

At any one time, the greater part of the blood volume is held in the smaller vessels of the peripheral circulation. There is therefore considerable scope for adaptive changes in this region as part of the response to blood loss. Two main aspects of the response to blood loss can be considered although the effects of each are complementary.

(1) *Selection of perfusion priorities*: the blood supply of less immediately vital organs is reduced to allow preferential perfusion of tissues where the function must be maintained at all costs, or where the margin of tolerance as far as oxygen supply is concerned is relatively low.
(2) *Reduction of the volume of the blood vascular system*: the closing down of large areas of the vascular bed reduces the capacity of the circulatory system. This permits the reduced volume of blood to provide adequate pressure and flow in the remainder of the circulatory system.

Normal blood flow and oxygen supply are maintained, as far as possible, to:

- The brain.
- The myocardium (coronary circulation).
- The adrenal cortex.

Reduced perfusion occurs in the kidneys, the skin, the gastrointestinal tract, muscle and bone.

Mechanisms for the circulatory rearrangements during blood volume loss

Not surprisingly, the controls for the vascular readjustments to blood loss are linked closely with those for determining the cardiac response to the same circumstances.

(1) Low blood pressure is recognized by *baroreceptors* in the aortic arch and carotid bodies. These 'notify' medullary vasomotor centres linked via the spinal cord to thoracic postganglionic nerve endings. Stimulation of this system results in liberation of adrenaline, which shuts down the precapillary arterioles thus reducing perfusion of cutaneous, muscular and visceral capillary beds. These signals are also potentiated by those from *chemoreceptors* in the aortic arch and carotid body sensing the low arterial oxygen content accompanying haemorrhagic shock.
(2) Psychic and emotional factors (pain, shock, fear) which are frequent accompaniments of the injured state can amplify the above signals and exaggerate the overall effect. As teleological adaptations for survival, these effects are probably beneficial, but they may make clinical assessment of the severity of injury more difficult.

The overall effect of these mechanisms is to produce *vasoconstriction* over large areas of the vascular bed. This elevates blood pressure at the expense of perfusion of some low-priority tissues, but maintains oxygenation of those organs which are most important in terms of ultimate survival.

Venous return and haemorrhagic shock

Maintenance of cardiac output depends entirely on an adequate return of venous blood to the right atrium. Haemorrhagic shock (or traumatic shock) may impede the normal mechanisms for maintaining venous return in various ways:

(1) Muscular pump activity is reduced as a result of immobilization.
(2) Prolonged untreated shock leads eventually to loss of venous tone and this is followed by retention and pooling of blood in an expanded venous volume.
(3) Chest injuries, haemothorax or positive pressure ventilation may abolish the 'suction effect' of inspiration which normally assists return of blood to the right atrium.

2.3 Restoration of Blood Volume from the Extracellular Fluid

Capillary function in shock

During normal tissue perfusion, water, electrolytes and some albumin leave the capillaries to enter the interstitial fluid. This takes place at the proximal, i.e.

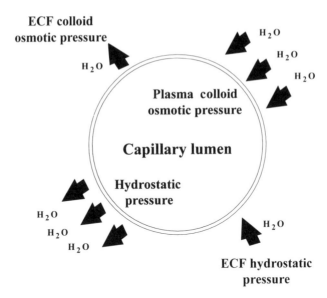

Figure 2   Influence of hydrostatic and oncotic pressure on fluid transport across the capillary endothelial membrane

arterial, end of the capillary where the *hydrostatic pressure* forcing water outwards exceeds the opposite combined effects of *plasma oncotic pressure* and *interstitial fluid pressure*. The reverse obtains towards the low-pressure venous end of the capillary where the oncotic pressure of plasma (largely due to albumin) ensures the return of most of the fluid (see Figure 2). The small amount of albumin, which is also leaked from the plasma, is returned through the system of lymphatics to re-enter the vascular system via the thoracic duct. Under normal circumstances, the final outcome is a small loss of water and albumin from the capillaries.

During hypotensive shock, this flow tends to be reversed. The greatly lowered intracapillary hydrostatic pressure results in an influx of extracellular water from the interstitium into the plasma. This is the most important natural mechanism for restoring plasma volume after haemorrhage. The response begins immediately and with massive blood losses; it is estimated that interstitial fluid can be returned to the vascular compartment at up to 1 l/h. The absorbed fluid is largely salt and water, which dilutes the plasma, reduces its oncotic pressure and in so doing progressively diminishes the stimulus for further influx. The oncotic pressure is, however, eventually restored by the return to the plasma of extra-cellular fluid albumin through the lymphatic system. During haemorrhagic shock the constricted precapillary arterioles, which are responsible for reducing blood flow in the cutaneous and visceral vascular beds, also lower the intracapillary hydrostatic pressure and, in consequence, enhance the return of extracellular fluid into the capillary system.

It is important, therefore, to appreciate that the 10 l or so of extracellular fluid with its content of albumin constitutes a readily and rapidly mobilized reservoir of fluid and protein to replenish sudden losses from the plasma volume. *Extra-*

cellular fluid is in effect an *internal transfusion supply* but one that *must be replenished* once resuscitation begins. This mechanism alone is capable of restoring a large part of the blood volume following moderate haemorrhage.

2.4   Respiratory Changes During Haemorrhage

Pulmonary ventilation increases both in frequency and in depth. These responses are due to the stimulation of medullary control centres by raised blood carbon dioxide tensions and lowered pH levels caused by deficient tissue perfusion and hypoxia. Anxiety also plays a part in increasing ventilation, but reduced blood oxygen levels are relatively less important.

2.5   The Role of the Kidney

The kidney occupies a central position with regard to maintenance of blood volume and pressure as a direct result of the regulation of salt and water metabolism. It seems surprising, therefore, to find the renal circulation apparently penalized during the circulatory readjustments resulting from haemorrhagic hypotension when the converse might have been expected. The paradox is probably explicable if the blood supply needs for salt and water metabolism are relatively small compared with the degree of blood perfusion required for effective excretion of waste metabolites.

Progressive hypotension leads to renal vasoconstriction and reduced blood flow. As a result, glomerular filtration rate and salt and water excretion all become reduced. *If severe hypotension is sustained, ischaemia, cortical necrosis and renal failure will ensue.* Before such drastic damage occurs normal renal physiological mechanisms are brought into action in an attempt to maintain circulatory function.

Pulse pressure is monitored in the afferent arteriole of the glomerulus; falling pressures lead to release of *renin* from the glomerular apparatus. Renin converts plasma angiotensinogen to *angiotensin*, a pressor agent maintaining blood pressure via its vasoconstrictor function. Renin also stimulates adrenal release of *aldosterone*, which enhances distal tubule sodium reabsorption. The increasing plasma sodium concentrations are detected by hypothalamic osmoreceptors, which in turn respond by releasing *antidiuretic hormone* to cause water reabsorption via the distal tubules. Hypothalamic antidiuretic hormone secretion is also stimulated by the hypotension and hypovolaemia accompanying the haemorrhagic episode. These three factors—renin, aldosterone and antidiuretic hormone—thus work together to restore plasma sodium, water and blood volume.

It is apparent, therefore, that conservation of renal function is necessary to allow these essential physiological responses during blood loss. It is also most important to remember that renal salt and water excretion provides a valuable safeguard against fluid overloading during intravenous therapy. Observation of an *adequate urine output and concentrating ability gives a valuable indication that resuscitative measures are successful.*

2.6   Oxygen Transport During Hypotensive Shock

A variety of adaptive mechanisms can be recruited to maintain tissue oxygenation during and following blood loss. In *chronic anaemia*, the reduced oxygen transport capacity of blood can be overcome by a combination of *increased circulation rate, increased capillary density* and *increased oxygen extraction from haemoglobin*. Synthesis of 2,3-diphosphoglycerate (DPG) is stimulated and this shifts the oxygen dissociation curve to the right, thereby facilitating oxygen offloading at tissue oxygen tensions. These oxygen affinity changes are reflected by a reduction in mixed venous oxygen tensions and an increase in the arteriovenous difference in the content of oxygen, indicating a greater degree of oxygen extraction by tissues. *Hyperventilation*, which is especially necessary during exercise, ensures adequate gas exchange even in the presence of accelerated circulation times. These changes in circulatory dynamics and oxygen affinity also occur after *acute blood loss* if blood volume, but not haemoglobin content, is maintained by transfusion of fluids other than blood. Clearly, the ability to sustain adequate oxygen delivery depends on the efficiency and integrity of the adaptive mechanisms described earlier. During haemorrhagic hypotension, acidosis and increased blood pCO_2 also act to displace the oxygen dissociation curve to the right, thereby facilitating oxygen release.

2.7   Energy Metabolism

Despite apparent wastefulness of energy utilization, the body metabolism of traumatized victims is diverted as best it can towards the maintenance of immediate energy needs. Protein catabolism releases amino acids for gluconeogenesis, and fats are likewise broken down to fatty acids and glycerol, leaving evidence in the form of ketone bodies and acidosis. Hyperglycaemia may occur, but the insulin release that would normally be expected to follow may be suppressed as a result of stress-induced catecholamine secretion.

2.8   Restoration of Red Cell Volume

The normal red cell mass is maintained by a steady-state cell renewal system in which regeneration balances age-related cell losses; these are usually of the order of 1% of the total red cell mass per day. Acute demands, such as posed by major haemorrhage, can increase red cell production up to 6–10 times if iron stores are adequate and nutritional and metabolic status is normal. This mechanism is triggered by deficient oxygenation of an endocrine tissue situated in the renal juxtaglomerular area. Hypoxia increases synthesis and release of the hormone *erythropoietin*; this stimulates erythroid stem cells in the bone marrow to accelerate red cell production. Although this process is initiated within hours, maximum red cell production rates are only of the order of 150 ml of red cells daily and this mechanism cannot therefore play a major part in recovery from acute haemorrhage. Unlike some animals, man has no significant pool of red cells available for instant release into the circulation.

3 THE PATHOLOGY OF SEVERE HAEMORRHAGIC SHOCK

The mobilization of extracellular fluid and albumin for plasma volume restoration and the distribution arrangements to conserve the blood flow to the most vital tissues are probably teleologically important adaptive measures ensuring survival after modest injury. In evolutionary terms, the fact that some of these effects may prejudice survival in otherwise already fatal injuries poses no additional problem. This is not so in resuscitation units where rescue of severely injured patients can be energetically pursued. Even if immediate resuscitation appears successful, patients may still be at risk from tissue damage sustained during the initial hypoxic episode. Severe hypoxic shock is one of the recognized causes of *multi-system organ failure* and *adult respiratory distress syndrome* (see chapter 13), for which often prolonged periods of ITU support may be necessary. Late trauma deaths due to these syndromes may occur days or even weeks following the initial injury.[1] It is therefore important to understand the complex derangements following as a consequence of massive injury and how blood transfusion management may help to prevent their occurrence.

3.1 Metabolic and Coagulation Derangements

Prolonged hypotension, and the resulting underperfusion of deprived regions of the circulation such as the visceral bed, leads to severe *anoxia* and *acidosis*. Anaerobic glycolysis leads to the formation of lactic acid, a major contributor to the acidosis. Under these circumstances arteriolar vasoconstriction can no longer be maintained; the precapillary arterioles relax, but postcapillary venules remain constricted. This causes stagnant pooling in a now flaccid and dilated capillary bed. The resulting slowing of blood flow causes cellular sludging and increased blood viscosity and this further impairs the circulation.

Disseminated intravascular coagulation begins to take place, with adherent and aggregating platelets and the formation of microthrombi. Anoxic capillary walls become highly permeable and leak albumin-rich fluid into the interstitium, causing oedema.

Prolonged hypotension of this degree will become irreversible unless treated promptly. The massive pooling of blood in the microvascular circulation deprives venous return and cardiac output, which compounds the hypotension.

Table 2 Consequences of prolonged hypotension

Renal failure and cortical necrosis
Cerebral anoxia
Myocardial anoxia
Disseminated intravascular coagulation

3.2 Hypoxic Damage to Cells

Tissue cells, injured by oxygen starvation, show a number of special metabolic disturbances which contribute in their own way to the total sum of hypoxic injury. Principal amongst these is *failure of the membrane cation pump* leading to loss of cellular potassium, while at the same time sodium and water passively diffuse inwards from the extracellular fluid. Cells therefore swell by absorption of extracellular water, thus reducing the amount available for restoration of plasma volume. The membrane cation pump is fuelled by ATP and the principal source of this high-energy phosphate is the citric acid cycle, which under normal conditions completes the end stages of glycolysis. Although smaller amounts of ATP are generated anaerobically in the early stages of glucose breakdown by the Embden–Meyerhof pathway, most of the cellular ATP is produced later on in the oxidative citric acid cycle. Entry into this terminal phase of glycolysis depends on the oxygen-dependent pyruate to acetylcoenzyme A reaction stage and this is therefore highly vulnerable during hypoxia.

3.3 Hypoxia and the Myocardium

Cardiac muscle has a capillary density well in excess of that of skeletal muscle, and this is a reflection of the fact that adequate oxygenation is absolutely vital to efficient performance. Muscle contraction requires ATP regeneration which, in turn, is dependent on oxidative phosphorylation. It is not difficult, therefore, to understand how a vicious circle of deleterious events occurs during the development of haemorrhagic shock. Hypotension and hypoxaemia prevent the efficient myocardial function that is essential to maintain blood pressure and perfusion.

3.4 Respiratory Complications: Adult Respiratory Distress Syndrome

Pulmonary damage comprising oedema, impaired gas exchange and perfusion abnormalities can occur primarily as a consequence of the original injury, be this severe haemorrhagic shock, septic shock or extensive burns. Pulmonary damage may also be aggravated by certain complications of transfusion such as micro-aggregate embolization, reduced plasma oncotic pressure or circulatory over-loading. Although a variety of precipitating factors are associated with the development of ARDS this condition is now recognized to be one manifestation of a syndrome of multi-system organ failure/septic shock syndromes, the complex causes of which are outlined in chapter 13.

3.5 Renal Disturbances

The incidence of acute renal failure following blood loss is greatly reduced by prompt and effective restoration of the circulatory fluid volume. Prolonged hypotension imposes severe renal vascular constriction which can lead to irreversible

Table 3 Clinical signs of blood loss

Pale clammy skin
Hypotension (particularly postural)
Tachycardia and increased cardiac stroke volume
Hyperventilation, low pCO_2 and respiratory alkalosis
Oliguria and concentrated urine
Anaemia (where haemodilution has had time to occur)

hypoxic damage. Less severe vasoconstriction may result in a reduced urine output which persists even after apparently successful volume replacement. Osmotic diuretics such as mannitol, gelatin solutions and low molecular weight dextrans, which are freely filtered but not reabsorbed by renal tubules, can be useful for maintaining diuresis and renal blood flow but are inadvisable when these are diminished. Maintenance of an adequate urine flow is an important indication that resuscitation is successful. The unavoidable lag between changes in renal circulation and the observed effect on urinary output must, however, be remembered during acutely changing circumstances.

3.6 Hypotension, Hypoxia and Atherosclerosis

Episodes of hypotension following haemorrhage may result in severe ischaemia or infarction of tissues supplied by atherosclerotic vessels. Cerebral and myocardial infarction are particular risks in such patients and add increased urgency to the need to restore effective perfusion.

4 THE CLINICAL SPECTRUM OF HAEMORRHAGE AND HAEMORRHAGIC SHOCK

The symptoms of haemorrhage are either those directly caused by blood loss, or those occurring indirectly as a result of the physiological compensations described in the preceding sections. Fear and anxiety exaggerate symptoms and may give a misleading impression of the degree of blood loss. Blood loss is not necessarily *external*; massive haemorrhage can take place into *internal tissues*, producing little outward evidence apart from *hypovolaemic shock*. In these patients it is important to be able to make the distinction between shock due to blood loss and that of cardiac or septic origin.

Anaesthesia can have potentially confusing hypotensive effects as a result both of relief of the pain and anxiety that potentiate sympathetic vasoconstriction and also of the general vasodilator properties of anaesthetic agents. Patients with mild, partially compensated hypovolaemia due to chronic blood loss and those in poor general condition, particularly the elderly or malnourished, may be dangerously exposed in this way.

Table 4   Consequences of blood loss

Slow chronic loss	Normovolaemic iron deficiency anaemia
	Haemodilutional anaemia
	Hypovolaemia/haemodilution
Rapid loss	Hypovolaemia

(Slow chronic loss ↓ to Rapid loss)

4.1   The Effect of the Rate of Blood Loss

The observable consequences of blood loss depend on its rate and duration.

(1) *Mild chronic blood loss* does not reduce the circulating blood volume, but produces a *haemodilutional anaemia* leading eventually to *iron deficiency* anaemia, when iron stores are exhausted. This is generally revealed when haemoglobin values reach 8–10 g/dl, at which point the extra cardiovascular and ventilatory responses required for even mild exercise make the patient aware that all is not well.

(2) *Subacute episodes* of *blood loss* accelerate the rate of change described above. *Hypovolaemic* symptoms, e.g. syncope and tachycardia, due to delayed replacement of plasma volume from extracellular fluid may occur transiently and are especially liable to be precipitated by exertion. *Postural hypotension* is a particularly important sign in difficult cases of suspected blood loss. Look for tachycardia (increase of 10 beats/min) or hypotension (fall of 15 mmHg BP) when performing head-down–head-raised manoeuvres. Chronic blood loss and the resulting *haemodilutional anaemia* reduce the ability of compensating mechanisms to cope with further acute bleeding episodes. This possibility should always be considered at the time of admission of acutely bleeding patients as it adds urgency to the need for red cell replacement.

(3) *Rapid blood loss* causes obvious hypovolaemia and hypotension. Signs and symptoms stem from this, or the various physiological mechanisms which are called into action as a result. *Acute haemorrhage of recent onset* will show hypotension and will typically show sympathetic autonomic compensatory effects. In contrast, a paradoxical bradycardia is sometimes seen after blood loss in the young and fit, and this can be misleading. In these patients hypotension from peripheral vasodilation, slowed pulse, nausea and loss of consciousness reflect an emotional rather than a physical reaction to blood loss. The signs and symptoms stem predominantly from a parasympathetic rather than sympathetic autonomic response and are transitory. In its milder form, the vasovagal attack or faint is sometimes seen in healthy blood donors, especially young people giving for the first time. It must be remembered that, immediately after acute blood loss, the haemoglobin will not have had time to be diluted by incoming extracellular fluid; nevertheless a substantial blood volume deficit may well have occurred.

4.2   Importance of the Volume of Blood Lost

Blood losses of the order of 10% of blood volume equate to that of normal blood donation and any symptoms will be those resulting either from the cause or from anxiety. Beyond this amount *tachycardia* and *postural hypotension* appear; 20% blood loss is usually associated with pronounced *tachycardia, weakness and thirst*. Losses of up to 30% of blood volume, in otherwise fit subjects, can be reasonably well accommodated by the normal compensating mechanisms pending resuscitative measures. Above this amount *confusion, restlessness and oliguria* are characteristic and progress to *anuria, air hunger and coma* if untreated. Over 50% blood loss will almost certainly exceed the ability to maintain pressure and perfusion unless resuscitation is prompt. If aortic pressures fall too low to support the coronary circulation any hope of recovery is lost. In a similar manner, central nervous system hypoxia will terminate the sympathetic mechanisms which maintain priority of perfusion of the most vital organs.

5   PRACTICAL ASPECTS OF RESUSCITATION AFTER BLOOD LOSS

Arrest of further bleeding and the *alleviation of hypoxaemic shock* are the primary objectives of resuscitation. Skilful management of severe blood loss is an art to be learnt at the bedside and in the operating theatre rather than from written texts, which can only serve as a guide to general principles. Actual regimens in successful practical use vary considerably according to individual practitioner's preferences. Many of the different and seemingly important choices have proved difficult to evaluate in acceptable randomized controlled circumstances.

Successful treatment of haemorrhage requires:

(1) Assessment of the *severity* of blood loss and of the patient's pre-existing physical condition.
(2) Decisions concerning the *urgency and choice* of resuscitative measures.
(3) *Monitoring of clinical signs and physical measurements* to allow the best choices to be made regarding continued treatment.

While the hypovolaemia of acute blood loss produces symptoms and signs common to all patients, their underlying physical condition must also be carefully evaluated as this also affects their chances of recovery and the selection of the best methods of treatment.

5.1   The Need for Urgent Restoration of Blood Volume

It is a cardinal principle that prompt restoration and maintenance of blood volume is of paramount importance; rectification of blood haemoglobin content is very much a secondary consideration, though it cannot of course be delayed indefinitely. In the initial phases, therefore, *administration of almost any intravenous fluid is infinitely preferable to delays due to difficulty in obtaining blood or plasma*. It should hardly be necessary to stress that treatment of an unrecordable blood pressure

Table 5 Acute blood loss

Determine:

  Cause
  Site
  Magnitude of blood loss

Assess patient's underlying physical condition

depends on the prompt establishment of intravenous lines and administration of fluids as rapidly as possible to restore volume in the vascular space. Despite this seemingly logical approach to resuscitation it has become recognized particularly in trauma surgery that too rigorous attention to restoration of circulatory normality must not stand in the way of prompt surgical repair of injuries. Hypotension in its own right diminishes continued haemorrhage into damaged tissues; restoration of circulation at the expense of attempts to repair areas of injury can be counter-productive and decrease survival chances.[2] Coordination of measures for restoration of the circulation with management of the repair of injury is essential. Fluid replacement should, however, match blood loss rates and should be maintained whenever surgical replacement is delayed.

Algorithms can be helpful in deciding at what point intravenous therapy should be instituted and the subsequent selection of either crystalloids, colloids, albumin or red cell replacement.[3] The objective of this difficult early phase of management is to minimize the duration of hypotension and prevent the onset of the late shock complications, i.e. renal failure, shock lung, circulatory failure and sepsis, which lead to later mortality.

5.2 Use of Crystalloids and Colloids

These are used in the initial stage of resuscitation before labile blood components can be obtained. Human albumin (4.5%) solution, isotonic saline, Ringer's lactate and synthetic colloids are the principal alternatives; despite extensive studies there is little evidence to support the preferential use of any one of them (their relative merits are considered in chapters 10 and 13). Resuscitation can certainly be achieved by crystalloid solutions alone even though this can lead to tissue oedema and extracellular fluid accumulation. This does not, however, appear to adversely affect clinical outcome.[4]

There are certainly no good physiological reasons to consider agents other than crystalloids as the sole replacement fluid for losses of the order of 20% blood volume.

Patients with *acute severe blood loss* of some hours' duration will show *hypovolaemia and haemodilutional anaemia* as well as an important extracellular fluid deficit. Water, salt and albumin will have been transferred to the plasma volume to replace losses and intravenous therapy should aim to replenish these.

An economical and logical approach for the treatment of such cases is to use a combination of crystalloids and synthetic colloids, e.g. 1.5 l colloid followed by crystalloid colloid mixtures in a 2:1 ratio.[5] This can be continued until haemo-dilution has resulted in a haemoglobin level around 10 g/dl,[6] at which point red cell replacement should begin. After more than 60% blood volume replacement the possibility of significant hypoproteinaemia and the need for a more sustained plasma expansion effect should be considered. (Plasma colloid osmotic pressure can be rapidly measured using a colloid osmometer.) At this point it may be beneficial to substitute albumin solutions in place of synthetic colloid (see chapter 10).

Low-volume resuscitation

Relatively recently there has been increasing interest in the value of low-volume (e.g. 6 ml/kg) hyperosmotic solutions given as bolus infusions for rapid primary resuscitation in trauma (see chapter 10). These agents seem to be particularly suitable for enabling paramedic teams to begin on-the-spot plasma volume restoration. The high osmotic/oncotic pressure of these materials draws water rapidly from the interstitium to the plasma volume. This ability to institute more effective pre-hospital resuscitation is claimed to relieve some of the pressure for the immediate 'scoop and run' of casualties to trauma units.[7]

5.3 Blood Transfusion During Acute Haemorrhage

Blood sample collection

Blood samples should be taken and dispatched promptly for blood grouping and cross-matching, full blood count (including platelets) and, where massive loss has occurred, for coagulation screen tests. These should be identified accurately (see chapter 25, section 3.1). A fail-safe system should exist for the identification of transfusion samples from emergency admissions.

The degree of urgency for transfusion should be accurately conveyed to the blood bank.

(1) Normal procedures for blood grouping, antibody screening and compatibility testing should be followed as far as practicable unless it is obvious that urgent and massive transfusion is likely.
(2) If emergency provision of blood is required this should be clearly indicated by the written request.

Use of uncross-matched group O blood for emergencies

The use of uncross-matched group O Rh-negative blood should be restricted to those patients who *must* receive red cells before the emergency provision of ABO and Rh D-compatible blood is possible.

Provision of uncross-matched blood

In extreme urgency the transfusion laboratory should be able to provide ABO and Rh D-identical blood shortly after receipt of the cross-match sample. (Whenever uncross-matched blood is released the donation number must always be recorded and a sample of donor red cells retained for subsequent compatibility testing.) *The ABO compatibility of issued blood units must always be confirmed by an immediate spin procedure.*

Emergency cross-match procedures

Where time permits an indirect antiglobulin cross-match should be performed unless antibody screening has already been done. An appropriate agreed shortening of the incubation time (e.g. 5 minutes for LISS (low ionic strength saline) techniques) should be used.

Non-identical ABO transfusion

Where blood stocks are likely to be insufficient, AB people should receive group A blood, and group B people should receive group O blood. Plasma (and therefore isoantibody)-depleted units are obviously to be preferred at least until one blood volume has been exchanged.

Compatibility testing during massive blood replacement

During massive transfusions elaborate procedures for compatibility testing of individual units become superfluous. Following determination of an *antibody screen* (chapter 25, section 2.4) continued issues of blood by *immediate spin cross-match* is entirely adequate. This procedure serves to ensure that no organizational error results in ABO incompatibility. It is most important to appreciate that the biggest step in assuring safety of transfusion is gained by avoidance of ABO incompatibilities. Further serological compatibility procedures make a comparatively small contribution to safety. Although important in routine transfusions, these considerations assume lesser significance in a haemorrhaging patient beset with a multiplicity of life-threatening complications.

Conservation of Rh D-negative blood stocks

If Rh-negative stocks are judged insufficient to cover the likely blood needs of an Rh-negative patient, a decision to use *Rh-positive blood* is best taken sooner rather than later. Priority for Rh D-negative blood is clearly highest for girls and women of childbearing age. It is, however, a serious misjudgement to allow the life of any patient to be jeopardized through inability to supply adequate amounts of Rh-negative blood. If extreme urgency demands it, Rh-positive blood should be dispatched and transfused without delay. The risk of anti-D sensitization is unimportant when faced with potentially catastrophic blood loss. It should be remembered that a small percentage of patients, particularly women, may have already been sensitized to the Rh D antigen. This should be readily revealed by antibody screening.

5.4   Choice Between Blood and Other Intravenous Fluids[8]

The general strategy should be to combine blood and other fluids to maintain the haemoglobin above 10 g/dl and the haematocrit over 0.30 or at an agreed lower value appropriate to the patient's clinical status.[6] Crystalloids, synthetic colloids, 4.5% albumin or (if coagulation failure occurs) fresh frozen plasma can usefully be combined with red cell transfusion under these circumstances (see chapter 11). Moderate haemodilution does not appear to be harmful for most surgical or trauma patients. In contrast, fear of underestimating blood loss may lead to over-transfusion with red cells and the increased blood viscosity may impair tissue oxygenation and place extra work demands on the heart. Surgical or traumatic blood loss may, indeed, be exacerbated by this state of iatrogenic polycythaemia. Fluid overload is always a risk during large transfusions and is usually shown by elevated jugular venous pressure and increased radiological heart size. Hypotension occurring from causes other than haemorrhage, e.g. septic shock or anaesthesia, should be treated, not by red cells, but by colloid or crystalloids which can be disposed of by more rapidly acting homeostatic mechanisms if too much is given.

Bleeding patients with *atheromatous vascular disease* present special risks; hypotensive episodes may be critically injurious to tissues already receiving a precarious oxygen supply. Blood volume and pressure maintenance are therefore of particular importance to those patients but changes in blood viscosity as a consequence of transfusion also affect tissue oxygenation. Some haemodilution may be beneficial in the presence of atheromatous vascular narrowing, but there is no firm agreement on this point. Certainly over-transfusion with red cell preparations will raise the viscosity and, despite increased blood oxygen content, tissue perfusion and oxygenation may be diminished.

Over 75% of all transfused patients receive no more than three units of blood during each transfusion episode; this figure probably differs little from country to country. Blood for these patients represents a major part of the total blood consumption need and it is therefore most important, for the sake of economy, to establish that the transfusion needs of these people can be met perfectly adequately by red cell concentrates in place of whole blood or even more conveniently (because of lower viscosity and faster flow rates) by red cells preserved in optimal additive solutions (see chapter 3). No scientific data have shown any appreciable coagulation disturbances, oncotic pressure problems, homeostatic difficulties or adverse preoperative recovery with the use of these materials for routine transfusions.

Minor blood loss (1 l or less than 20% of blood volume)

For this degree of loss in a previously healthy adult, use of blood or plasma is unnecessary. The risks of transfusion, though small, outweigh any conceivable benefit that would be conferred by blood or plasma administration. Crystalloids will suffice since these obviate the physiological need to restore lost volume from the extracellular fluid; up to three or four times the lost volume may be required.

Replacement with red cells is only necessary when the initial haemoglobin values are below 11.0 g/dl. Red cell transfusion should be given more readily to the elderly or in the presence of pulmonary or coronary disorders where undue haemodilution would be ill advised.

Moderate amounts of blood loss (1–2 l or 20–60% of blood volume)

Prompt administration of crystalloids or synthetic colloid solutions (e.g. 2 l over 0.5–1.0 hour) will stabilize an otherwise precarious state of hypovolaemia, but red cell preparations will then be necessary to replace past losses in addition to balancing the effects of any continued haemorrhage. A commonly accepted practice is to maintain haemoglobin/haematocrit levels around 10.0 g/dl or 0.30 respectively. Red cells (two packs per litre lost) supplemented with crystalloids or colloid combinations will be suitable. Although whole blood remains a common preference (on the basis that whole blood is lost) there are no scientific data to support this view. Surgical misgivings regarding the use of red cell concentrates as replacement for modest blood loss have largely been allayed by the repeated inability to distinguish between the clinical outcomes comparing patients given whole blood with those receiving red cell concentrates.[9–11]

Red cells can therefore be adequately supplied as concentrates or optimal additive preserved units.

Serious haemorrhage (exceeding 60% of blood volume loss)

Blood loss of this order of magnitude may raise anxieties regarding plasma protein depletion. Theoretical calculations and observations on plasma exchange patients show these fears to be largely unfounded. Steady loss of 3 l of blood

Table 6 Blood loss replacement strategy

Volume lost (% of blood volume)	Preferred replacement material
Below 20	Crystalloids/synthetic colloid
20–60	Crystalloids/synthetic colloid + red cell concentrates
60–100	As above + consider albumin for high-risk patients
Over 100	Consider need to supplement with FFP and/or platelets etc.

Selection depends on rate of loss and nature of haemostatic disturbances.

Table 7 Traditional haematological replacement targets during treatment of blood loss

Blood volume	Normal
Haemoglobin	> 10.0 g/dl
Haematocrit	> 0.30
Plasma protein	Above 50 g/l
Platelets	Above $50 \times 10^9/l$
PT, PTT	Below 1.5 × control

replaced only by red cells and crystalloid–colloid combinations would not be expected to reduce plasma proteins to less than 50% of initial values. Even this is a cautious estimate as it discounts the return of extravascular albumin via the lymphatic system and also the synthesis and release of coagulation factors and other proteins. Nevertheless, blood replacement of this magnitude is often but unjustifiably supplemented with albumin or fresh frozen plasma. This practice represents treatment of a non-existent clinical problem. More rational and prudent practice would be to identify those groups of patients in whom creation of a low plasma oncotic pressure could be hazardous. These include *malnourished patients*, and those with *hypoproteinaemia, oedema, sepsis, burns* or with *pre-existing or sustained shock*. Resuscitation of such patients should preferentially be with red cell concentrates supplemented with albumin preparations, until the nature of the primary abnormality of fluid and protein maldistribution is understood.

Massive blood loss (greater than total blood volume replacement)

Massive blood loss and replacement are associated with a range of additional problems. These are considered in chapter 12.

5.5 Resuscitation Objectives

It might at first sight seem self-evident that management of severe blood loss and replacement should entail restoration of near-normal circulatory conditions. The conventional approach to management has relied upon clinical assessment, e.g. a lack of evidence of excess *sympathetic activity*, maintenance of *normal cerebration*, a normal *pulse rate* and *systolic blood pressure* and a *urine flow of at least 30 ml/h* as an indication that resuscitation is adequate. This approach was combined with maintenance of *near-normal haematological indices* (see Table 7). This strategy works adequately for transfusion replacement of relatively moderate blood loss. Nevertheless, it has been shown that for more severe problems blood replacement needs will be underestimated. Conventional resuscitation objectives may seem to have been adequately met, but only because compensatory mechanisms have obscured the overt clinical manifestations of shock, e.g. hypotension, oliguria and pale, clammy skin. Investigations frequently show such patients to have evidence of oxygen lack (e.g. intestinal mucosal hypoxaemia, anaerobic metabolism and lactic acidosis). Some evidence now suggests that the outcome of severely traumatized patients can be improved by a more energetic approach to oxygen delivery assessment.[12] These conclusions follow observations that critically injured survivors tended to maintain higher values for cardiac output (e.g. cardiac index (CI, 1/min per square metre), *oxygen delivery* (DO_2, ml/min per square metre) and *oxygen consumption* (VO_2, ml/min per square metre)). Management protocols have been developed to ensure that these performance values are maintained at supranormal levels.[13] It is claimed that non-survivors failing to achieve such performance values are more likely to succumb to multiple organ failure and other shock-related complications (see chapter 13).[14]

Measurement of oxygen delivery, calculated as the product of cardiac output and arterial oxygen content, reflects the rate of oxygen supply to tissues and provides an indication of overall circulatory performance. The intention of this more energetic resuscitation policy is to ensure that VO_2 is not limited by poor oxygen delivery. Proof of this problem can be obtained by increasing DO_2 progressively until no further gains in VO_2 occur. This can be achieved by combining red cell replacement with colloids and use of inotropic agents (e.g. dopamine as a cardiac stimulant).[12] Experience gained from the use of this newer approach has cast doubt on the reliability of traditional measures of resuscitation success, e.g. pulmonary capillary wedge pressure measurements, CVP measurements and haematological values (see sections 5.6 and 5.7). Pulmonary arterial cannulation and arterial lines are required for these more invasive oxygen transport measurements.

5.6 Haemoglobin/Haematocrit Targets During Blood Replacement

The long-established concept of an optimal haemoglobin/haematocrit target, e.g. 10.0/0.30, during blood replacement is being increasingly challenged. Haemoglobin values must be considered in the context of total blood volume and overall oxygen supply capability. Tissue oxygen utilization (VO_2) must be maximized; however, if blood volume is maintained, quite low haemoglobin concentrations do not appear to be a disadvantage. Indeed oxygen transport is facilitated by reduction in blood viscosity and the resultant increase in cardiac output.[15]

When haemoglobin concentrations are reduced oxygen consumption is sustained by increasing the proportion of oxygen extracted. Merely increasing oxygen transport capacity by increasing haemoglobin values does not necessarily ensure higher oxygen consumption. In one study involving adequately volume-resuscitated shock patients, tissue oxygen utilization could not be improved by increasing haemoglobin values above 8.3 g/dl as a means of increasing DO_2.[16] Another study involving paediatric patients identified a haemoglobin value of 10.2 g/dl above which no further improvements in tissue oxygen utilization could be demonstrated.[17] Data such as these have been utilized in the USA National Blood Resources Education Program, which advises that 'adequate oxygen-carrying capacity can be met by a haemoglobin of 7.0 g/dl (haematocrit value of approximately 21%) or less when the intravascular volume is adequate for perfusion'. Reliable evidence for the safety of surgery in the presence of reduced haemoglobin concentrations is provided by the numerous studies on Jehovah's Witnesses.

Even under these extreme conditions, mortality figures no greater than 0.5–1.5% have been recorded for a range of surgical procedures for which transfusion is usually regarded as essential.[18] There is, however, some evidence to caution against too great a reliance on overall measurements of *whole-body* tissue oxygen utilization. Higher rates of myocardia, ischaemia and cardiac morbidity were recorded in high-risk vascular patients where haematocrit levels were below 28%.[19] Similarly, increased mortality where haemoglobin values were below 10.0 g in patients with sepsis, cardiac disease and substantial blood loss has been demonstrated.[15] In practical terms, therefore, the capacity to mobilize compensatory oxygen delivery systems, the presence of other pathology, e.g. sepsis or coronary insufficiency, and the quality of blood volume restoration all affect the degree to which any given patient can tolerate low haemoglobin values. The degree to which haemodilution can be permitted is ultimately an individual clinical decision. The choice of the traditional target value for haemoglobin/haematocrit (10.0 g.dl/0.30) could either be regarded as unnecessarily high or alternatively as a relatively safe compromise where there is uncertainty regarding a patient's fitness. As a workable, practical measure, it seems prudent and safe to retain the traditional 10.0 g.dl/0.30 red cell transfusion trigger for those patients in whom there is reasonable suspicion that cardiovascular or pulmonary performance may be limited. For critically ill patients with sepsis, ARDS or other reasons for raised oxygen requirements, near-normal haemoglobin values may be safer.[6]

5.7 Clinical Investigation and Monitoring

At the same time as resuscitation begins the *site* and *cause of blood loss* must be determined. The cause may often be relatively obvious but cases of difficulty may require an exhaustive search (see Table 8). Careful monitoring of transfusion therapy is necessary to ensure improvement rather than deterioration in the patient's condition. Clinical experience, skill and judgement are essential in order to select the appropriate monitoring strategy and interpret the overall pattern of changes shown by clinical signs and the results from monitoring equipment.

The intensity of the monitoring procedure depends on the anticipated difficulty of the management problem. Monitoring of blood loss and the success of resuscitation measures is usually carried out by recording the following observations:

(1) *Measurement of blood loss*: accurate measurement can be very difficult and the conclusions therefore potentially misleading. However, under certain circum-

Table 8 Investigations for unexplained acute blood loss

Endoscopy
Aspiration and lavage of body cavities
X-ray/tomography
Angiography (where bleeding is brisk)
Explorative surgery

stances, e.g. during surgery, the exercise is worth undertaking and considerable experience has been gained as to the best approach to various problems.

(a) *Swabs*: these can be weighed dry, then again after blood contamination, to give an idea of the weight of blood absorbed. Alternatively, an estimate of blood loss can be made from measurement of potassium and haemoglobin recovered in the washings.[20]

(b) *Surgical drapes*: these will contain partially dried blood, stained areas and portions of clotted blood. Washing systems have been devised to try to overcome the problems of measuring the quantity of blood on these materials but the results have not been very successful. The experienced judgement of theatre staff probably enables a better estimate.

(c) *Blood lost in suction apparatus or drains*: estimates of the volume will be misleading if this is mixed with irrigation fluids or is allowed to clot. If an anticoagulant is added to the reservoir bottles, haemoglobinometry or red cell counts[21] can be performed from the contents using instruments designed for the particularly low readings that are likely. A relatively simple apparatus for estimating paediatric losses has been described.[22]

(d) Blood lost from fractures into injured limbs can be substantial.[23] Amounts range from up to 800 ml in the forearm to around 2 litres for pelvic and femoral fractures. Careful measurements of limb circumference help.

During elective surgery, a relatively simple formula can be used for calculating the blood loss allowable before the lowest acceptable haemoglobin (Hb) value is reached[24] (assuming isovolaemic plasma volume replacement):

Allowable blood loss

$$= \text{Estimated blood volume}^* \times \frac{\text{Initial HB} - \text{Lowest acceptable Hb}}{\text{Average Hb}\dagger}$$

For example, where the total blood flow = 5 l, initial Hb = 12 g/dl and minimum tolerable Hb = 8.0 g/dl, 2 l of blood loss can be permitted.

(2) *Haemoglobin or haematocrit measurements*: these can only be interpreted in the context of preceding values. Changes in blood count are slow indicators of blood loss. Up to 24 hours may be required before haemodilution allows any accurate degree of assessment of red cell volume loss.

(3) Clinical observation of *blood pressure, pulse, respiration and temperature*: these should be charted to enable early recognition of deterioration.

(4) *Monitoring cutaneous and internal body temperatures*: the restriction of cutaneous blood flow during shock results in a fall in skin temperature relative to internal blood temperatures. A temperature difference of less than 5 °C suggests absence of serious circulatory problems.

---

*75 ml/kg serves as a working approximation.
†The average haemoglobin is the average of the initial and the lowest acceptable haemoglobin concentration.

(5) Measurement of *urinary output and concentrating ability* (specific gravity or osmolarity): over 30 ml urine output per hour (0.5 ml/kg per hour), and a specific gravity of over 1018 or 500 mOsm/l should be obtained.

(6) *Central venous pressure (CVP) monitoring*: values up to, but not exceeding, 15 cm of saline confirm satisfactory right atrial filling pressure and that the heart is not placed in a state of failure through over-transfusion. Low values, below 5 mm of saline, probably indicate a deficiency of venous return to the heart which will prevent an adequate cardiac output. In massively transfused patients, use of balloon-tipped catheters inserted into the pulmonary vessels allows measurement of CVP, cardiac output and *pulmonary capillary wedge pressures* (PCWP, approximating to left atrial pressure). These can be invaluable in allowing the precise metering of transfusion fluid therapy. The recognition of hypovolaemia is assisted by observing the CVP or PCWP response to bolus fluid replacement. Unsustained increases in pressures following doses of 5–10 ml/kg over 10 minutes usually indicate that more fluid is required. Measurement of *mixed venous oxygen tension* can be undertaken at the same time and this shows whether the oxygen supply to peripheral tissues is adequate.

(7) *Assessment of tissue oxygen utilization*: in severely traumatized and shocked patients clinical assessments of oxygen supply are usually supplemented by a variety of invasive or non-invasive procedures.[25]

Pulse oximetry enables non-invasive monitoring of arterial oxygen partial pressures based on the spectroscopic difference between oxygenated and de-oxygenated haemoglobin. Although of proven value, it will be less effective in states of anaemia, severe shock, peripheral vasoconstriction and hypothermia.

Direct measures of cardiac function, acid–base analysis, oxygen transport and tissue oxygen utilization are increasingly used as a resuscitation guide (see section 5.5) but these entail pulmonary and systemic arterial catheterization.

(8) *Electrocardiography (ECG)* is of little value during routine situations but does provide a warning against *hyperkalaemia* combined with *hypocalcaemia*, which may occur in massive transfusions.

(9) *Blood volume measurements*: these would be valuable if the available techniques permitted repeated precise determination of blood volume during blood loss and replacement. Unfortunately, the error in isotopic blood volume measurements, even under the best circumstances, is high. This error becomes even greater when attempts are made to perform blood volume monitoring during intensive resuscitation. Errors occur as a result of imperfect reinjection of labelled blood, the irregular rates of blood loss, and the prolonged circulation times required to achieve perfect mixing when there are relatively static regions of the circulation. These difficulties are especially pronounced in those very patients for whom such information would be most needed. The expected blood volume, red cell mass and plasma volume can be predicted from body weight or preferably from normograms derived from height and weight (body surface area). These estimates are less reliable in the presence of gross obesity, extreme malnutrition and accumulation of oedema or fluid in serous cavities. Calculation of the expected red cell volume can be useful in estimating the red cell deficit that requires replacement. Taking average figures of, say, 30 ml of red cells per kg (1100 ml/m^2) for males and 25 ml/kg (840 ml/m^2) for females

and multiplying these by the measured haemoglobin or haematocrit (if these have fully stabilized after blood loss) expressed as a fraction of the normal, will give an approximation of the remaining red cell mass and of the deficit to be made good.

REFERENCES

1 Messmer, K. and Arfors, K.E. (1988) Can primary resuscitation be improved? In: Vincent, J.L. (ed.), *Intensive Care and Emergency Medicine*, Vol. 5, pp. 13–17. Berlin: Springer-Verlag.

2 Evans, R.C. and Evans, R.J. (1992) Accident and emergency medicine. *I. Postgrad. Med. J.*, **68**: 714–734.

3 Hopkins, J.A., Shoemaker, W.C. and Chang, P.C. (1983) Results of a clinical trial in the use of emergency resuscitation algorithm. *Crit. Care Med.*, **11**: 621.

4 Virgilo, R.W., Rice, C.L., Smith, D.E. *et al.* (1979) Crystalloid vs. colloid resuscitation: is one better? *Surgery*, **85**: 129–139.

5 Ramsay, G. (1988) Intravenous volume replacement: indications and choices. *Br. Med. J.*, **296**: 1422–1423.

6 Lundsgaard-Hansen, P. (1992) Treatment of acute blood loss. *Vox Sang.*, **63**: 241–246.

7 Gold, C.R. (1987) Pre-hospital advanced life support vs 'scoop and run' in trauma management. *Emergency Med.*, **16**: 797–801.

8 Lundsgaard-Hansen, P. (1980) Component therapy of surgical hemorrhage: red cell concentrates, colloids and crystalloids. *Bibl. Haematol.*, **46**: 147–169.

9 Lundsgaard-Hansen, P., Koch, S., Lindt, R., Senn, A. and Tschirren, B. (1981) Influence of a blood component program on postoperative complication rates: a retrospective study in 372 patients. *Vox Sang.*, **41**: 193–200.

10 Robertson, H.D. and Polk, H.C. (1975) Blood transfusions in elective operations: comparison of whole blood versus packed red cells. *Ann. Surg.*, **181**: 778–783.

11 Schorr, J.B. and Marx, G.F. (1970) Transfusion trends. *Anaesth. Anal.*, **49**: 646–651.

12 Shoemaker, W.C., Kram, H.B. and Appel, P.L. (1990) Therapy of shock based on pathophysiology, monitoring, and outcome prediction. *Crit. Care Med.*, **18**: S19–S25.

13 Fleming, A., Bishop, M., Shoemaker, W. *et al.* (1992) Prospective trial of supranormal values as goals of resuscitation in severe trauma. *Arch. Surg.*, **127**: 1175–1181.

14 Fiddian-Green, R.G., Haglund, U., Gutierrez, G. and Shoemaker, W.C. (1993) Goals for the resuscitation of shock. *Crit. Care Med.*, **21**: S25–S31.

15 Spence, R.K. (1991) The status of bloodless surgery. *Transfusion Med. Rev.*, **5**: 274–286.

16 Dietrich, K.A., Conrad, S.A., Cullen, A.H. *et al.* (1990) Cardiovascular and metabolic response to red blood cell transfusion in critically ill volume-resuscitated nonsurgical patients. *Crit. Care Med.*, **18**: 940–944.

17 Mink, R.B. and Pollack, M.M. (1990) Effect of blood transfusion on oxygen consumption in pediatric septic shock. *Crit. Care Med.*, **18**: 1087–1091.

18 Kitchens, C.S. (1991) Are transfusions overrated? Surgical outcome of Jehovah's Witnesses. *Am. J. Med.*, **94**: 117–119.

19 Nelson, A.H., Fleisher, L.A. and Rosenbaum, S.H. (1993) Relationship between post operative anemia and cardiac morbidity in high-risk vascular patients in the intensive care unit. *Crit. Care Med.*, **21**: 860–866.

20 Freedman, M. (1984) A new indicator dilution method for the estimation of surgical blood loss. *Anaesthesia*, **39**: 826–831.

21 Boliston, T.A. (1984) Determination of blood loss during transurethral surgery by cell counts on irrigation fluid. *Ann. R. Coll. Surg. Engl.*, **66**: 94–95.

22 Wilkinson, D.J. and Redmond, J. (1984) Measurement of blood loss in children. *Anaesthesia*, **39**: 72.

23 More, D.G. (1984) Initial assessment of acute haemorrhage. *Anaesth. Intens. Care,* **12**: 206–211.

24 Gross, J.B. (1983) Estimating allowable blood loss: corrected for dilution. *Anaesthesiology,* **58**: 277–280.

25 Evans, R.C. and Evans, R.J. (1992) Accident and emergency medicine. II. *Postgrad. Med. J.,* **68**: 786–799.

12

Transfusion for Massive Blood Loss

Massive haemorrhage following trauma or surgery is an extreme emergency; it demands rapid assessment of treatment priorities and a coordinated teamwork approach involving a variety of clinical disciplines. The danger of imminent loss of life can create considerable tensions between those attempting to treat the haemorrhage, those producing blood or blood components and the staff providing laboratory services. These circumstances can easily combine to result in mistakes that can endanger the patient, or cause waste of scarce transfusion materials without securing discernible clinical benefit. Each patient presents unique problems; standardized inflexible protocols for management are therefore not applicable. It is, nevertheless, worthwhile defining the general principles of management so that the most effective therapy can be instituted promptly and the dangers resulting from clinical indecisiveness can be avoided.

Delayed control of blood loss, coupled with *inadequate blood volume replacement*, is the patient's greatest enemy. Even before the patient reaches hospital resuscitation facilities, emergency measures can be instituted that may be life saving. Application of *tourniquets*, rapid administration of *intravenous fluids* and *oxygen administration* all increase the likelihood that a traumatized patient survives to reach the resuscitation area. The patient must not be allowed to suffer irreversible or protracted shock with the attendant risks of *multi-system organ failure* (see chapter 10). However, repair of damaged tissue is also important, and too great an emphasis on immediate restoration of haemodynamic normality before securing haemostasis and surgical repair is now recognized to reduce the chances of survival (see chapter 11).

Despite the tensions and drama inherent in the management of massive haemorrhage, it is important to define the problems to be faced, to identify areas where unjustified therapy should be curtailed and to attempt to clarify principles of transfusion management that have obtained common agreement. There is, in this topic, a considerable diversity of opinion regarding management. It must, however, be appreciated that established proof of the efficiency of many frequently advised regimens is much less substantial than commonly assumed. The reasoning behind much of this area of transfusion practice is based more on benefits that are hoped for than those that have been conclusively proven.

1 DEFINITION OF MASSIVE TRANSFUSION

This is somewhat arbitrary, but is commonly accepted to entail transfusion of *an amount equal to the total blood volume* during a relatively short period. This is usually taken to be of the order of 3 hours, but a more conservative definition would extend the time period to 24 hours. The underlying principle of importance is that *transfusion replacement is being administered at a rate which potentially exceeds the ability of homeostatic mechanisms to maintain all the important aspects of blood composition at safe levels.* The ability to tolerate massive blood replacement will obviously depend to a considerable extent on the age and clinical condition of the patient.

Despite fully justified clinical concern for the patient's condition, logical analysis and planning of transfusion therapy are essential, otherwise valuable resources are wasted, and therapeutic materials given that are ineffective or even dangerous. It is, in fact, not easy to produce clinically significant alterations in blood composition during transfusion. Even assuming no homeostatic mechanisms and no 'reserves', stepwise rapid loss and replacement of the blood volume alter blood constituents in a fairly predictable manner. For example, in an adult with a blood volume of 5l the predicted Factor VIII levels remaining if lost blood is replaced by stored blood assumed to be devoid of the original Factor VIII activity can be calculated to be 60% after 2.5l and is still as high as 35% after an amount equal to the blood volume has been transfused.

Limiting the definition of massive transfusion to situations in which the blood volume has been exchanged completely has, therefore, a theoretical basis and has also been found to be a workable practical definition.

The management strategy outlined is directed towards traumatized patients who, for example, arrive in casualty exsanguinating, or towards surgical or obstetric patients presenting with sudden uncontrollable haemorrhage. It should be emphasized that, unless there are pre-existing abnormalities of haemostasis or plasma protein composition, haematological problems should not be expected for transfusion rates less than mentioned above.

2   AIMS OF TREATMENT

The blood transfusion strategy should be to maintain blood composition within limits that are safe with regard to *haemostasis, blood oxygen-carrying capacity, oncotic pressure and plasma biochemistry*. Transfusion should, therefore, maintain reasonable homeostasis and not of itself contribute to further deterioration.

Potentially catastrophic blood loss demands instantaneous transfusion but it is axiomatic that haemostasis be identified and secured at the earliest opportunity. Massively transfused patients, as expected, show increased morbidity; but this is in part attributable to the progressively increased difficulties in maintaining perfusion of critical organs and freedom from the complications of transfusion as time progresses. *Urgent volume replacement is of much greater immediate importance than restoration of haemoglobin level.*

3   RISK FACTORS FOR COMPLICATIONS

Massively transfused patients do not form a homogeneous group in which complications can be anticipated in a predictable manner. Conservative management protocols must take account of the possibility that pre-existing high-risk factors may not have been accurately identified. It must be recognized, however, that these problems may accelerate the appearance of transfusion complications.

Prolonged hypotension and shock predispose to disseminated intravascular coagulation and adult respiratory distress syndrome. Delayed treatment of shock is probably the most important factor predisposing to problems during resuscitation.

Adult respiratory distress syndrome is believed to be more likely in patients with persisting congestive cardiac failure, sepsis and those who are either under-transfused or over-transfused.

Extensive tissue damage particularly involving *head injuries* can also be associated with coagulation disturbances. Patients with severe head injuries may also be at risk of dangerous cerebral oedema if plasma oncotic pressure is allowed to fall excessively.

Patients with *hepatic* or *renal failure* may not only have abnormalities of haemostasis or plasma proteins but may also have impaired metabolic responses to the citrate, potassium or glucose infused with stored blood.

4   PROBLEMS OF MASSIVE TRANSFUSION

4.1   Blood Volume Replacement

Many of the complications of massive transfusion are aggravated by either under- or over-transfusion. Judgement of the adequacy of this is a skilled clinical matter,

Table 1 Potential problems following massive transfusion

Platelet depletion
Coagulation factor depletion
Increased blood oxygen affinity
Hyperkalaemia and hypocalcaemia
Hypothermia following administration of cold blood
Acid–base disturbances
Hyperglycaemia
Pulmonary damage from microaggregates in stored blood
Altered plasma oncotic pressure

discussion of which is beyond the scope of written texts. As a minimum, normal systolic pressures, a urine output of at least 30 ml/h, haematocrit values of 0.30 and, where applicable, a stable level of consciousness are indicative of acceptable blood transfusion replacement. For *high-risk patients*, transfusion therapy is tailored towards maximizing tissue oxygenation and for this measurements of cardiac output, oxygen transport and tissue oxygen utilization are employed (see chapter 11).

4.2 Thrombocytopenia[1–4]

Blood stored for several days is devoid of functioning platelets; dilutional thrombocytopenia is therefore to be anticipated during extensive blood replacement. The refrigeration of blood appears to have a deleterious effect on platelet function, although it is believed that some clinically effective platelets are still present in blood up to 24 hours after collection. Theoretical predictions as well as clinical observations indicate that at least 1.5 blood volumes (e.g. 7–8 l for adults) of stored blood must be transfused before significant dilutional thrombocytopenia is likely. This will not, however, be true if *disseminated intravascular coagulation* occurs (see below) or if the patient has *pre-existing thrombocytopenia* for other reasons.

It has been shown that the platelet counts in massively transfused patients generally fall more slowly than would be expected as a result of dilution.[5] The rate of fall does *not* appear to be influenced by prophylactic platelet administration, nor is there any evidence that microvascular bleeding can be prevented. Indeed, impaired haemostasis during massive blood replacement is very likely to be due to acquired *platelet dysfunction*, particularly in patients with sustained acidosis or hypothermia (see sections 4.7 and 4.8).[6] Prevention of these complications may be the best means of preventing protracted haemorrhage.[7]

Platelet counts should be maintained above 50×10^9/l. During cardiac bypass surgery (see chapter 14), as well as in some other instances of massive transfusion, apparent thrombocytopenic bleeding may occur at counts higher than this, probably because of an acquired functional defect.

Since platelet concentrates are often in short supply, their use, when vigorous blood loss from surgical wounds is still in progress, is wasteful unless successful surgical haemostasis is in sight.

4.3 Coagulation Factor Depletion[1,2]

Despite common assumptions, clinically significant reductions of coagulation factor concentrations are not a frequent occurrence. Stored whole blood contains adequate amounts of all coagulation factors, except for Factors V and VIII, which decay during storage.[8] Deficiencies of even these factors are less of a problem than commonly supposed.[9]

Factors V and VIII concentrations of over 20% have been reported in 21-day stored ACD blood. Factor VIII is also an acute-phase protein; synthesis and release are stimulated by the stress of trauma and surgery. The remaining coagulation factors are reasonably stable in stored blood and should not contribute to disordered haemostasis. Clearly then for purely dilutional reasons only mild reductions in total coagulation performance are to be expected following haemorrhage and stored blood replacement. Because of their much reduced plasma content, use of optimal additive preserved red cells will produce a greater dilutional effect.

Disseminated intravascular coagulation (DIC) must be considered as the most likely cause of excessive bleeding and abnormal haemostasis test results. In severe examples there may be widespread microvascular bleeding from all injured surfaces, together with significantly abnormal laboratory results, in particular thrombocytopenia, hypofibrinogenaemia and elevated fibrinogen degradation products. *DIC is a likely consequence of delayed or inadequate resuscitation and is probably the explanation for platelet counts and clotting test results that are worse than expected for the volume of transfusion given.*

Excessive bleeding may reflect haemostatic failure requiring corrective therapy. However, prophylactic use of blood components, or 'formula' replacement of a proportion of fresh blood or platelets interspersed with bank blood, has been abandoned as being wasteful and ineffective.[10] The need for coagulation factor (usually fresh frozen plasma or cryoprecipitate) or platelet therapy should where possible be supported by laboratory evidence. This might take the form of platelet counts below $50 \times 10^9/l$ (or levels falling towards that figure) fibrinogen $<0.8\,g/l$ or of partial thromboplastin and prothrombin times which are either prolonged to greater than 50% over control values or which show progressive deterioration.

Undoubtedly pressures exist to give immediate treatment for the assumed haemostatic problem, particularly when results of laboratory investigations are not readily available. Samples for haemostasis studies must nevertheless be collected. Coagulation or platelet count results are sometimes inconclusive during what appear to be clear cases of microvascular bleeding, and in these instances therapy may be justified on clinical grounds alone. Laboratory tests may, on occasion, indicate a severity of haemostatic function that suggests the earlier choice of therapy to have been inappropriate or totally inadequate. It seems reasonable, however, when fresh components are available, to recommend their use on the basis of a presumptive diagnosis; but this does not preclude laboratory monitoring to provide more specific guidance to therapeutic needs.

4.4 High Oxygen Affinity of Stored Blood

The increased oxygen affinity of 2,3-diphosphoglycerate (DPG)-depleted stored blood (see chapter 4, section 1.1) becomes that of the patient's blood as rapid exchange transfusion proceeds. Thus either cardiac output and tissue perfusion must rise, or tissue oxygen tensions must fall to maintain oxygen offloading. Transfusion of high-affinity blood might, therefore, be expected to prejudice tissue oxygenation and increase cardiopulmonary workload, and this may be dangerous in critically ill patients who may be poorly equipped to cope with this additional problem. A theoretically convincing case for use of close-to-collection-date blood can easily be advanced, but clear-cut evidence of value in this clinical setting is hard to come by. It seems likely that this effect will be of most importance in:

(1) Patients with *severe anaemia*, in whom 'exchange' with blood which is less able to deliver oxygen may make tissue oxygen supply even more precarious.
(2) Where there is concern regarding the efficiency of blood supply to *grafted* or *anastomosed tissues*.
(3) Patients with *arteriosclerotic narrowing* of *cerebral* or *myocardial blood vessels*. Cardiac muscle has such an avid demand for oxygen that even under normal circumstances its needs are only satisfied by a very high level of oxygen extraction. This is normally obtained by reducing coronary venous oxygen tensions to the lowest tolerable. A combination of atherosclerotic coronary arteries, low coronary perfusion pressures and a left-shifted oxygen dissociation curve could, in theory, be dangerous.

Objective proof, however, that disordered oxygen affinity presents clinical risks is scanty, although there is some evidence that even top-up transfusions to chronically anaemic patients result in better tissue oxygenation when fresh blood is used.[11] Cardiac surgery patients transfused with blood of low oxygen affinity also appear to need less increase in cardiac output during the early postoperative recovery phase.

While this evidence of the importance of oxygen affinity is awaited, it seems reasonable to use recently collected red cell units (e.g. less than 1 week of age) particularly, for example, where arteriosclerotic vascular disease or poorly vascularized tissue anastomoses are problems. Absolutely fresh blood (e.g. less than 24 hours old) is *not* indicated for this reason alone.

Elevated plasma phosphate levels from the anticoagulant solution (either ACD or CPD) promote *in vivo* DPG regeneration, as also does citrate and the alkalosis resulting from its metabolism. DPG regeneration begins within a few hours and is usually complete within 24–48 hours following transfusion. DPG is not, of course, the only determinant of oxygen affinity. Increased carbon dioxide, increased temperature and lowered pH all improve tissue oxygen delivery as a result of reduced oxygen affinity, while the converse also applies. The final net effect of all these changes during transfusion is hard to predict, but they are probably best reflected by the *in vivo* P_{50} of the patient's blood, in contrast to the standard P_{50} which largely reflects changes in the concentration of DPG alone.

The objective of transfusing blood with normal or even increased P_{50} is to:

(1) Obviate the need for cardiovascular or pulmonary compensations which are in themselves costly in terms of energy requirements.
(2) Safeguard patients in whom cardiopulmonary function lacks the reserve capacity to cope with extra demands.

As a further example of the complexity of the oxygen supply equation, it must be appreciated that maintaining a right-shifted oxygen dissociation curve is theoretically only of value when blood can be oxygenated normally in the lungs. Where alveolar oxygen tensions drop this decrease in oxygen affinity becomes a disadvantage as haemoglobin cannot be fully saturated. This fact is readily apparent from chapter 3, Figure 2.

4.5 Hypocalcaemia

The citrate in anticoagulant fluids binds ionized calcium and potentially lowers plasma calcium levels. This is much less of a problem than might be expected because the healthy adult liver metabolizes citrate at rates equal to one unit of blood transfused every 5 minutes. This capacity cannot always be assumed and neonates (see chapter 20) and hypothermic patients are especially vulnerable to citrate toxicity. Hypocalcaemia does not have a clinical effect on blood coagulation; neuromuscular effects are more likely and very uncommonly patients may show a transient tetany. The major consequence of lowered calcium levels is due to its synergism with high potassium levels in disturbing cardiac function (see below).

4.6 Hyperkalaemia

The plasma potassium content of blood increases during storage and may reach over 80 mEq/l. High K^+ and low Ca^{2+} (together with hypothermia and acidosis) combine to impair myocardial performance and could eventually cause cardiac arrest in diastole. Clinical evidence of poor haemodynamic responses to apparently adequate transfusion therapy is a pointer to this metabolic problem. Features include persistent hypotension with poor pulse pressure and elevated central venous pressure. Hyperkalaemia is, in practice, not a common problem during transfusion of adults unless large amounts of blood are being given very quickly. This may, in part, be a consequence of the renal tubular exchange of K^+ for H^+ that takes place during alkalosis (see below: pH disturbances).

Prevention depends best on ECG monitoring and warning signs include:

• Prolonged P–R interval.
• QRS widening.
• Peaking of T waves.

Patients at risk include:

(1) Those with *impaired renal function* (either pre-existing or due to unrelieved vasoconstriction). Normally the kidney responds to haemorrhagic hypotension by sodium retention and potassium secretion.
(2) Patients with *internal bleeding*, for example into the gastrointestinal tract (K^+ from haemolysed blood is reabsorbed).

Remedies:

- For hyperkalaemia, insulin and glucose can be administered intravenously.
- For patients with chronic renal failure, give potassium-absorbing calcium-loaded ion-exchange resins.

Prevention of hypothermia (see section 4.8) is probably the most effective measure for avoidance of effects due to hyperkalaemia and hypocalcaemia. Because of fluctuations in plasma protein concentrations, total plasma calcium measurements are unreliable indicators of hypocalcaemia; ionized calcium measurements give a better guide. Where clinical and electrocardiographic evidence suggests hypocalcaemia, 5 ml of 10% calcium gluconate (proportionately less for children) should be given at 5-minute intervals intravenously until the ECG is normal. The advice formerly given, that calcium should be administered after transfusion of predetermined amounts of blood, is unsafe.

4.7   Acid–Base Disturbances

Lactic acid—the end-product of red cell glycolysis—in the blood pack could theoretically contribute to the overall acidosis of hypoxic shocked patients. In practice, however, transfusion alleviates acidosis as a result of improved tissue perfusion and relief from hypoxia. The arterial pH should be monitored during massive transfusion. If acidosis cannot be counteracted by control of ventilation and improved tissue perfusion it may be necessary to add sodium bicarbonate to intravenous fluids.

Citrate metabolism generates bicarbonate and a metabolic alkalosis is found to be the later effect of large transfusions.

4.8   Hypothermia

Unwanted cooling of the body may result from rapid infusion of blood and other fluids. Blood warmers should be used for rates of infusion exceeding one unit every 10 minutes and correspondingly less for children. The choice, calibration and maintenance of blood warmers are important if damage to blood is to be avoided, yet adequate warming and flow rates achieved. A review of blood warmer performance concluded that equipment utilizing the counter-current principle was more efficient at very high flow rates (> 250 ml/min) than that utilizing a water-bath or dry heat.[12]

Excessive cooling of patients may also result from prolonged exposure or evaporation of fluid lost during surgery. Hypothermia slows citrate metabolism, potentiates the harmful cardiac effects of hyperkalaemia and low calcium, and reduces oxygen release from haemoglobin. Platelets function less well and this may lead to excessive bleeding. Shivering to keep warm consumes energy and oxygen and also demands increased cardiac output.

4.9 Adult Respiratory Distress Syndrome

The aetiology of this condition is not well understood and the importance of various proposed preventative measures remains highly controversial. Certain of the recognized predisposing factors have been mentioned elsewhere (chapter 13). Under- or over-transfusion should if possible be avoided. The plasma oncotic pressure should, if possible, not fall below 20 mmHg (normally associated with serum albumin concentrations below 30 g/l). Hypoproteinaemia will not occur as a result of transfusion unless excessive amounts of crystalloids have been given.

Corrective action requires albumin concentrate (20 g/100 ml) as a bolus dose; one bottle normally increases serum albumin concentrations by 5 g/l.

Unless buffy coat-depleted red cells are used, microaggregate filters are advisable during massive transfusion (but not when platelets are being administered).[13]

5 BLOOD TRANSFUSION POLICIES

(1) *For massive uncontrolled haemorrhage*, where blood is being lost at a rate equal to that which can be replaced, there is no point in attempting to replace blood components to maintain haemostatic competence. Major blood vessel bleeding must be stemmed surgically. Stored whole blood, red cell concentrates, synthetic colloids or crystalloids should be used to maintain blood volume and pressure and haemoglobin/haematocrit values at least above 10.0 g.dl/0.30. Use of fresh blood, plasma or platelets in this setting would be pointless. Blood replacement needs exceeding 0.2 l/h are usually taken to constitute a clear indication for surgical investigation of the cause of the haemorrhage.

(2) When the rate of blood loss is substantially lessened and obvious major vessel bleeding is being, or has been, attended to, it becomes worthwhile attempting to rectify any haematological abnormalities. Platelet counts and coagulation tests should be performed as pointers to the scale of intervention required.

Component therapy is particularly indicated where:

(1) Bleeding is presumed to be due to deficient haemostasis rather than from major vessel injuries. This conclusion should be supported by both clinical and laboratory results.

(2) A specific need for components, e.g. platelets or cryoprecipitate, is disclosed by laboratory results but red cell replacement is not required.

Disseminated intravascular coagulation necessitates more energetic therapy. Platelet concentrates (one pack per 10 kg), fresh frozen plasma (12 ml/kg) or cryoprecipitate (1–1.5 packs per 10 kg) should be given to replace deficiencies of haemostatic factors, particularly fibrinogen, Factor VIII and platelets.

Fresh whole blood versus component therapy for replacement of massive haemorrhage

Massive blood loss has traditionally been recognized as a situation in which the calls for the use of fresh blood as a means of preventing or correcting haemostatic failure have been most strident. The popularity of the modern, and fully justified, practice for component therapy has, to a large extent, coincided with the concept that use of fresh whole blood (e.g. transfused unrefrigerated and soon after collection) is an outdated non-specific and wasteful practice. If issued prior to completion of microbiological test results the patient would be placed at further and quite unjustified extra risk of infection. It is almost certainly true that the extraordinary faith sometimes placed by the theatre team in the elixir of life, as provided by warm freshly collected blood, is misplaced. This area of contention is likely to remain for some time to come; however, the tensions between surgical teams and haematologists during these stressful episodes should be minimized by the provision of a prompt investigational service accompanied by adequate therapeutic support, professional interest and advice.

REFERENCES

1 Counts, R.B., Haisch, C., Simon, T.L., Maxwell, N.G., Heimbach, D.M. and Carrico, C.J. (1979) Hemostasis in massively transfused trauma patients. *Ann. Surg.*, **190:** 91–100.

2 Mannucci, P.M., Federici, A.B. and Sirchia, G. (1982) Hemostasis testing during massive blood replacement: a study of 172 cases. *Vox Sang.*, **42:** 113–123.

3 Noe, D.A., Graham, S.M., Luff, R. and Sohmer, P. (1982) Platelet counts during rapid massive transfusion. *Transfusion*, **22:** 392–395.

4 Russell, W.J. and Tunbridge, L.J. (1982) Platelet counts in stored donor blood. *Anaesth. Intens. Care*, **10:** 271–273.

5 Reed, R.L., II, Heimbach, D.M., Counts, R.B. *et al.* (1986) Prophylactic platelet administration during massive transfusion: a prospective, randomised, double-blind clinical study. *Ann. Surg.*, **203:** 40–48.

6 Ferrara, A., MacArthur, J.D., Wright, H.K. *et al.* (1990) Hypothermia and acidosis worsen coagulopathy in the patient requiring massive transfusion. *Am. J. Surg.*, **160:** 515–518.

7 Lesile, S.D. and Toy, P.T. (1991) Laboratory hemostatic abnormalities in massively transfused patients given red blood cells and crystalloid. *Am. J. Clin. Pathol.*, **96:** 770–773.

8 Nilsson, L., Hedner, U., Nilsson, I.M. and Robertson, B. (1983) Shelf-life of bank blood and stored plasma with special reference to coagulation factors. *Transfusion*, **23:** 377–381.

9 Lovric, V.A. (1984) Alterations in blood components during storage and their clinical significance. *Anaesth. Intens. Care*, **12:** 246–251.

10 Wilson, R.F., Dulchavsky, S.A., Soullier, G. and Beckman, B. (1987) Problems with 20 or more blood transfusions in 24 hours. *Am. Surg.*, **53:** 410–417.

11 Napier, J.A.F. (1980) Effect of age and 2,3-DPG content of transfused blood on serum erythropoietin. *Vox Sang.*, **39:** 318–321.

12 Uhl, L., Pacini, D. and Kruskall, M.S. (1992) A comparative study of blood warmer performance. *Anesthesiology*, **77:** 1022–1028.

13 Wenz, B. (1993) Massive blood transfusion: the blood bank perspective. *Transfusion Sci.*, **14:** 353–359.

13
Blood Transfusion and the Adult Respiratory Distress Syndrome

1 DEFINITION

Adult respiratory distress syndrome (ARDS, shock lung syndrome) is now an uncommon, but nevertheless serious, complication of major trauma and transfusion. It should, however, be remembered that ARDS can also occur as a consequence of a variety of severe metabolic, toxaemic or allergic disorders which may exist as complications in the transfused patient.[1,2] The clinical syndrome comprises:

- Respiratory distress.
- Increased lung compliance (stiffness) which necessitates a greater energy expenditure to maintain ventilation.
- Hypoxaemia which is not relieved by oxygen.
- Bilateral diffuse consolidation shown by X-ray examination.

There may also be concurrent failure of hepatic, renal, gastrointestinal or cardiovascular function. These features together constitute the syndrome currently described as *multi-organ system failure* or sometimes as *septic shock*.

The pulmonary functional disturbances stem from widespread *interstitial and alveolar oedema coalescing to form large areas of lung that are perfused with blood but cannot be ventilated.* Shunting of blood through these areas results in substantial admixture of desaturated 'venous' blood into that returning to the systemic circulation. As a result the *arterial oxygen tension is reduced.* The primary abnormality in ARDS appears to be *damage to pulmonary capillary endothelial cells* which greatly increases their permeability to proteins. Leakage of protein leads to loss of the transcapillary colloid oncotic pressure gradient; the water diffusion that follows causes flooding of the interstitium and alveoli. The causative mechanisms of pulmonary endothelial damage and indeed the generalized capillary endothelial damage responsible for ARDS and end organ failure are highly complex. Irrespective of the apparent precipitating cause, e.g. shock, sepsis, burn injury or massive blood transfusion, the pathological process seems to centre around damage to the monocyte macrophage system cells, which in turn become activated and produce an exaggerated inflammatory response.

Initiators of the macrophage response which have been recognized include:

(1) *Endotoxin*: this is most obviously aetiological when sepsis is clinically apparent but is also likely to be an injurious agent in covert microbiological infections or from gastrointestinal bacteria no longer constrained within the bowel lumen as the mucosal barrier becomes damaged by ischaemia.

(2) *Complement activation products* either from classical or alternate pathway activation. $C3_a$ and $C5_a$ are recognized to directly provoke the monocyte macrophage inflammatory response but also have a direct damaging effect on neutrophils[3] (see below).

The macrophage activation response appears to involve release of a series of cytokine inflammatory mediators of which tumour necrosis factor (TNF) and interleukins 1 and 6 (IL-l, IL-6) are examples. These cytokines, presumably produced in pathological excess, as well as complement activation products and bacterial endotoxin, appear to mediate the widespread tissue damage. Mechanisms of this damage include:

(a) *Endothelial injury*: this increases capillary wall permeability exposing *collagen* and initiating contact activation systems and fibrinolytic systems.

(b) *Disseminated intravascular coagulation (DIC)*: this can occur directly as a consequence of prolonged *hypotensive shock.* The thrombotic process leads to progressive microvascular occlusion which causes further damage to the capillary circulation. Local release of fibrinolytic (proteolytic) enzymes from the microthrombi may also contribute to the further capillary damage.

(c) *Platelet activation*: this further enhances the pathological thrombotic process.

(d) *Neutrophil damage*:[4] activated and damaged neutrophils, high numbers of which are normally lodged in the marginal pool of the pulmonary circulation, are thought to play a dominant role in the pulmonary component (ARDS) of multi-organ system failure. Damaged neutrophils aggregate and lodge as emboli in the pulmonary capillaries. These then liberate destructive proteases or superoxide radicals which are also toxic to capillary endothelial cells.

1.1 Blood Transfusion as a Cause of Adult Respiratory Distress Syndrome

Although ARDS is now recognized to represent the end result of damage caused by a highly complex pathologically exaggerated inflammatory response to injury, there is also concern over the possible role of blood transfusion in the severity of its manifestation. Arguments revolve around:

(1) The importance of the microaggregates of stored blood in disrupting lung perfusion through multiple microembolization.
(2) Whether crystalloid infusions, by lowering plasma colloid osmotic pressure, enhance the transcapillary fluid flux and thereby predispose to ARDS.
(3) Whether albumin, by maintaining plasma colloid osmotic pressure, facilitates retention of plasma volume and water, prevents fluid loss into the interstitium and protects against the development of ARDS.
(4) Whether, in contrast, leakage of transfused albumin through damaged capillaries into interstitial fluid reduces the colloid osmotic pressure gradient and thereby creates an intractable state of pulmonary oedema.

These arguments are considered below.

1.2 Microaggregates in Stored Blood[5–7]

Storage of blood in any anticoagulant results in progressive accumulation of aggregated particles of fibrin, leucocytes and platelets. These particles vary in size from $10\,\mu m$ upwards, but the majority are too small to be trapped by the usual $170\,\mu m$ mesh filters present in most standard blood administration sets. Development of aggregates begins shortly after collection and increases with storage time. Within the first 5 days particles are small but numerous; as time goes on their size increases, as does the total weight of filterable material, which reaches around $0.5\,g$ dry weight by 35 days of storage. The microaggregate content of stored blood has generally been assessed by determination of the weight of material trapped on filters or, alternatively, by measuring the amount of pressure required to force blood containing microaggregates through a $20\,\mu m$ screen filter (screen filtration pressure). Newer techniques have utilized optical or laser light-scattering methods to measure the numbers of microaggregate particles present in stored blood.

1.3 Microaggregate Embolization

The initial reports of multiple emboli, histologically identical to the microaggregates present in stored blood, in the lungs of massively transfused battle casualties offered persuasive evidence of their aetiological role in ARDS. Morbidity and mortality correlated with the numbers of transfused blood units but also, not surprisingly, with the degree of initial injury and the severity of other complications. There is, however, no evidence that microaggregates in stored blood

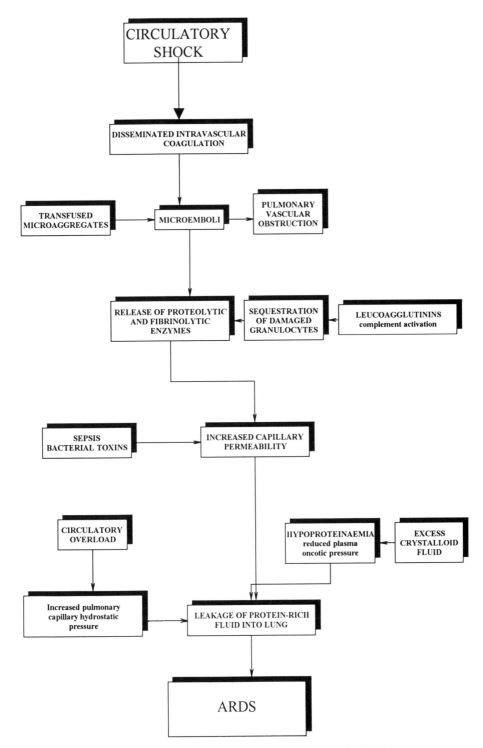

Figure 1   Relationship between circulatory shock transfusion and ARDS

present such a serious risk to lung function during massive transfusion that blood administration should in any way be curtailed. The apposite observation that bleeding patients were more likely to die from the blood they did not receive restored a degree of balance to the argument being propounded that blood transfusion was, in its own right, seriously contributing to avoidable morbidity and mortality.

Minor lung dysfunction as a result of microembolization can certainly be demonstrated by sophisticated pulmonary function studies even in routine surgical patients receiving modest amounts of blood. In the overwhelming majority of patients these pass completely clinically unnoticed, are of transient duration and do not provide a justification for expensive prophylactic measures.

Microaggregate filters undoubtedly remove this debris from transfused blood and, from human studies, probably reduce the incidence of measurable pulmonary functional abnormalities in massively transfused patients.

The clinical risk of ARDS in most studies involving more modestly transfused surgical patients is small and remains unchanged by the use of filters. For moderate blood replacement (up to six or seven units of blood) microaggregate blood filters have not, in the main, been shown to significantly affect pulmonary function and certainly have not reduced the already small risk of clinically evident lung problems. Despite the relative paucity of data regarding their protective role in preventing lung damage, conflicting opinions are, nevertheless, firmly expressed regarding the indications for their use.[8]

1.4 Use of Microaggregate Filters

Removal of microaggregates can be efficiently accomplished by filtration of transfused blood through screen (woven polyester mesh) or depth (packed synthetic fibre) microaggregate filters. These replace the standard administration set filter which has a 170 μm filter mesh. Screen filters usually have a mesh size of around 40 μm and remove particles by physical obstruction. Depth filters are variously claimed to remove particles in excess of 20–40 μm and work by adsorption of microaggregates. In view of the paucity of evidence for the benefit of microaggregate blood filtration for other than massive transfusions, it seems reasonable to discourage their use until at least 50% blood volume replacement has occurred with conventional red cell components. Buffy coat-depleted red cells in optimal additive solution contain so little filterable material that microaggregate filters are unnecessary. It is believed that fresh platelets will be removed by depth filters although stored platelet concentrates, possibly because of a storage-related functional defect, appear to pass through filters without loss. Microaggregate filters have several drawbacks. Microaggregate filtration adds to the expense of transfusion. Filter blockage and slow infusion rates usually necessitate a replacement of the filters after every four to five blood units. During emergency resuscitation, the impediment to blood flow may be of greater consequence to the patient than an unquantifiable risk from microaggregate damage. There is no clear evidence to support the routine use of filters during the small red cell replacement transfusions commonly given during the neonatal period (see chapter 20). Their use during large-scale paediatric transfusions (around 60 ml/kg) or for clinically more complex problems should follow the same guidelines as for adults. Filters with small priming volumes are available for paediatric use.

1.5 The Importance of Plasma Colloid Osmotic Pressure and the Influence of Albumin or Crystalloid Infusion[9-13]

The choice between the use of crystalloids or albumin solution for resuscitation has proved extremely difficult to resolve. Crystalloids are cheap, easily available in unlimited quantities and are effective for blood volume restoration. As disadvantages it is recognized that they cause extracellular fluid accumulation, lower the plasma colloid osmotic pressure and might, though this is debated, predispose to pulmonary oedema. Albumin is expensive, but it maintains colloid osmotic pressure and should, on theoretical grounds, protect against pulmonary oedema and ARDS.

ARDS is almost certainly multifactorial in origin; there is, in fact, considerable doubt as to whether the choice of non-red cell resuscitation fluids in any way affects the likelihood of its occurrence. The fact that no clear consensus has emerged amongst many that have studied this problem possibly suggests that the plasma albumin concentration is certainly not a major determinant in the appearance of clinically significant pulmonary disorders. The debate is largely concerned with whether albumin, which should in theory maintain plasma colloid osmotic pressure and protect against fluid egress from pulmonary capillaries, does in fact have this effect. Proponents of this view believe that a reduction in plasma albumin and oncotic pressure following crystalloid infusion permits a drift of salt and water into extracellular fluid spaces, thereby contributing to pulmonary dysfunction.

The basic facts regarding the differences between crystalloids and albumin in affecting serum albumin levels, colloid osmotic pressure, extracellular fluid expansion and tissue oedema are not in doubt. What is unclear is the relevance of these to the appearance of the symptom complex of ARDS. *Particularly vulnerable patients in whom this choice might be important are the elderly and malnourished, and those debilitated or with renal failure or pre-existing pulmonary insufficiency.* Uncertainty surrounds the significance of low plasma colloid osmotic pressures (COP) when found in transfused patients. The low oncotic pressure seen in experimental and many clinical circumstances is not usually associated with pulmonary damage and it is by no means agreed that it has a major causative role in ARDS. It is likely that low COP would lead to fluid loss only when combined with pulmonary capillary endothelial damage. In that sense the maintenance of plasma COP can only be seen as worthwhile insofar as it might be a safety factor raising the threshold at which pulmonary oedema can develop for other reasons. To add further complication to the argument, data have been produced to show that albumin, far from being protective, may sometimes be harmful in this context. Transfused albumin has been shown to leak through damaged capillary membranes and cause a reduction in the oncotic pressure differential between the plasma and interstitial fluid. The resulting protein-rich oedema fluid may be even more difficult to shift than before. Fortunately the lymphatic drainage system is

Table 1 Transfusion and ARDS

Prompt treatment of shock by effective resuscitation
Awareness of high-risk patients
Appropriate use of microaggregate filters
Supplement crystalloids with albumin to maintain COP greater
    than 20 mmHg, albumin greater than 30 g/l or serum protein
    greater than 50 g/l
Avoid circulatory overloading

usually capable of removing these protein-rich fluid transudates. Failure of this normal function of the lymphatic system, coupled with increased permeability of the alveolar capillary endothelial cells, is probably an important determinant of ARDS. Clinical observations have shown that patients given albumin need longer periods of ventilatory support and higher levels of inspired oxygen tension to maintain adequate arterial oxygen saturation and this is assumed to be indicative of a degree of ARDS.

In general it seems that the balance of support now favours use of crystalloids for the early stages of resuscitation after blood loss. Albumin solutions do not seem to confer the advantages at first anticipated and certainly have not been clinically shown to protect the lungs from ARDS. Albumin infusions as well as synthetic colloids do, however, lessen the overall volume of fluid required for volume replacement compared with the use of crystalloids, although this might appear to be an expensive remedy for a clinical problem of debatable significance. It is, however, widely believed that albumin or synthetic colloids in some form should be used in combination with crystalloids to prevent undue lowering of the colloid osmotic pressure. This goal may be of greater importance for patients with pre-existing plasma protein deficiencies.

2 MANAGEMENT OF ADULT RESPIRATORY DISTRESS SYNDROME/MULTI-SYSTEM ORGAN FAILURE

This depends on skilful transfusion therapy of acute and massive blood loss as discussed in chapters 11 and 12, and also on cardiorespiratory supportive measures which are beyond the scope of this book. In general, severe ARDS will require increased inspired oxygen tensions to maintain pO_2 above 60–70 mmHg and also mechanical ventilation with positive end expiratory pressure which assists in the inflation of waterlogged alveoli.

Cardiac output, oxygen transport and utilization studies assist in the transfusion management of patients with septic shock. For example, red cell supplements can be used as one means of stepwise increasing oxygen transport, while simultaneously confirming oxygen utilization shows a proportionate increase. Using such an approach it has been shown that some patients benefit from modest increases of haemoglobin in the 8.0–10.0 g/dl range.[13]

The recent recognition of the important endothelial damaging effect of cytokine inflammatory mediators in ARDS and multi-system organ failure has led to great interest in the possibilities of neutralizing their pathological effects. Monoclonal antibody against endotoxin (anti-HA-1A) has, for example, been used in patients with septic shock. While no universally convincing proof of benefit has emerged, there is evidence that certain subgroups of patients, e.g. those with evidence of Gram-negative infection, particularly when shocked on admission, do show a reduction in mortality rates. Monoclonal antibodies against TNF and IL-1 receptor are also under investigation for use in similar circumstances.

REFERENCES

1 Sinclair, S. and Singer, M. (1993) Intensive care: reviews in medicine. *Postgrad. Med. J.*, **69**: 340–358.
2 Leading article (1986) Adult respiratory distress syndrome. *Lancet*, **i**: 301–303.
3 Williamson, L.M., Sheppard, K., Davies, J.M. and Fletcher, J. (1986) Neutrophils are involved in the increased vascular permeability produced by activated complement in man. *Br. J. Haematol.*, **64**: 375–384.
4 Windsor, A.C.J., Mullen, P.G., Fowler, A.A. and Sugerman, H.J. (1993) Role of the neutrophil in adult respiratory distress syndrome. *Br. J. Surg.*, **80**: 10–17.
5 Snyder, E.L. and Bookbinder, M. (1983) Role of microaggregate blood filtration in clinical medicine. *Transfusion*, **23**: 460–467.
6 Symposium on microfiltration of blood and pulmonary functions (1980) *Vox Sang.*, **39**: 46–59.
7 Bredenberg, C.E., Collins, J.A., Fulton, R.L., McNamara, J.J., Solis, R.T. and Walker, B.D. (1977) Does a relationship exist between massive blood transfusions and the adult respiratory distress syndrome? If so, what are the best preventive measures? International forum. *Vox Sang.*, **32**: 311–320.
8 International Forum (1986) When is the microfiltration of whole blood and red cell concentrates essential. When is it superfluous? *Vox Sang.*, **50**: 54–64.
9 Lowe, R.J., Moss, G.S., Jilek, J. and Levine, H.D. (1977) Crystalloid vs colloid in the etiology of pulmonary failure after trauma: a randomised trial in man. *Surgery*, **81**: 676–683.
10 Weaver, D.W., Ledgerwood, A.M., Lucas, C.E., Higgins, R., Bouwman, D.L. and Johnson, S.D. (1978) Pulmonary effects of albumin resuscitation for severe hypovolemic shock. *Arch. Surg.*, **113**: 387–392.
11 Virgilio, R.W., Rice, C.L., Smith, D.E. *et al.* (1979) Crystalloid vs colloid resuscitation: is one better? *Surgery*, **85**: 129–139.
12 Shires, G.T., Peitzman, A.B., Albert, S.A., Illner, H., Silane, M.F. and Perry, M.O. (1983) Response of extravascular lung water to intraoperative fluids. *Ann. Surg.*, **197**: 515–519.
13 Steffes, C.P., Bender, J.S. and Levison, M.A. (1991) Blood transfusion and oxygen consumption in surgical sepsis. *Crit. Care Med.*, **19**: 512–517.

14

Cardiopulmonary Bypass Surgery

1   INTRODUCTION

The specialty of cardiac surgery has traditionally placed heavy demands on blood transfusion services for all forms of components. This situation seems likely to continue unabated as the emphasis shifts from a workload of valve replacements and repair of congenital defects towards addressing the potentially enormous demand for coronary bypass grafts as treatment for ischaemic heart disease. Fortunately, cardiac surgery teams have become progressively more economical in their use of blood; typical figures of 10 or more units per case in the early 1970s have now been reduced to around one-half to one-third of that amount.[1,2]

Enormous advances in blood conservation techniques, for example, pre-operative haemodilution, red cell salvage and use of pharmacological agents (see chapter 15) can be applied during cardiac surgery to further reduce transfusion needs. Blood replacement needs reported in surveys clearly vary according to case mix; however, an American study showed the greatest variation to occur between hospitals, suggesting that locally prevailing historical practices, attitudes and knowledge have the greatest influence on blood usage.[3] Several surveys suggest use of plasma or platelets on a routine prophylaxis basis or for poorly substantiated reasons, to be not infrequent.[1,2]

That there is scope for further improvement has been shown by the demonstration that even cardiac surgical procedures on Jehovah's Witnesses[4] can be performed without blood. Improved surgical techniques and the lower frequency of massive transfusions have now removed the need for fresh blood or components in any form as a routine requirement. However, despite the undoubted advances in surgery and transfusion management, around 3–5% of patients suffer severe haemorrhage and in many cases reoperation is necessary in an attempt to stop the bleeding. These patients are at risk from the added problems of massive transfusion (chapter 12) and in particular, because of the bypass circulation-induced neutrophil damage (see section 1.3), are prone to respiratory damage and multisystem organ failure (see chapter 13).

Cardiopulmonary bypass (CPB) surgery presents a combination of special circumstances which may influence transfusion management. These principally include:

(1) Use of a large-volume extracorporeal circulation.
(2) Exposure of the circulating blood to large areas of foreign surfaces.
(3) Controlled haemodilution.
(4) Exposure to blood–gas interfaces.
(5) Mechanical trauma of recycled blood.
(6) Heparinization.
(7) Hypothermia.

In addition to the particular problems posed by cardiac surgery there are, of course, the potential risks of any of the complications that may follow massive blood loss and replacement.

1.1 Pre-operative Condition of the Patient

(1) *Pre-operative coagulation* and *platelet studies* are commonly performed and may show a high incidence of abnormalities. Unless particularly pronounced these abnormalities do not seem to be predictive of increased post-operative loss.[5]

Of rather greater importance in forecasting the likelihood of excessive blood loss is an abnormal *clinical history* or *symptomatic evidence of a haemorrhagic tendency*. Despite this, the routine pre-operative assessment of haemostatic function, in many surgical centres, includes at least the determination of:

• Platelet count.
• Partial thromboplastin time.
• Prothrombin time.

In addition, bleeding time measurements, fibrinogen assay and tests of fibrinolytic performance are sometimes recommended.

Excessive bleeding is particularly liable in patients with *liver disease* including those with congestion or cirrhosis secondary to *tricuspid valve damage*.

(2) Patients receiving oral *anticoagulation* may have this replaced by heparin over several days preceding surgery. If this is considered likely to make stable anticoagulant control too difficult, fresh frozen plasma, given just prior to surgery, can be used to titrate the prothrombin time to an acceptable level for the immediate post-operative period. Aspirin or other cyclooxygenase inhibitors affecting platelet function may also have been taken pre-operatively by

patients undergoing myocardial revascularization procedures. Their effects may persist for up to a week and have been shown to be associated with higher peri-operative blood losses.[6]

(3) Patients with *erythrocytosis* due to *cyanotic congenital cardiac defects* (e.g. tetralogy of Fallot) are liable to have abnormalities of their haemostatic mechanism and excessive operative bleeding.[7-9] The high blood viscosity also adversely affects tissue oxygen supply. Pre-operative venesection to reduce the haematocrit is advised or, as an alternative, a greater degree of haemodilution is employed so that the intra-operative haemoglobin is lowered to the same extent (below 10.0 g/dl) as for non-polycythaemic patients.[9] In view of their high operative mortality, cyanotic polycythaemic children frequently have a preliminary shunting operation performed to relieve hypoxia and reduce polycythaemia so that surgical correction may be performed more safely at a later date.[7]

(4) In common with many surgical procedures *repeat operations* are frequently associated with excessive blood loss.

1.2 Bypass Procedure

Priming solutions and haemodilution

Crystalloid solutions (e.g. physiological saline with or without dextrose, Ringer's lactate solution) or crystalloid supplemented with albumin or plasma are now preferred for priming the extracorporeal circulation. Albumin is sometimes included in the priming solution cocktail in the expectation that it will be absorbed onto plastic surfaces and improve biocompatibility of the CPB circuit lining. It has not, however been possible to substantiate this benefit.[10] Heparin, mannitol, bicarbonate or dextrans are sometimes also added to the priming solutions.[11] The former practice of using whole blood to fill the extracorporeal circulation was found to result in less satisfactory perfusion, a higher rate of renal and pulmonary complications and larger amounts of mechanical damage to blood components. Crystalloid–colloid combinations are now used instead; these are generally administered at doses of around 20 ml/kg with the objective of reducing the haemoglobin and haematocrit to below 10.0 g/dl and 0.30, respectively. Calculations, taking into account the extracorporeal volume (1500–2000 ml) and the patient's predicted blood volume (70 ml/kg) allow estimations of the likely haematocrit during surgery. The haematocrit (Hct) will change according to the relation:

$$\text{Hct during bypass} = \text{Initial Hct} \times \frac{\text{Blood volume}}{\text{Blood volume} + \text{Extracorporeal volume}}$$

This relationship will be disturbed by loss of some of the transfused fluid into the extracellular space and there will, therefore, be some degree of underestimation of the haematocrit. Red cell concentrates should be administered before or during bypass to maintain a haematocrit of around 0.25.

Heparinization

This is required to prevent coagulation in the extracorporeal circuit. Doses of 200–300 IU (or 2–3 mg) per kilogram body weight are given either using standardized dosage regimens or, preferably, on the basis of clotting time measurements. The *activated whole-blood clotting time* (ACT) is popular for this purpose and can be performed as and when required in the operating theatre. This test is a version of the whole-blood clotting time in which contact activation is standardized and the endpoint can be determined automatically. As with the whole-blood clotting times, 2.5-fold prolongation (usually equivalent to a measured clotting time of 400 seconds) over pre-heparinization times is regarded as acceptable. If the clotting time is performed both before and immediately following heparinization, a dose–response curve can be constructed which enables an estimate to be made of the heparin concentration in subsequent samples. This is useful when the dose of protamine for heparin neutralization is to be calculated.

Heparin neutralization

This takes place following bypass and is accomplished by protamine administration in doses of the order of 1–2.0 mg/100 IU of heparin given intravenously slowly over 10 minutes. Precise dosage is best determined by calculations from the results of ACT tests or from heparin titration assays.[12]

Under-treatment leads to a risk of bleeding from heparin rebound, which can be a dangerous cause of post-operative bleeding.

1.3 Transfusion Problems During Cardiac Surgery

Excessive blood loss

During bypass, the haemostatic status is entirely determined by the level of heparinization. Excessive bleeding following bypass or, later, during recovery occurs in some patients and presents diagnostic and therapeutic problems. Generally, 'excessive bleeding' is defined as:

- Continued losses of around 200 ml/h.
- Or more dramatic onset of bleeding at any time.
- Or generalized oozing from all sites.

Laboratory tests must help in decisions as to whether reoperation or corrective therapy is required. The following haematological diagnostic possibilities must be considered:

(1) *Heparin rebound* indicating the need for further protamine.[12] This phase of relapsing hypocoagulability, usually 1–1.5 hours after apparently successful neutralization of heparin, has been ascribed to reappearance of heparin from the tissues into the circulating blood. Heparin rebound is now an uncommon problem with modern protocols for heparin titration and neutralization.

(2) *Dilution of coagulation factors* through extensive use of red cells and asanguineous fluids. In practice, as discussed in chapter 13, coagulation factor dilution is rarely the predominant cause of a bleeding problem.

(3) *Thrombocytopenia* and/or *platelet functional disorders*: for reasons discussed below, some alterations of this nature are to be expected. Severe depletion causing bleeding and requiring treatment is unusual.

(4) Unrecognized *pre-existing haemostatic defects*.

(5) *Disseminated intravascular coagulation* and/or *fibrinolysis*: Some of the coagulation changes following bypass are dilutional in origin although other influences must be operating since levels of all factors are not equally affected. Factor V shows the most substantial reduction; others are not depressed to clinically significant levels and all show recovery over the first 24–48 hours.[8,13]

It is obviously important to note whether the patient has received pre-operative *vitamin K antagonist anticoagulants. Disseminated intravascular coagulation* and *fibrinolysis* may occur for the same reasons as in other massively transfused surgical patients. Thromboplastic or fibrinolysis-activating substances released from damaged tissues may combine in their damaging effects on haemostasis. The beneficial effects of aprotinin in reducing blood loss seem to suggest that excessive fibrinolysis has been under-recognized as a cause of excessive bleeding.

Thrombocytopenia or *platelet functional abnormalities* (see below) are also likely contributing factors towards abnormal bleeding. Management of irrepressible bleeding following cardiac surgery is acknowledged to be fraught with tensions in the race against time to identify both cause and remedy. There is understandable reluctance to undertake re-thoracotomy when the possibility of haemostatic failure has not been convincingly excluded. It is in these circumstances that pressures to use 'fresh blood', even delivered warm from the most accessible donors, are sometimes sought. The approach to management of escalating blood loss is as for massive transfusion (chapter 12). It has been clearly shown that prophylactic fresh blood transfusions or prophylactic platelet concentrates do not affect transfusion requirements, post-operative blood losses or haemostatic parameters.[14] Whether a separate case can be made for surgery in infants remains to be resolved. One study has shown use of relatively fresh whole blood (< 48 hours post collection) to result in less post-operative blood loss but only where complex surgery was undertaken.[15]

Laboratory analysis of suspected abnormalities may include:

- Heparin assay/protamine titration.
- Thrombin time, reptilase time.
- Fibrinogen and FDP assay.
- Platelet count and bleeding time.
- Prothrombin and partial thromboplastin time.

Treatment of abnormal findings (in bleeding patients) requires combinations of blood components, e.g. platelet concentrates (1 pack/10 kg), fresh frozen plasma (12–15 ml/kg), cryoprecipitate (1–1.5 packs/10 kg), depending on individual circumstances.

Abnormal results do not necessarily indicate bleeding and should not automatically mandate treatment. Normal results (or results showing only insignificant abnormalities) in excessively bleeding patients point to the need for reoperation to secure haemostasis.

Damage to blood in the bypass circuit

CPB procedures expose the blood to unusual mechanical stresses as well as prolonged contact with foreign surfaces. Contact activation of the coagulation system and platelets is a normal physiological response although it contributes to haemostatic failure in the CPB setting. Early models of roller pumps appeared to cause mechanical *red cell haemolysis* although this problem has been minimized by improvements in design. Red cells are also particularly easily damaged by manoeuvres such as suction recovery of shed blood (the injurious effect seems to depend upon the frothing of air and blood mixtures). Oxygenation units also cause some lysis, the more commonly used bubble type being rather worse than membrane oxygenators. The difference between these two systems is small and may be unimportant compared with the amount of damage caused by the blood pumps which becomes worse with prolonged perfusion.[16] Platelets are also damaged by similar mechanisms.[17] Probably the most clinically significant problem arising during CPB is the *platelet functional defect* resulting from activation following repeated contact with foreign surface materials, or possibly also from ADP released from damaged red cells. It has been shown that aggregation responses to ADP, ristocetin and collagen are reduced and bleeding times may also be prolonged following bypass procedures.[18-20]

The increases found in plasma levels of platelet factor 4 and β-thromboglobulin may be indicative of α-granule release. Platelet functional impairment is supposedly proportional to the duration of CPB; its effects, however, are temporary and recovery is largely complete within an hour or so following surgery. *Platelet counts commonly fall* to around 50% preoperative values and may remain reduced for 4–5 days.[8,13] This reduction does not necessarily indicate a risk of bleeding or, on its own account, require correction. However, bleeding during or post bypass, when platelet counts are not reduced to levels normally considered significant (e.g. 100×10^9/l) is usually taken to indicate the possibility of platelet functional defect and to justify platelet concentrate replacement. Treatment restores abnormal bleeding times as well as clinical haemostasis. Attempts have been made to use desmopressin to bolster von Willebrand factor and hence platelet function or, alternatively, prostacyclin to protect against foreign surface-induced activation damage. Neither approach has yielded convincing benefits.

Hypoproteinaemia, low plasma oncotic pressure and tissue oedema resulting from use of crystalloids in the extracorporeal circuit

In the absence of pre-existing pulmonary disease, and if tissue perfusion is adequate, the transient period or reduced plasma oncotic pressure appears to be unimportant. If necessary, oedema formation can be minimized by inclusion of colloids in the solution used for haemodilution.[21]

Microaggregate formation in the extracorporeal circulation

This was a serious problem during early extracorporeal procedures. Thrombo-plastic agents from damaged blood components and extensive contact activation by foreign surface materials combine to cause microcoagula and emboli in blood being returned to the systemic circulation. This showed clinically as multiple organ dysfunction, cerebral, retinal and renal effects being particularly evident. The problem is now controlled by microaggregate filtration of blood before reinfu-sion.

Abnormal complement activation[22,23]

CPB surgery, extracorporeal membrane oxygenation and haemodialysis are each characterized by prolonged exposure of the blood to the foreign surfaces of the plastic disposable equipment. In both conditions it appears that activation of the complement system occurs; this has been linked with neutrophil injury, neutropenia and, in the case of CPB surgery, to multiple organ dysfunction as a result of sequestration of very large numbers of terminally damaged neutrophils throughout body tissues. Extracorporeal circuits appear to cause complement activation—whether by classic or alternative pathway is so far not fully resolved; depressed haemolytic complement (CH_{50}) capacity has been shown as well as some evidence of activation of complement components (C3d, C5a and Ba). Neutrophils can be shown to be damaged *in vitro* by these products and similar abnormalities *in vivo* have been found. For the same reasons, neutropenia is sometimes seen during haemodialysis and, very occasionally, extensive leuco-sequestration occurs in the lungs where liberation of granulocyte proteases causes respiratory distress syndrome (see chapter 13). This cannot happen while on bypass since the lungs are not perfused, but neutrophil sequestration and tissue damage (due to C3–C5–C9 conversion) are seen occasionally in other par-enchymal organs and in the lungs following re-establishment of circulation.

Hypothermia and cold antibodies

Hypothermia, which entails cooling of the body to around 28 °C and sometimes to even lower temperatures by means of heat exchangers incorporated into the bypass circuit, reduces tissue oxygen requirements and prevents ischaemic damage. The use of hypothermia is probably the only justification for performing room temperature compatibility testing (see chapter 25, section 2.3). In considering hypothermic surgery for patients with cold antibodies, an important fact to be determined is the highest temperature at which the antibody can be shown to react *in vitro*. It may be possible to conclude that the antibody will be harmless[24] or that haemolysis will not occur if the degree of hypothermia is limited.[25] Plas-mapheresis has been used for one patient with cold agglutinins.[26] Very cold (e.g. 4 °C) cardioplegic electrolyte solutions, used to prevent myocardial ischaemia during bypass, will cause autoagglutination in the presence of high-titre cold agglutinins, but the problem has been shown to be surmountable by pre-flushing the myocardial vascular bed with warmed (37 °C) solution to remove red cells.[27]

1.4 Blood Conservation Measures During Cardiac Surgery

CPB surgery is one area where there has been great interest in techniques for reducing use of blood and blood components. The main principles of this are covered in chapter 15. Approaches of particular value in cardiac surgery include:

(1) *Return of blood to the circulation following termination of the bypass procedure*: the bypass circuit contains an important volume of red cells which can be retrieved for return to the patient's circulation.[28] Following bypass a brisk diuresis should ensue as crystalloids are lost and the haematocrit will rise as the hypervolaemia is corrected. Haematocrits of 0.28–0.32 are acceptable; lower values will again require red cell concentrate supplementation. As a result of the hypervolaemia, there may initially be a restricted need for intra-venous fluids, but as this period is particularly characterized by haemody-namic instability, hypotensive episodes may occur which will require red cells, albumin or plasma according to individual circumstances.[29]

(2) *Collection of autologous platelet-rich plasma prior to surgery*: for patients not pre-treated with aspirin this approach has some rationale as a means of protecting the patient's platelets from the damaging effect of CPB circulation. Whether this is a beneficial and cost-effective measure for prevention and management of the minority of patients who develop serious haemorrhage related to platelet dysfunction remains to be seen.

(3) *Pharmacological approaches to reducing blood loss*: the most energetic attempts to reduce surgical blood loss by pharmacological means have been pioneered in CPB surgery. The principal agents examined include desmopressin (DDAVP),[30,31] prostacyclin (PGI$_2$)[32] and aprotinin.[33] Aprotinin used *prophylacti-cally* was first shown to curtail blood loss in high-risk patients. Subsequently, it was shown to be effective for reducing blood loss in low-risk routine proce-dures and also aids in the control of established peri-operative haemorrhage. Pharmacological strategies for controlling blood loss are beginning to have a more widespread application in surgery and are considered more fully in chapter 15.

(4) *Fibrin sealant* (see chapter 7, section 2.5): fibrin sealant can assist haemostasis when applied topically to openly bleeding exposed surfaces.

REFERENCES

1 Russell, G.N., Peterson, S., Harper, S.J. and Fox, M.A. (1988) Homologous blood use and conservation techniques for cardiac surgery in the United Kingdom. *Br. Med. J.*, **297**: 1390–1391.
2 Goodnough, L.T., Johston, M.F.M. and Toy, P.T.C. (1991) Variation in transfusion prac-tice in coronary bypass surgery. *JAMA*, **265**: 86–90.
3 Surgenor, D.M., Wallace, E.L., Churchill, W.H., Hao, S.H.S., Chapman, R.H. and Collins,

J.J. (1992) Red cell transfusions in coronary artery bypass surgery (DRGs 106 and 107). *Transfusion*, **32**: 458–464.

4 Sandiford, F.M., Chiariello, L., Hallman, G.L. and Cooley, D.A. (1974) Aorto-coronary bypass in Jehovah's Witnesses: report of 36 patients. *J. Thorac. Cardiovasc. Surg.*, **68**: 1–7.

5 Ramsey, G., Arvan, D.A., Stewart, S. and Blumberg, N. (1983) Do preoperative laboratory tests predict blood transfusion needs in cardiac operations? *J. Thorac. Cardiovasc. Surg.*, **85**: 564–569.

6 Boldt, J., Zickmann, B., Herold, C., Dapper, F. and Hempelmann, G. (1992) The effects of preoperative aspirin therapy on platelet function in cardiac surgery. *Eur. J. Cardiothorac. Surg.*, **6**: 598–602.

7 Kirklin, J.W., Blackstone, E.H., Kirklin, J.K. *et al.* (1983) Surgical results and protocols in the spectrum of tetralogy of Fallot. *Ann. Surg.*, **198**: 251–260.

8 Inglis, T.C., Mc.N., Breeze, G.R., Stuart, J., Abrams, L.D., Roberts, K.D. and Singh, S.P. (1975) Excess intravascular coagulation complicating low cardiac output. *J. Clin. Pathol.*, **28**: 1–7.

9 Milam, J.D., Austin, S.F., Nihill, M.R., Keats, A.S. and Cooley, D.A. (1985) Use of sufficient hemodilution to prevent coagulopathies following surgical correction of cyanotic heart disease. *J. Thorac. Cardiovasc. Surg.*, **89**: 623–629.

10 Boldt, J., Zickman, B., Ballesteros, B.M., Stertmann, F. and Hempelmann, G. (1992) Influence of five different priming solutions on platelet function in patients undergoing cardiac surgery. *Anesth. Analg.*, **74**: 219–225.

11 Miller, D.W., Jr, Binford, J.M. and Hessel, E.A. (1982) Results of a survey of the professional activities of 811 cardiopulmonary perfusionists. *J. Thorac. Cardiovasc. Surg.*, **83**: 385–389.

12 Pifarre, R., Sullivan, H.J., Montoya, A. *et al.* (1989) Management of blood loss and heparin rebound following cardiopulmonary bypass. *Semin. Thromb. Haemostasis.*, **15**: 173–177.

13 Moriau, M., Masure, R., Hurlet, A. *et al.* (1977) Haemostasis disorders in open heart surgery with extracorporeal circulation. *Vox Sang.*, **32**: 41–51.

14 Wasser, M.N.J.M., Houbiers, J.G.A., Amaro, J.D. *et al.* (1989) The effect of fresh versus stored blood on post-operative bleeding after coronary bypass surgery: a prospective randomized survey. *Br. J. Haematol.*, **72**: 81–84.

15 Manno, C.S., Hedberg, K.W., Kim, H.C. *et al.* (1991) Comparison of the hemostatic effects of fresh whole blood stored, stored whole blood, and components after open heart surgery in Children. *Blood*, **77**: 930–936.

16 Tabak, C., Eugene, J. and Stemmer, E.A. (1981) Erythrocyte survival following extracorporeal circulation: a question of membrane versus bubble oxygenator. *J. Thorac. Cardiovasc. Surg.*, **81**: 30–33.

17 van den Dungen, J.J.A.M., Karliczek, G.F., Benken, U., Homan, van der Heide, J.N. and Wildevuur, C.R.H. (1982) Clinical study of blood trauma during perfusion with membrane and bubble oxygenators. *J. Thorac. Cardiovasc. Surg.*, **83**: 108–116.

18 Harker, L.A., Malpass, T.W., Branson, H.E., Hessel, E.A. and Slichter, S.J. (1980) Mechanisms of abnormal bleeding in patients undergoing cardiopulmonary bypass: acquired transient platelet dysfunction associated with selective α-granule release. *Blood*, **56**: 824–834.

19 Edmunds, L.H., Jr, Ellison, N., Colman, R.W. *et al.* (1982) Platelet function during cardiac operation: comparison of membrane and bubble oxygenators. *J. Thorac. Cardiovasc. Surg.*, **83**: 805–812.

20 O'Brien, J.R., Etherington, M.D., Shuttleworth, R.D. and Davison, S. (1984) Platelet and other tests followed sequentially for 14 days after operation. *Clin. Lab. Haematol.*, **6**: 239–245.

21 Reed, R.K., Lilleaasen, P., Lundberg, G. and Stokke, O. (1985) Dextran 70 versus donor plasma as colloid in open heart surgery under extreme haemodilution. *Scand. J. Clin. Lab. Invest.*, **45**: 269–274.

22 Cavarocchi, N.C., Pluth, J.R., Schaff, H.V. *et al.* (1986) Complement activation during

cardiopulmonary bypass: comparison of bubble and membrane oxygenators. *J. Thorac. Cardiovasc. Surg.*, **91**: 252–258.

23 Collett, B., Alhaq, A., Abdullah, N.B. *et al.* (1984) Pathways to complement activation during cardiopulmonary bypass. *Br. Med. J.*, **289**: 1251–1254.

24 Kurtz, S.R., Ouellet, R., McMican, A. and Valeri, C.R. (1983) Survival of MM red cells during hypothermia in two patients with anti-M. *Transfusion*, **23**: 37–39.

25 Leach, A.B., van Hasselt, G.L. and Edwards, J.C. (1983) Cold agglutinins and deep hypothermia. *Anaesthesia*, **38**: 140–143.

26 Klein, H.G., Faltz, L.L., McIntosh, C.L., Appelbaum, F.R., Deisseroth, A.B. and Holland, P.V. (1980) Surgical hypothermia in a patient with cold agglutinin: management by plasma exchange. *Transfusion*, **20**: 354–357.

27 Blumberg, N., Hicks, G., Woll, J. *et al.* (1983) Successful cardiac bypass surgery in the presence of a potent cold agglutinin without plasma exchange. *Transfusion*, **23**: 363.

28 Newland, P.E., Pastoriza-Pinol, J., McMillan, J., Smith, B.F. and Stirling, G.R. (1980) Maximal conservation and minimal usage of blood products in open heart surgery. *Anaesth. Intens. Care*, **8**: 178–182.

29 Weisel, R.D., Burns, R.J., Baird, R.J. *et al.* (1983) Optimal postoperative volume loading. *J. Thorac. Cardiovasc. Surg.*, **85**: 552–563.

30 Weinstein, M., Ware, J.A., Troll, J. and Salzman, E. (1988) Changes in von Willebrand factor during cardiac surgery: effect of desmopressin acetate. *Blood*, **71**: 6.

31 Salzman, E.W., Weinstein, M.J. Weintraub, R.M. *et al.* (1986) Treatment with desmopressin in acetate to reduce blood loss after cardiac surgery. *N. Engl. J. Med.*, **314**: 1402–1406.

32 Fish, K.J., Sarnquist, F.H., van Steennis, C. *et al.* (1986) A prospective, randomized study of the effects of prostacyclin on platelets and blood loss during coronary bypass operations. *J. Thorac. Cardiovasc. Surg.*, **91**: 436–442.

33 Hunt, B.J. and Yocoub, M. (1991) Aprotinin and cardiac surgery: reduces perioperative blood loss. *Br. Med. J.*, **303**: 660–661.

15

Autologous Transfusion and Blood Conservation

1 INTRODUCTION AND OVERVIEW

It has now become generally accepted within modern transfusion practice that the use of *allogeneic blood transfusion* should be reduced to the essential minimum. The impetus for change has been largely fuelled by increased recognition of the viral infection risks of transfusion, although ironically conventional transfusion of volunteer donor blood has never been safer than it is today. In addition, concerns at present poorly substantiated that transfusions are associated with increased post-operative infection risk or with a greater likelihood of cancer recurrence have also led to caution in the use of allogeneic blood.

1.1 Benefits of Blood Conservation Measures

Autologous transfusion and to a variable extent blood conservation measures in general have a number of advantages:

(1) There are reduced risks of transmitted viral infections. The advent of AIDS provided, not surprisingly, considerable impetus to the development of autologous transfusion programmes. Anxieties about the risks of AIDS have led to

increasing requests from patients for autologous transfusion arrangements to be made to cover their expected needs. Their fears undoubtedly have some foundation but have generally been greatly exaggerated by popular media coverage. The risks of acquiring transmitted infection from volunteer blood are extremely small—certainly far less than the general perception and indeed in most developed countries transfusion risks are small in comparison with those faced in general by patients requiring surgery and anaesthesia or treatment for their primary pathology. Nevertheless, autologous transfusion does offer an increment in safety if carefully managed. Arrangements must be made to ensure that the even more dangerous risks of damaged or bacterially contaminated blood packs or of mistaken identity do not occur. These are new problems to be faced for hospitals where regular blood collection is not a routine activity.

Arising from the same public concern has been pressure to collect blood from family and friends of patients (known as directed donor programmes) in the hope that this might provide greater safety. These schemes also suffer from the drawbacks described above. It is also worth bearing in mind that there is no guarantee that the actual level of safety will be greater than transfusion using random volunteer donations. The consequence of transfusion-related mishap, when blood has been donated by friends or family members, could be far worse!

(2) Alloimmunization against blood components is avoided; so too are haemolytic or other allergic reactions arising from exposure to various forms of cellular or protein alloantigens.

(3) Autologous transfusion programmes are useful if blood shortages are prevalent.

(4) Autologous transfusion is frequently used to replace blood loss during bone marrow donation.

(5) One of the most important indications for autologous transfusion is the management of patients having antibodies to high-frequency antigens, e.g. anti-Kp^b and anti-$P + P_1 + p^k$ or Oh (Bombay) patients with anti-A,B and anti-H. Some patients lacking high-frequency antigens may not be immediately recognized at the time of their first transfusion although the problem will eventually emerge if they become immunised. To avoid this problem, relatives found to have the same rare blood group could, if they need blood, be given phenotypically identical red cells or autologous transfusion in order to avoid immunization.

(6) Jehovah's Witnesses may accept autologous transfusion provided their blood remains in continuity with their own circulatory system. The proposal to use autologous transfusion must be discussed with them on an individual basis. Surgery, trauma and obstetric blood loss pose immense problems for those involved in the management of Jehovah's Witnesses. Various combinations of haemodilution and blood salvage autologous transfusion may be permitted[1-4] or transfusion may be refused absolutely.[5] The medicolegal position is considered in chapter 25, section 9.

(7) Because the patient's own blood is being returned, the routine cross-matching workload of the hospital transfusion laboratory is reduced.

(8) Red cell salvage procedures provide immediate support and do not require the instantaneous response from the hospital blood bank, and for major blood losses lessen the drain on blood bank stocks.

(9) Autologous transfusion avoids the alleged problem of increased post-operative infections and enhanced risks of tumour recurrence (see Chapter 23, section 4.4) associated with allogeneic blood transfusion.

There are several ways of minimizing the need for conventional blood transfusion. These include:

(1) *Adherence to strict transfusion criteria.*

   Critical assessment of the 'surgical' haematocrit: the commonly accepted requirement for a haemoglobin of 10.0 g/dl and haematocrit of 0.30 has been rightly challenged as being unnecessarily cautious. Informed opinion has suggested that decisions about transfusion should be made on the basis of a careful assessment of the patient's fitness and cardiopulmonary status. It is now recognized that for many patients values of Hb 8.0 g/dl and Hct 0.25 are acceptable, provided careful attention is paid to perioperative care and blood volume replacement (see chapter 11, section 5.6).

(2) *Pharmacological and anaesthetic approaches to reduction of blood loss*: Blood loss and the need to transfuse can be considerably affected by the nature of surgical and anaesthetic techniques, e.g. hypotensive surgery,[6] epidural and spinal anaesthesia have been found to minimize blood requirements.[7] In addition various pharmacological agents can reduce surgical blood loss. Most successful has been the use of aprotinin during cardiac surgery, but other materials such as DDAVP (see section 4) have received attention.

(3) *Autologous transfusion*: various peri-operative transfusion manoeuvres can lessen the use of allogeneic donor blood. These include:

   (a) Pre-operative haemodilution: this entails removal of a substantial proportion of the red cell volume prior to surgery, replacing this with asanguineous fluid. The collected blood units are then available to replace operative losses.

   (b) Pre-deposit blood banking: during which a patient donates and has stored on their behalf, blood units in advance of elective surgery.

   (c) Red cell salvage procedures: these entail recovery of blood shed surgically or immediately post-operatively which is then returned via a conventional transfusion procedure.

Each of these transfusion techniques has particular merits. With enthusiastic commitment on the part of surgeons, anaesthetists and haematologists, various combinations are possible with the ultimate objective of avoiding completely the use of allogeneic blood.[8] These alternatives are considered below in more detail

2 PRE-OPERATIVE HAEMODILUTION

Haemodilution refers to purposeful reduction of the haemoglobin concentration prior to surgery.[7,9] This has the aim of:

(1) Reducing blood viscosity.
(2) Reducing the operative red cell losses as a consequence of the reduced haematocrit.
(3) Providing a bank of freshly collected autologous whole blood for return when surgery is complete.

A typical procedure entails collection of 'two to three units' (approx. 1350 ml) simultaneously with the replacement of crystalloids or colloids. If crystalloids are used, three times the volume removed must be returned (see chapter 10, section 1). Haemodilution carried out under supervision of an experienced anaesthetic team has been shown to be safe, provided patients with contraindications such as congestive cardiac failure or atherosclerotic disease are excluded.

2.1 Blood Viscosity and Oxygen Transport

Conventionally accepted target values for haemodilution require reduction of the haemoglobin to around 10.0 g/dl and the haematocrit to 0.3. Oxygen transport, it has been shown, will then increase as a result of increased cardiac output.[10]

Haemodilution is, of course, an artificial state of anaemia and tissue oxygenation can only be maintained if an increase in arteriovenous oxygen extraction occurs (tissue oxygen tensions must fall in order to achieve this) or if blood flow increases. Increased blood flow and tissue perfusion are dependent at least on maintenance and preferably on expansion of the circulating blood volume. This may present difficulties if surgical blood loss becomes excessive.

It seems likely that cardiac output and blood flow can be increased reliably in those with relatively healthy cardiovascular responses and for these patients there would be no problem in maintaining tissue oxygenation. The overall reduction in blood viscosity following haemodilution results in improved venous return which, in turn, increases cardiac output. Experimental data have been produced showing that maximum blood flow occurs at a haematocrit of around 0.3;[11] this appears to be as much as 20% in excess of that at normal blood count levels. Whether the improved blood flow occurs equally in all tissues and under different conditions of physiological stress is by no means established. Indeed, studies on isolated intestinal segments showed blood flow to be optimal at a haematocrit as high as 0.49,[12] although oxygenation was not in fact substantially reduced unless the haematocrit fell below 0.25. In the treatment of patients, however, *blood volume* appears to be the most critical determinant; provided hypovolaemia is avoided, tissue oxygenation is strongly related to arterial pO_2 and is not influenced by the haematocrit.[13]

The clinical benefits of haemodilution in routine surgical and anaesthetic practice are, however, not universally understood or accepted.[14]

In the face of conflicting data and varied opinions it is not easy to formulate definite conclusions. For some practitioners it is difficult to accept that the normal haemoglobin and haematocrit do not represent an evolutionarily selected ideal which, in modern life, would be also most befitting a surgical patient. However, it is quite clear from many years' experience in cardiac surgery, the surgical management of patients with renal failure and anaemia and from the more recent application of haemodilution to other surgical fields that the practice is safe. Economy of blood use and avoidance of the risks of blood administration are extremely important current issues. When these are taken into consideration it seems clear that moderate haemodilution should be practised more widely.

There are several clinical circumstances (see sections 2.2 and 2.3) in which a degree of caution is appropriate.

2.2   Recurrent Haemorrhage as a Contraindication to Haemodilution

Where there is a risk of further haemorrhage, any state of anaemia, even if therapeutically induced, may render the patient at a relative disadvantage. Since some of the reserve cardiac capacity has already been taken up by the compensation for anaemia, the patient's ability to surmount extra unanticipated problems such as alterations in oxygen supply, fluctuations in blood pressure, sudden blood loss, temperature changes, infections or anaesthetic problems may well be reduced.

2.3   Haemodilution and Vascular Disease

A particularly controversial matter is the value of haemodilution in patients with atherosclerotic arterial disease. Moderate haemodilution and the resulting reduction in blood viscosity could, in theory, be beneficial in the presence of fixed stenotic coronary vessels. In this instance, it is essential that coronary blood flow increases in order to compensate for the reduced blood oxygen content; the coronary sinus pO_2, which is normally very low, precludes any substantial increase in arteriovenous oxygen extraction. Cardiac output will, in fact, be automatically increased during haemodilution because of the lower blood viscosity and this may be achieved without a corresponding increase in actual myocardial workload and energy consumption. The increased cardiac output is achieved largely as a result of increased ventricular stroke volume; the heart rate remains unchanged. However, any further increases in cardiac output that may be required, e.g. to combat perioperative problems, will depend on increased heart rate and, therefore, on a substantial increase in myocardial oxygen supply. If this is not forthcoming because of restricted coronary perfusion, myocardial ischaemia, impaired myocardial function and defective systemic oxygen transport will be the result. It seems, therefore, that this group of patients merits a particularly cautious approach to the use of haemodilution.

2.4   Indications

Haemodilution is probably safest and most suited to younger patients judged to be free from cardiopulmonary pathology, cerebrovascular disease, hypertension or

Table 1 Surgical haemodilution

Exclude coronary or cerebral vascular disease, hypertension or hypovolaemia
Confirm that the pre-operative haemoglobin and haematocrit are adequate
Maintain high inspired oxygen tension during anaesthesia
Replace operative blood losses with colloid or crystalloids until haemoglobin/haematocrit
  reach 10.0 g.dl/0.30. Transfuse red cells only at this point.
Give post-operative iron replacement

hepatic problems. The usual target value of 10 g/dl haemoglobin for planned haemodilution may allow many fit patients with completely normal preoperative blood counts to have modest degrees of blood loss (e.g. 20–30%) replaced by asanguineous fluid alone in the interests of both safety and economy. Use of a more pronounced degree of haemodilution or haemodilution in other clinical circumstances may best be restricted to centres with special interests and experience in anticipating and managing any problems that may occur. Haemodilution, in which replacement of crystalloids or synthetic colloids has been inadequate, may predispose to orthostatic hypotension during the post-operative period as a result of the relatively short period of time that plasma volume can be maintained with these agents.

3 AUTOLOGOUS TRANSFUSION

Autologous blood collection, either pre-deposit or intraoperative salvage, should only be considered for operative procedures for which, usually by reference to the hospital Maximum Blood Order Schedule (MBOS) list (chapter 25, section 6) transfusion is likely to be needed. Use of autologous transfusion for procedures not normally requiring blood is wasteful, and participation in a pre-deposit programme will also place the donor at unnecessary risk. Unfortunately, but perhaps not surprisingly, surveys have shown that a substantial number of autologous transfusion procedures are unnecessary.[15,16] The patients concerned have been shown to have lost too little blood to require transfusion in any form. A further and costly consequence of over-use of autologous transfusion is the need to discard unused collections.[15]

3.1 Pre-surgical (Pre-deposit) Blood Collection

The patient's fitness to donate must be carefully evaluated and balanced against the particular indication for autologous transfusion. Serologically 'untransfusable' patients require special consideration as there may be no other logistically feasible source of blood. It has been said that patients who are considered to be fit enough for surgery are, by the same criteria, also fit enough for a judiciously planned blood collection programme. Patients with any degree of refractory bone marrow failure are clearly unsuitable as they will be unable to replace the blood donated.

In general, it must be emphasized that it is unrealistic to attempt to apply the fitness criteria pertaining to normal blood donors to those donating blood for autologous use.

Eligibility criteria

In some countries guidelines for autologous pre-donation have been prepared[17] and these describe the degree of relaxation advisable under the individual circumstances. In particular:

(1) *Haemoglobin* values down to 11.0 g/dl are probably acceptable. Pre-deposit collection should not normally be considered where the haemoglobin is below 10.0 g/dl.
(2) *Age:* elderly patients have been shown to tolerate pre-deposit programmes safely provided that careful assessment is made particularly of their cardiovascular and pulmonary status.[18-21] From the haematological point of view, pre-deposit programmes are also acceptable for *children*, provided that suitable adjustment of the collection volume (< 12% blood volume) and anticoagulant quantity are made. The child should of course be willing and cooperative and parental consent is required.
(3) *Pregnancy*: there seems to be little advantage to be gained from routine pre-deposit arrangements during pregnancy. Transfusion needs are unpredictable and infrequent, and non-usage of collected units is likely.[15]

    Although there is little risk as far as the mother is concerned,[22] blood donation is considered to be hazardous to the fetus particularly in the first and third trimesters. Problems recorded in late pregnancy have included fetal bradycardia, premature delivery and maternal hypotension.[23] Certainly pre-deposit donation is contraindicated in pregnancies complicated by impaired placental blood flow and/or intrauterine growth retardation, including hypotension, preclampsia etc.[17]
(4) Patients with *cardiovascular disease* need careful specialist assessment before being accepted for pre-deposit donation. Studies have established the safety of pre-deposit programmes for such patients.[19-21]

    The consequences of prolonged post-donation hypotension, a possible complication for all blood donors, must be considered. In particular stenosis in any critical area of arterial supply results in ischaemia during episodes of hypotension. Caution is also necessary in patients receiving beta-blockers and angiotensin-converting enzyme (ACE) inhibitors, both of which attenuate the peripheral vascular response to hypovolaemia. For such patients it should be remembered that in the UK the risks from conventional transfusion are so small that it seems unnecessary to subject patients with some degree of cardiovascular instability to risks of blood donation which are at present poorly quantified.
(5) Volunteer donors with a history of *epilepsy* are not normally accepted because of the recognized risk of recurrences and it might be wise to adopt a similar caution with regard to autologous donations.

Blood collection procedures

Collection of a small stock of conventionally refrigerated stored blood is often adequate to cover minor bleeding risks, and can be carried out without special facilities. The following procedures have been found useful.[24]

Two units of blood are taken: the first 10–14 days preoperatively, and the second 3–7 days before operation. It may be desirable to give the patient an iron supplement in the preoperative period. If more than two units are required a careful predeposit schedule must be devised. Blood can technically be stored for at least 42 days in optimal additive solutions and this sets the timing of the start of the collection schedule. The last donation of the collection series should be obtained no closer than 3 days prior to surgery. To enable accumulation of a sufficient total to cover major surgery 'leap-frog' procedures have in the past been found useful. Currently under evaluation are pre-deposit schedules involving the use of recombinant human erythropoietin (rHuEPO).[25,26]

Doses of around 300 IU/kg are used twice weekly as a marrow stimulant. This has been shown to:

(1) Enable collection of a larger number of blood units within the time available.
(2) Ensure the haemoglobin concentration of the patient and that of the donated units is maintained at an acceptable level.
(3) Result in an actively proliferating erythron, thus enhancing the endogenous response to red cells lost over the surgical period. rHuEPO has been shown to be safe and effective, and licensing approval for its use to enhance pre-deposit collections is anticipated. The accelerated erythropoiesis is, however, dependent on an adequate iron supply and it appears that neither mobilization from body iron stores nor oral iron therapy can reliably support the needs for erythropoiesis.[28]

Accordingly parenteral iron, e.g. ferrous saccharate in doses of 100 mg elemental iron per donation removed, has been found to be necessary.[26]

The donor's haemoglobin should be monitored; collection can usefully be continued as long as haemoglobin values remain above 11.0 g/dl, haematocrit 0.34.

For pre-deposit autologous transfusion programmes to succeed, good communications must be established between the blood bank staff and the patient's physician. Full information and consent are necessary on the part of the patient. Cancelled surgery will, of course, present major problems since the collected units may pass beyond their expiry date.

An efficient and secure organization is necessary to prevent the return of red cell units to the wrong patient. The blood pack should be accurately labelled as described in chapter 25, section 3.1. The donor can also be asked to add his or her signature to the blood pack label confirming that the identity details are correct. Blood packs should be stored in a specially designated area clearly separated from volunteer donations.

Not infrequently the collected autologous blood units are not required either during or following surgery. This non-use rate (approx. 37% in a multi-centre US survey)[15] obviously increases the cost of pre-deposit programmes as compared with conventional voluntary donations. A contentious issue concerns the possible re-use of autologous pre-deposit units for other patients.[29] In the UK this is not permitted; autologous units will not in general have been collected under circumstances which meet the specification for blood donations for general use.[27] Indeed it cannot be claimed that autologous donors offer their blood with the same impartiality with regard to risk factors as is expected of random voluntary donors. Certainly a higher incidence of positive viral markers has been observed in autologous donors compared to conventional donors.

Laboratory testing for autologous donations

It has been argued that, provided a secure system of labelling is in operation such that autologous units will only be returned to their intended recipient, the conventional test procedures applied to voluntary donations are unnecessary. While this might be strictly true, in the UK autologous units are handled in a similar manner to conventional donations. Full blood grouping, antibody screening and microbiological examination for all mandatory markers is carried out. This is justified for several reasons:

(1) Autologous recipients may need supplemental transfusion with conventional bank blood. This justifies the need for grouping and antibody screening.
(2) Because of the finite, although small risk of organizational errors or laboratory accidents, most blood bank supervisors prefer to exclude any donations with positive markers for viral infectivity that could constitute a hazard to other patients or to staff. Autologous donors should therefore be counselled regarding the intended performance of these microbiological screening tests on their donations.

3.2 Blood Salvage Procedures

Blood shed during surgery can be recovered for reinfusion into the patient provided that it can be gathered into a tissue cavity which allows use of suction or drainage catheters. These re-utilization procedures, normally described as 'blood salvage procedures', are usually performed intra-operatively. However, for certain vascular and orthopaedic procedures, blood recovered in drains during the immediate postoperative period can also be returned for transfusion. Blood salvage procedures should only be performed when the predicted blood loss would normally necessitate replacement by transfusion. The cost-effectiveness of red cell salvage procedures as compared with voluntary allogeneic donations has been a matter of contention. Certainly within the UK, salvage techniques are likely to be more expensive, and a USA study could only demonstrate near cost equivalence when transfusion needs were high.[30] The criteria to be met for utilizing autologous transfusion are therefore those for transfusion generally.

Blood salvage techniques

Two main approaches are utilized:

(1) *Single-use, disposable collection canisters* (e.g. Solcotrans): using these devices systemic heparinization of the patient is necessary. The aspirated blood is collected into ACD anticoagulant in a collection canister, and can then be reinfused through a microaggregate filter without further manipulation. Infused blood will contain activated platelets, partially coagulated/defibrinated plasma, and some haemolysis from red cell damage may be evident. At the volumes conventionally collected and transfused these do not appear to cause discernible clinical effects, although plasma haemoglobin levels and fibrinogen degradation products can be shown to be increased. These devices are relatively simple to use and entail no capital outlay. It is essential that a system exists to ensure the collection canister is labelled appropriately to guarantee return to the correct recipient. Reinfusion must also take place within an agreed time; this is usually 6 hours from the start of the collection process. A similar system is also available for post-operative orthopaedic use, and this does not necessitate systemic heparinization.

(2) *Automated or partially automated salvage systems*: these devices, exemplified by the Haemonetics 'cell saver'[31,32] autologous blood recovery system, are now becoming popular means for performing intra-operative blood salvage. Blood is collected by aspiration from 'clean' operative sites, centrifugally washed, filtered and the red cells are held ready for reinfusion. Red cells equivalent to a single unit can typically be processed in around 3 minutes with standard equipment, but larger machines are now available with sufficient processing capacity for coping with, for example, the needs of liver transplantation surgery.

Intra-operative autotransfusion has proved to be particularly suitable for blood recovery during cardiovascular surgical procedures. However, almost any operative procedure providing suitable access for the suction catheter can benefit from red cell salvage procedures, the main exception being those in which there is faecally contaminated blood loss. Haemostatic abnormalities have not been a problem even following autotransfusion of around 4 l of washed cells.[33] Because only washed cells are returned to the circulation, systemic anticoagulation is unnecessary.

Red cells that are not immediately reinfused should be stored under refrigeration for no longer than 6 hours. This limit is necessary because saline-washed red cells lack nutrients to support glycolysis and also because the collection procedure carries an unavoidable risk of bacterial contamination. After this time unused packs should be discarded. It is important to ensure that blood packs are accurately labelled with the patient's identification details and the date and time of collection.

Practical considerations

There are various potential problems to be considered with automated intra-operative blood salvage procedures in which systemic anticoagulation is not utilized:

(1) The red cells must usually be washed and filtered to remove *tissue fragments, fat emboli,* and *microaggregates* of leucocytes and platelets.
(2) *Partially coagulated plasma,* containing activated clotting factors, must be removed. Salvaged plasma may also show undesirable activation of the complement and kinin systems.
(3) *Mechanical haemolysis* of red cells: high suction pressure, roller pumps, frothing of the blood and 'skimming' suction actions are damaging. If these are avoided survival of reinfused red cells will be normal.
(4) *Air embolization* was a risk during earlier procedures. The design of modern automated red cell salvage systems appears to have eliminated its occurrence.
(5) Red cells alone will be reinfused. There may, therefore, be an additional need for transfusion of conventional blood bank plasma components (see chapter 12).
(6) *Bacterial infection*: it was formally believed that blood should only be recovered from *clean operative sites*, e.g. the peritoneal cavity, thorax or mediastinum. Experience has shown that this is not essential.[34]

    The red cell washing and plasma removal will achieve some partial reduction in bacterial contamination. It is, however, most important that red cell return is prompt. Clearly contaminated collection sites, e.g. in proximity to foci of infection, must be avoided.
(7) *Tumour cell dissemination*: the possibility that metastatic spread might be facilitated has traditionally been viewed as a contraindication to blood salvage procedures. It now seems evident that this fear was ill founded. Tumour cells may be unavoidably disseminated via the circulation during surgery, but the return of salvaged blood will not compound the problem.
(8) A continuous rota of trained staff is required to operate the equipment if full and economic use is to be made of its potential.
(9) Capital and disposable costs may result in all but the most extensive transfusions being more expensive than conventional donor transfusions.

4 PHARMACOLOGICAL MEASURES FOR BLOOD CONSERVATION[35]

Attempts to understand the haemostatic impairment occurring in cardiac surgery have shown the importance of *activation damage* to *platelet function* and of *fibrinolysis* as factors leading to excessive blood loss. These factors may be operative in a wide variety of other surgical procedures, in particular those in which it is necessary to transfuse large volumes of blood over an extended period of time, e.g. vascular surgery, hepatic transplantation, or spinal fusions for scoliosis. It seemed logical therefore to investigate pharmacological agents which might attenuate these adverse changes. The principal agents studied include:

(1) *Desmopressin (DDAVP)*: DDAVP increases plasma concentrations of high molecular weight von Willebrand factor (see chapter 8) and via this mechanism improves platelet function and corrects the bleeding time prolongation in various conditions (e.g. uraemia, cirrhosis and cardiac surgery). DDAVP has been examined in cardiopulmonary bypass surgery as well as other surgical situations in which high blood loss are problematic. Although there has been some initial evidence of improved blood loss rates, the early promise does not seem to be borne out in more extended studies.[36]

(2) *Platelet function-inhibiting agents*: principal amongst these has been prostacyclin. Although platelet functional inhibition might seem illogical as a means of ultimately preserving platelet function, prostacyclin has been proposed as a protective agent against the pathological platelet activation occurring in cardiopulmonary bypass circuits. While this might be true, clinically evident reductions in transfusion requirements have not been confirmed.

(3) *Aprotinin*: use of aprotinin has yielded convincing evidence of reduced blood loss in cardiac surgery,[37,38] hepatic transplantation,[39] spinal fusion, as well as in other surgical problems. Aprotinin is a peptide functioning as a serine protease inhibitor. In this context its principal actions are:

  (a) Direct *inhibition of plasmin*, thereby controlling abnormal fibrinolysis.
  (b) *Inhibition of kallikrein*, an activator of the complement cascade and of the *contact phase of coagulation* (XII–XIIa), and also of *tissue plasminogin activator* blocking its effect as an inflammatory mediator (see chapter 13).

It also appears that aprotinin has a *platelet-sparing* role during cardiac bypass procedures since the bleeding time prolongation seems to be reduced. Despite these physiological observations, the precise role of aprotinin in improving haemostasis in these various circumstances is not entirely clear. The benefits of aprotinin, however, now seem well established and it is being examined over an increasingly wide range of surgical situations.[39–41]

REFERENCES

1 Harris, T.J.B., Parikh, N.R., Rao, Y.K. and Oliver, R.H.P. (1983) Exsanguination in a Jehovah's Witness. *Anaesthesia*, **38**: 989–992.
2 Sandiford, F.M., Chiariello, L., Hallman, G.L. and Cooley, D.A. (1974) Aorta–coronary bypass in Jehovah's Witnesses: report of 36 Patients. *J. Thorac. Cardiovasc. Surg.*, **68**: 1–7.
3 Gollub, S. and Bailey, C.P. (1966) Management of major sugical blood loss without transfusion. *JAMA*, **198**: 149–152.
4 Clarke, J.M.F. (1982) Surgery in Jehovah's Witnesses. *Br. J. Hosp. Med.*, **27**: 497–500.
5 Bonakdar, M.I., Echous, A.W., Bacher, B.J., Tabbilos, R.H. and Peisner, D.B. (1982) Major gynecologic and obstetric surgery in Jehovah's Witnesses. *Obstet. Gynecol.*, **60**: 587–591.
6 Sharrock, N.E., Mineo, R., Urquhart, B. and Salvati, E.A. (1993) The effect of two levels of hypotension on intraoperative blood loss during total hip arthroplasty performed under lumbar epidural anaesthesia. *Anesth. Analg.*, **76**: 580–584.
7 Moller, L., Steady, H.M., Korten, K.W. and Turner, R.H. (1982) Blood conservation in revision arthroplasty. In: Turner, R.H. (ed.), *Revision Total Hip Arthroplasty*, pp. 343–357. New York: Grune & Stratton.
8 Tulloh, B.R., Brakespear, C.P., Bates, S.C. *et al.* (1993) Autologous predonation, haemodilution and intraoperative blood salvage in elective abdominal aortic aneurysm repair. *Br. J. Surg.*, **80**: 313–315.

9 Atallah, M.M., Abdelbaky, S.M. and Saied, M.M.A. (1993) Does timing of haemodilution influence the stress response and overall outcome? *Anesth. Analg.*, **76**: 113–117.

10 Messmer, K.F.W. (1987) Acceptable haematocrit levels in surgical patients. *World J. Surg.*, **11**: 41–46.

11 Marshall, M. and Bird, T. (1981) *Blood Loss and Replacement*. London: Edward Arnold.

12 Shepherd, A.P. and Riedel, G.L. (1982) Optimal haematocrit for oxygenation of canine intestine. *Circ. Res.*, **51**: 233–240.

13 Chang, N., Goodson, W.H., Gottrup, F. and Hunt, T.K. (1983) Direct measurement of wound and tissue oxygen tension in postoperative patients. *Ann. Surg.*, **197**: 470–478.

14 Lundsgaard-Hansen, P. (1979) New clothes for an anaemic emperor. *Vox Sang.*, **36**: 321–336.

15 Renner, S.W., Howanitz, P.J. and Bachner, P. (1992) Preoperative autologous blood donation in 612 hospitals: a college of American Pathologists' Q-Probes study of quality issues in transfusion practice. *Arch. Pathol. Lab. Med.*, **116**: 613–619.

16 Goodnough, L.T., Verbrugge, D., Vizmeg, K. and Riddell, J., IV. (1992) Identifying elective orthopaedic surgical patients transfused with amounts of blood in excess of need: the transfusion trigger revisited. *Transfusion*, **32**: 648–653.

17 British Committee for Standards in Haematology Blood Transfusion Task Force (1993) Guidelines for autologous transfusion. I. Pre-operative autologous donation. *Transfusion Med.*, **3**: 307–316.

18 McVay, P.A., Andrews, A., Kaplan, E.B. *et al.* (1990) Donation reactions among autologous donors. *Transfusion*, **30**: 249–252.

19 Mann, M., Sacks, H.J. and Goldfinger, D. (1983) Safety of autologous blood donation prior to elective surgery for a variety of potentially 'high-risk' patients. *Transfusion*, **23**: 229–232.

20 Spiess, B.D., Sassetti, R., McCarthy, R.J., Narbone, R.F., Tuman, K.J. and Ivankovich, A.D. (1992) Autologous blood donation: haemodynamics in a 'high-risk' patient population. *Transfusion*, **32**: 17–22.

21 Domen, R.E., Hnat, H. and Panasiuk, M. (1992) Autologous blood donation by patients with cardiovascular disease. *Vox Sang.*, **63**: 137.

22 O'Dwyer, G., Mylotte, M., Sweeney, M. and Egan, E.L. (1993) Experience of autologous blood transfusion in an obstetrics and gynaecology department. *Br. J. Obstet. Gynaecol.*, **100**: 571–574.

23 Tabor, E. (1990) Potential risks of blood donation during pregnancy for autologous transfusion. *Transfusion*, **30**: 76.

24 Harden, P.A. (1982) Autologous transfusion. *Asian Pacific Regional Blood Transfusion Newsletter*, **2**.

25 Goodnough, L.T., Price, T.H., Rudnick, S. and Soegiarso, R.W. (1992) Preoperative red cell production in patients undergoing aggressive autologous blood phlebotomy with and without erythropoietin therapy. *Transfusion*, **32**: 441–445.

26 Mercuriali, F., Zanella, A., Barosi, G. *et al.* (1993) Use of erythropoietin to increase the volume of autologous blood donated by orthopaedic patients. *Transfusion*, **33**: 55–60.

27 Red Book Reference (1993) *Guidelines for Blood Transfusion Services in the UK*. London HMSO.

28 Biesma, D.H., Kraaijenhagen, R.J., Poortman, J., Marx, J.J.M. and van de Wiel, A. (1992) The effect of oral iron supplementation on erythropoiesis in autologous blood donors. *Transfusion*, **32**: 162–165.

29 Polesky, H.F. (1988) Is blood from autologous donors safe for others? *Transfusion*, **28**: 204.

30 Solomon, M.D., Rutledge, M.L., Kane, L.E. and Yawn, D. H. (1988) Cost comparison of intraoperative autologous versus homologous transfusion. *Transfusion*, **28**: 379–382.

31 Chant, A.D.B. and Thompson, J.F. (1986) Autotransfusion with salvaged blood. *Br. J. Surg.*, **79**: 389–390.

32 Dale, R.F., Lindop, M.J., Farman, J.V. and Smith, M.F. (1986) Autotransfusion, an experience of seventy six cases. *Ann. R. Coll. Surg. Engl.*, **68**: 295–297.

33 Keeling, M.M., Gray, L.A., Brink, M.A., Hillerich, V.K. and Bland, K.I. (1983) Intraoperative autotransfusion. *Am. Surg.*, **197**: 536–541.

34 Ezzedine, H., Baele, P. and Robert, A. (1991) Bacteriologic quality of intraoperative autotransfusion. *Surgery*, **109**: 259–264.

35 Hunt, B.J. (1991) Modifying perioperative blood loss. *Blood Rev.*, **5**: 168–176.

36 Jobes, D.R. and Ellison, N. (1992) Pharmacology of hemostasis in the surgical patient. *Anesth. Analg.*, **75**: 317–318.

37 Covino, E., Pepino, P., Iorio, D., Marino, L., Ferrara, P. and Spampinato, N. (1991) Low dose aprotinin as blood saver in open heart surgery. *Eur. J. Cardiothorac. Surg.*, **5**: 414–418.

38 Hunt, B.J. and Yacoub, M. (1991) Aprotinin and cardiac surgery: reduces perioperative blood loss. *Br. Med. J.*, **303**: 660–661.

39 Smith, O., Hazlehurst, G., Brozovic, B. *et al.* (1993) Impact of aprotinin on blood transfusion requirements in liver transplantation. *Transfusion, Med.*, **3**: 97–102.

40 Valentine, S., Williamson, P. and Sutton, D. (1993) Reduction of acute haemorrhage with aprotinin. *Anaesthesia*, **48**: 405–406.

41 Taylor, K.M. (1992) Aprotinin therapy and blood conservation: extending the indications. *Br. J. Surg.*, **79**: 1258–1259.

16
Management of Patients with Burns

1 PATHOPHYSIOLOGY OF BURNS INJURY

1.1 Fluid and Protein Losses from the Plasma

Severe burns cause *hypovolaemic shock* and *circulatory failure*. If untreated these contribute to *renal and pulmonary failure* and also predispose to *sepsis* in the damaged tissues. The hypovolaemia results from massive leakage of fluid and plasma protein from the vascular compartment into the interstitial tissues. The plasma protein loss occurs because capillary endothelial cells both at burn-damaged areas and also at sites distant from the injury become abnormally permeable. The leakage of plasma protein reduces the oncotic pressure difference between plasma and interstitial fluid and this permits water loss into the interstitium. The problem can be exacerbated by the very high catecholamine secretion occurring in burns injury which causes venous constriction, leading in turn to increased capillary hydrostatic pressures and greater fluid loss. Failure of the cell membrane cation pump also accompanies severe shock and cells therefore absorb water and sodium and leak potassium ions. It is easy, therefore, to see how the badly burned patient can suffer from severe maldistribution of water, electrolytes and plasma protein.

Large amounts of water are lost externally from burn areas and this aggravates the hypovolaemia. Fluid losses of up to $200 \, \text{ml/m}^2$ per hour may occur which exceed 10-fold the normal evaporation rate from the skin. Haemoconcentration will therefore occur unless these losses are made good. The amount of evaporative losses depends greatly on the degree of skin injury, the type of dressings applied and the ambient temperature and humidity. Hypovolaemic shock also causes hyperventilation which again increases fluid loss.

1.2 Haematological Changes[1]

Anaemia may occur in cases of severe burns, from blood loss as well as from haemolysis of heat-damaged erythrocytes. Intravascular haemolysis can be a contributing factor to the renal failure and disseminated intravascular coagulation seen in patients with burns. Burned patients show an increase in protein catabolism and possibly later a reduction in protein synthesis. As a result, *immunoglobulin levels* and *immune responses*[2] may be depressed, predisposing to infection, particularly of the exposed and damaged surface areas. Temporary impairment of bone marrow function is common and is probably also a consequence of deranged protein synthesis. The burns injury alone is sufficient to disturb haemopoiesis but the problem can be worsened when protracted sepsis occurs. The bone marrow impairment, not surprisingly, slows the recovery from blood loss or haemolysis.

1.3 Pulmonary Damage

Inhalation injury is probably the leading cause of death in badly burned patients now that modern fluid resuscitation regimens have improved the outlook from circulatory failure. However, caution is necessary to ensure that neither untreated hypovolaemia nor over-hydration due to excessive crystalloid use aggravate the risk of pulmonary injury.[3]

2 FLUID REPLACEMENT

Intravenous fluid replacement plays an important part in the management of patients with severe degrees (generally over 10% of body surface in children and 15% of body surface in adults) of burn injury. The principal aim of treatment is the prevention of uncompensated shock and its consequences. This entails the restoration and maintenance of plasma volume by means of intravenous crystalloid or colloid infusions. A large number of different regimens have been described, none of which have been universally accepted as being superior. Differences in the popularity of the various fluid replacement regimens probably reflect differences in the availability of particular intravenous preparations as well as other differences in the circumstances and problems affecting the management of patients in burns centres around the world. An obvious difference is the preference within the UK to utilize protein solutions at the initial stages of management, whereas in the USA crystalloids form the mainstay of treatment during the first few hours. None of the published fluid regimens serve as more than a guide to the early phases of management; as time goes on the volume and composition of replacement therapy must be determined by conscientious monitoring of the clinical progress.

2.1 Choice of Fluid Replacement Regimen[4]

Crystalloids or colloids?

Crystalloids have been advocated, certainly in the USA, as the sole replacement fluid during the first few hours, on the basis that the pathological leakage of proteins through damaged capillary walls renders albumin therapy of no particular advantage. Capillary permeability particularly in non-burn areas begins to recover after 8–12 hours and, by that time, albumin or plasma therapy can be shown to be more useful. Return of capillary membrane function is followed by reabsorption of protein and fluids into the vascular space. Proponents of crystalloid regimens have claimed on the basis of controlled trials that no benefit can be shown by administration of albumin during the first 24 hours.[5] Indeed the albumin-treated patients accumulated larger amounts of pulmonary oedema despite having lower overall fluid requirements. Alternatively, it can be argued that the plasma protein loss justifies replacement right from the start. Proponents of either view are able to show successful results with each of their advocated approaches. Accordingly, regimens exist beginning with crystalloids alone,[6] utilizing mixtures of crystalloids with synthetic colloids, crystalloids with albumin or use of albumin or plasma alone.[8] Crystalloid solutions (e.g. Ringer's lactate or Hartmann's solution; see chapter 10, section 1) are considered entirely satisfactory as the sole resuscitation fluid for moderate burn injury in young fit subjects.

The choice between use of crystalloids or colloids in the early resuscitative period remains unresolved. The ambient temperature and humidity and the temperature of both the body and the burn surface and the type of dressing affect the choice of transfusion fluids to cover haemodynamic, evaporative and metabolic needs.

The need for blood components

Full-thickness burns produce a loss of red cells either directly in the burn tissues or, as a result of immediate thermal damage, in other areas of the circulation. It may therefore be necessary to transfuse blood during the resuscitation period; this is usually at an approximate rate of 1% blood volume for each 1% of surface area of deep burn damage. Transfusion of red cells will often be required to correct a more slowly developing anaemia due to a milder degree of erythrocyte damage, though this need only becomes apparent after the first few days. There are claims that neutrophil function is impaired after burns injury; this may be a consequence of the reduction in fibronectin levels which have been reported. These neutrophil defects appear to be correctable (*in vitro*) with fresh plasma; there may therefore be a role for fibronectin therapy in the form of fresh frozen plasma or cryoprecipitate, although this remains so far unproven. Granulocytes have been used to help combat serious infections but again no controlled trials have been reported. The role of specific immunoglobulin, e.g. to combat *Pseudomonas* infection, is currently being investigated.

How much fluid?[8]

Loss of plasma volume in burned patients is predominantly shown by haemoconcentration; measurement of the haematocrit therefore provides a useful guide to the volume of replacement fluid needed. Extensive haemolysis will, of course, make conclusions based on this measurement less reliable.

The volume of infused fluid is initially selected according to the formulae based on body weight (or surface area) and the percentage of the surface area with definitive burn injury (i.e. excluding erythema). Widely used protocols include the following:[5-7]

(1) 4 ml crystalloid/kg per cent burns over the first 24 hours, adding colloids later.
(2) 1 ml 5% albumin+1 ml crystalloid/kg per cent burns during the first 24 hours, reducing by half over the next 24 hours.

Initial rates of fluid loss can be massive and in all regimens it is generally necessary to administer the first half of the 24-hour allocation within the first 8 hours.

When crystalloids are used for resuscitation much larger volumes (e.g. × 3–4) must be administered and extracellular fluid accumulation is greater than with use of albumin. This has not been shown to be a clinical problem; pulmonary oedema is said to be rather less likely than it is following albumin administration. It has been claimed recently that the need for such large volumes of crystalloid solutions can be reduced by increasing the sodium content of the fluid to as much as 250 mEq/l.[9] Although peripheral oedema appears to be minimized and the plasma volume better maintained, the regimen requires further clinical study.

Addition of synthetic colloids (see chapter 10 section 3), e.g. dextran 40 (which promotes an osmotic diuresis—particularly useful if haemoglobinuria is present) or dextran 70, also reduces the volume of fluid needed and the amount of tissue oedema formation. Fluid loading is tolerated far less well by the elderly; for these patients regimens containing albumin at more modest infusion rates may be safer than the more aggressive Parkland formula. Once capillary integrity has recovered, protein colloids (e.g. 5% albumin) are certainly required and these must often be given in very large quantities. During the recovery phase excess tissue fluids will be mobilized and excreted provided that renal function is satisfactory.

3 CLINICAL AND LABORATORY OBSERVATIONS

Subsequent management must depend on the clinical response because individual patients, even those with similar degrees of burn injury, vary in the physiological responses. It will usually be necessary to reassess the fluid replacement needs no less frequently than every 12 hours. The replacement regimens referred to earlier provide initial guidance only and do not represent rigid rules. The following observations are usually made:

- Blood pressure

Urine volume and concentrating power ($>0.5–1.0$ ml/kg per hour and specific gravity >1018) should be maintained.

- Haemoglobin and haematocrit.
- Serum protein concentration or colloid osmotic pressure.
- Serum electrolytes.
- Acid base balance.

Clinical observation enables assessment of peripheral perfusion and freedom from shock.

Severely burned patients require monitoring of circulatory performance along the lines described for massive blood loss and replacement (see chapter 13), although even in severe cases circulatory failure develops more slowly. The more invasive measures become necessary only when neglect or delay in providing treatment has occurred. These measurements might include pulmonary capillary wedge pressure and cardiac output, arterial and mixed venous oxygen tensions, assessment of pulmonary compliance, intrapulmonary shunting and tissue oxygen consumption.

REFERENCES

1   Lawrence, C. and Atack, B. (1992) Haematologic changes in massive burn injury. *Crit. Care. Med.*, **20**: 1284–1288.
2   Wood, J.J., Rodrick, M.L., O'Mahony, J.B. *et al.* (1984) Inadequate interlukin 2 production: a fundamental immunological deficiency in patients with major burns. *Ann. Surg.*, **200**: 311–318.
3   Herndon, D.N., Langner, F., Thompson, P., Linares, H.A., Stein, M. and Traver, D.L. (1987) Pulmonary injury in burned patients. *Surg. Clin. North Am.*, **67**: 31–46.
4   Demling, R.H. (1987) Fluid replacement in burned patients. *Surg. Clin. North Am.*, **67**: 15–29.
5   Goodwin, C.W., Dorethy, J., Lam, V. and Pruitt, B.A. (1983) Randomized trial of efficacy of crystalloid and colloid resuscitation on hemodynamic response and lung water following thermal injury. *Ann. Surg.*, **197**: 520–531.
6   Baxter, C.R. and Shires, G.T. (1968) Physiological response to crystalloid resuscitation of severe burns. *Ann. NY Acad. Sci.*, **150**: 874–894.
7   Watson, J.S., Walker, C.C. and Sanders, R. (1977) A comparison between dried plasma and plasma protein fraction in the resuscitation of burn patients. *Burns Incl. Ther. Inj.*, **3**: 108–111.
8   Milner, S.M., Hodgetts, T.J. and Rylah, L.T.A. (1993) The burns calculator: a simple proposed guide for fluid resuscitation. *Lancet*, **342**: 1089–1091.
9   Monafo, W.W., Halverson, J.D. and Schechtman, K. (1984) The role of concentrated sodium solutions in the resuscitation of patients with severe burns. *Surgery*, **95**: 129–135.

17

Autoantibodies and Autoimmune Haemolysis

Most of the recognizable antibodies in blood or tissue fluids have specificities clearly directed against exogenous antigenic materials. These immunogenic substances share in common the property of differing immunochemically from the blood or tissue antigens of the individual who produced them and the antibodies they stimulate therefore discriminate in their reactions between self and non-self antigens. This mechanism forms an important component of the immunological defence system against invading microorganisms. Under certain pathological circumstances this efficient arrangement is disturbed, and endogenously reactive *autoantibodies* are produced which, when directed against blood cells, can have the same destructive effects as those described earlier (chapter 2, section 5) for alloantibodies. It appears likely that this malfunction is a consequence of diminished activity of a part of the suppressor T lymphocyte system whose normal role is to confine immune responses to those recognizing foreign or 'non-self' antigens alone.

The management of autoantibody (autoimmune) haematological disorders affects the work of the blood bank in various ways. Autoantibodies against blood cells present problems to the blood bank as regards both diagnosis of the pathological condition and also the provision of any necessary transfusion treatment. They may also interfere with, and as a consequence lead to errors during, routine serological testing. For some conditions there may be a place for autoantibody removal by plasmapheresis therapy and these disorders are discussed in chapter 19.

The principal conditions of concern include:

- autoimmune haemolytic anaemias (AIHA);
- autoimmune (idiopathic) thrombocytopenia (ITP); and less commonly
- autoimmune neutropenia.

Aplastic anaemia may sometimes appear to result from autoimmune activity against marrow precursor tissues; this possibility is particularly of relevance during the management of patients by bone marrow transplantation when the pre-graft immunosuppression alone has sometimes appeared to be curative.

1 CRITERIA FOR DIAGNOSIS

The presence of autoantibodies against peripheral blood cells does not always signify the presence of a clinically significant destructive process. There may at times be no evidence whatsoever of *in vivo* cell destruction; alternatively, haemolysis may occur but only to such a limited extent that it can be fully compensated for by extra bone marrow proliferative activity.

For a diagnosis of autoimmune haemolysis the following evidence should be sought:

(1) Evidence of immunological attack to the cell line concerned: this takes the form of *cell-bound immunoglobulin*, usually IgG, much less commonly IgA, and/or *complement*, particularly the components C3d and C4d. Red cells show positive direct antiglobulin results; platelets may have surface-bound immunoglobulin demonstrable by various antiglobulin-based test procedures (radio-labelled antiglobulin, immunofluorescence or enzyme-linked antiglobulin techniques).

   Cell-bound immunoglobulin is not necessarily indicative of an autoimmune haemolytic state. Around one in 4000 healthy blood donors, for example, have a positive direct red cell antiglobulin test unassociated with any other features indicative of haemolysis.

(2) The presence of *free antibody* in the serum: high-affinity antibodies with optimal temperatures of reaction at 37 °C may be largely cell bound (e.g. those often found in autoimmune haemolytic anaemias), very little remaining in the serum. Cold-reactive red cell autoantibodies are always easily demonstrable in the serum and sometimes they are present in extremely high titre.

   Unfortunately neither the titre of serum antibody nor the strength of the antiglobulin reactions provide any reliable guide to the clinical severity of the haemolytic state.

(3) Evidence of *peripheral blood cell destruction*: this takes the form of:

   (a) Morphological features of *cell injury*. Typically seen are spherocytic red cells (particularly in the case of 'warm' antibody AIHA), or erythrocytes misshapen as a result of phagocytosis and loss of membrane areas that have been covered with immunoglobulin or complement. In cold agglutinin haemolytic anaemias blood films often show conspicuous red cell agglutinates.

(b) Signs of *regeneration* of immature cells to replace those lost from the blood. This shows as polychromasia of red cells (due to residual RNA in reticulocytes) or large megathrombocytes in ITP.

(c) *Hyperplasia* of the appropriate precursor cell line in the bone marrow.

(4) For haemolytic anaemias *biochemical* evidence of red cell degradation is provided by unconjugated hyperbilirubinaemia and increased urobilinogen excretion. In cases of intravascular haemolysis there will be haemoglobinuria, urinary haemosiderin and absent serum haptoglobins.

(5) Diminished red cell survival can be demonstrated by labelling autologous red cells with radioisotopes.

2 RED CELL AUTOANTIBODIES

Red cell autoantibodies usually react against the majority of normal blood samples as well as the patient's own red cells. There may be antibody specificity against identifiable but ubiquitous antigens, e.g. anti-I, anti-H, anti-HI. These typically 'cold'-reacting antibodies show graded reactions according to the antigen content of the test cells. Autoanti-H, for example, reacts with diminishing strength against cells of group O, A_2 and A_1 in proportion to their residual H antigen content—a reflection of the fact that this precursor material is consumed during biosynthesis of the blood group A and B polysaccharides. 'Warm' antibodies usually react against all test cells but may show a degree of apparent specificity in terms of a preference for cells bearing particular Rh antigens. Apparent autoanti-e antibodies are a frequent example of this phenomenon.

2.1 Asymptomatic Low-titre Cold Antibodies

These antibodies, which are of no clinical significance, are ubiquitous in normal sera. The antibodies can cause laboratory problems when clotted blood samples are stored refrigerated; binding of the cold reacting IgM antibody to red cells is followed by complement uptake to the stage of C3d and C4d. This complement persists on the red cells, even after washing, and leads to positive direct antiglobulin results that can be clinically misleading or cause serologically erroneous conclusions.

2.2 Cold Haemagglutinin Disease: High-titre 'Cold' Antibodies

Clinical and pathological features

Occasional patients' sera are found to contain very high-titre cold antibodies and these are highly likely to produce clinically apparent symptoms. The antibodies are IgM in type and cause direct agglutination of red cells, particularly at temperatures below 37 °C.

Anticoagulated blood samples cooled to room temperature frequently show so much macroscopic red cell agglutination that it is easily visible to the naked eye.

If the antibody has a high binding affinity and agglutinates at the temperature of exposed peripheral skin capillaries (these are frequently as low as 30 °C) red cell agglutination occurs *in vivo*. These red cell agglutinates cause sludging and disrupt perfusion, causing *ischaemia, cyanosis* and sometimes even *gangrene* of the digits. These are symptoms of Raynaud's phenomenon. Agglutinates disperse in the circulation following rewarming, but complement components will remain cell bound, and the direct antiglobulin test will be positive. Sublytic complement uptake (as far as C3b binding) leads to reticuloendothelial entrapment of red cells and *extravascular haemolysis*. Acute episodes of haemolysis may take place; these are often clearly precipitated by cold exposure. Alternatively, and more usually, anaemia due to a low-grade chronic haemolytic process may occur. Minimally affected cells may escape haemolysis and natural plasma C3 and C4 inactivators (e.g. C3b INA) convert cell-bound C3b and C4b to C3d and C4d respectively, which can be detected by direct antiglobulin testing. Monospecific sera can be used to identify the presence of C3d and C4d on the cell surface; these components may persist for weeks after a sensitizing episode. Severe chilling may cause enough complement activation to produce *intravascular haemolysis* and frank *haemoglobinuria*. This is brought about by sequential uptake of the terminal components of the complement sequence, namely C5a through to C9, creating the 'membrane attack unit' which enzymatically penetrates the cell membrane and leads to cell lysis.

Cold autoagglutinins usually show specificity within the I/i antigen system. Most are anti-I, reacting therefore against virtually all adult red cells but showing lower titres against cord red cells, because in these the I antigen has not yet developed. Chronic cold haemagglutinin disease (CHAD) with monoclonal anti-I cold agglutinins is often *idiopathic* although it is sometimes associated with underlying *lymphoid malignancies*. Acute episodes of cold agglutinin haemolysis due to anti-I (polyclonal) frequently follow *Mycoplasma pneumoniae* infection. Haemolytic anaemia due to anti-i antibodies is most typically found as an uncommon complication of *infectious mononucleosis*; these postinfective haemolytic anaemias usually resolve spontaneously. Steroids are most frequently used for treatment of severe acute haemolysis; in chronic disease their use is less rewarding. Transfusion management is considered in chapter 4, section 3.3.

Laboratory features

(1) Cold antibodies cause *direct agglutination* of red cells at low temperatures. This activity is expressed in terms of the *titre* causing agglutination; very high titres (e.g. up to or exceeding 64 000) are not unusual. The temperature (e.g. 4 °C, 22 °C, 30 °C, etc.) at which the highest titres occur is referred to as the *thermal amplitude*; this is of direct clinical relevance as it appears to correlate with the likelihood of clinically evident haemolysis.

(2) The *specificity* in terms of the I/i antigen system is assessed by comparing titres using both adult and cord blood cells. Antibodies which show IH activity, rather that I alone, will react preferentially with group O red cells compared with group A cells.

(3) The direct *antiglobin test* is positive and is usually due to cell-bound C3d and C4d. *Indirect tests* using the patient's serum will also be positive either because of complement binding or from the heavy coating of IgM antibody persisting after washing. This is sometimes sufficient to cause agglutination of the cell suspension even without addition of antiglobulin reagents.

(4) *Blood grouping and antibody screening problems*: as the patient's serum usually causes direct agglutination of all cell suspensions the ABO serum groups cannot easily be determined and antibody screening and cross-matching tests involving low-temperature saline tests will be impossible. Even if agglutination is avoided by performing tests at 37 °C, complement binding may obscure the results of antiglobulin tests during antibody screening or cross-matching. If there is a sufficient coating of autoantibody on the patient's red cells they will agglutinate spontaneously, thus invalidating the results of ABO cell typing.

There are several ways of overcoming these problems. Washing the red cells with warm (e.g. 45 °C) saline usually removes sufficient IgM antibody to allow cell grouping. Such warm washed cells can be used to auto-absorb cold antibody from the serum to allow a search for other alloantibodies. Antibody studies can also be accomplished more easily if strict attention is paid to performing and keeping all tests at 37 °C. The direct antiglobulin test should be performed on blood collected warm into EDTA to prevent *in vitro* complement binding. These same cells, washed in warm saline, are also suitable for ABO typing and for other antigen studies.

2.3 Paroxysmal Cold Haemoglobinuria

Paroxysmal cold haemoglobinuria describes a clinical syndrome caused by an IgG autoantibody distinguished by its unique *in vitro* behaviour. When blood samples from such patients are cooled, autoantibody is bound; this dissociates on rewarming but not before a haemolytic level of complement binding is acquired. This causes sufficient red cell lysis for haemoglobin to be easily visible in the plasma, especially when the plasma is compared with an unchilled sample. The principle of this process of biphasic antibody uptake, and complement binding is employed diagnostically in the *Donath–Landsteiner test*, during which fresh patient's serum is incubated, as described above, with test red cell suspensions. The Donath–Landsteiner antibody reacts against virtually all red cells but, in fact, has specificity within the P blood group system (see chapter 2, section 4.5). There may be sufficient residual complement on the unhaemolysed patient's cells to give a *positive direct antiglobulin test*.

Paroxysmal cold haemoglobinuria is rare but *typically* follows as a complication of various *acute infections in children*. *Haemolysis* may be severe and accompanied by *gross haemoglobinuria* but is usually self-limiting and followed by permanent recovery. High doses of steroids are usually given during the acute phase. Transfusion is rarely needed, except for very severe anaemia, which is fortunate since serologically compatible units will not be obtainable.

2.4   Autoimmune Haemolysis due to Warm Antibodies

Clinical and pathological features

Haemolytic anaemias of this category are caused by IgG autoantibodies show-ing optimum serological reactions at body temperatures, in distinction to the 'cold' antibodies discussed above. *The direct antiglobulin test should be positive*; monospecific antiglobulin reactions can be used to demonstrate the presence of either IgG, IgG together with complement (predominantly C3d and C4d) or com-plement alone.

Very rare cases do not appear to have sufficient cell-bound immunoglobulin (e.g. at least 200–400 molecules) to show a positive direct antiglobulin test by standard antiglobulin techniques. In these instances increased cell-bound immu-noglobulin can sometimes be demonstrated by quantitative radiolabelled or enzyme-labelled antiglobulin-based assays.

Warm autoantibodies may cause *severe fulminant haemolysis* or at the other extreme of the clinical spectrum merely produce *positive direct antiglobulin* tests without any evidence of accelerated red cell destruction. Haemolysis, when it occurs, is due to reticuloendothelial clearance of red cells damaged by immunoglobulin or complement as described for alloantibodies (chapter 2, section 5).

Clinical associations of warm autoimmune haemolytic anaemias include other autoimmune conditions (e.g. *systemic lupus erythematosus, idiopathic thrombocyto-penia*), and lymphoid malignancies such as *chronic lymphocytic leukaemia*. About 20% of patients treated with *α-methyldopa* develop an apparently identical condition. Most cases of autoimmune haemolysis are *idiopathic* and remain unexplained despite prolonged follow-up. In general, acute illness is followed by spontaneous or steroid-accelerated remission. Some cases persist as sub-acute or chronic haemolysis requiring continued steroid therapy. Splenectomy, by removing the prime site of haemolysis, improves a proportion of chronic cases.

Serum studies

In contrast to cold antibody haemolytic anaemias, it may not be possible to demonstrate free autoantibody in the serum; autoantibodies are more likely to be found if enzyme-treated test cells are used for screening, these being more suitable for detection of the residual low-affinity antibodies in the serum. Eluates from the red cells, however, should contain high-affinity antibody species. Both eluates and sera should be examined against cell panels for evidence of specificity; when present this generally shows as a preference for certain Rh genotypes (e.g. anti-e). Specificity may be more apparent from the reactions of the patient's serum against the cell panel than it is from the eluted antibodies, which are of higher affinity and may react to a greater extent with all cells tested. An indication of relative specificity can also be obtained by titration of the sera or eluates against the cell panel.

Coincidental alloantibodies

It has been claimed that these can be demonstrated in 30–40% of all cases,[1,2] anti-C and anti-K being the most frequent finding.[1]

The risk of forming alloantibodies in patients with autoimmune haemolytic disease is influenced by *previous pregnancies* and by *blood transfusions* just as it is in patients with other anaemias.[2] These alloantibodies are hard to detect in the presence of warm autoantibodies but an attempt should nevertheless be made because they will have the same haemolytic potential during transfusion as those found in other patients. Their presence is revealed when specific antibodies, demonstrated as described above, are directed against antigens not carried on the patient's own red cells. These will usually occur against a background of autoantibody reacting to some degree against all red cells including, of course, the patient's own cells. A search for alloantibodies can be made by using the patient's own cells, after first freeing them from bound autoantibody, as a reagent to absorb out autoantibodies from the serum. This approach cannot, of course, be used in patients who have recently been transfused; the period of a few days immediately following a transfusion would in any case be a bad time to look for alloantibodies as they may have been absorbed *in vivo*. Various approaches have been used to assist the detection of alloantibodies. The patient's own cells can be used for autoabsorption after repeated warm saline washes, treatment with chloroquine,[3] or dithiothreitol–papain (ZZAP).[4] If the patient's phenotype has been established, normal cells of an identical phenotype can be used for absorption of 'autoantibody' provided these cells are also negative for the clinically significant antigen systems the patient lacks.

Transfusion of patients with warm autoimmune haemolysis

Blood transfusions are only given when absolutely necessary on clinical grounds. Frequently no donor cells are found that are compatible; provided no alloantibodies can be found, the customary practice is to give the *least incompatible units*.[5] The most common alternative, applicable when no evidence for specificity exists, is to transfuse blood of the *same Rh genotype* as that of the recipient. Before embarking on transfusion an attempt should always be made to determine the Rh genotype of the patient; this task will be made easier if the bound autoantibody from the red cells is removed. It is most important to remember that the opportunity to determine the genotype accurately will be lost after the first transfusions have been given. The post-transfusion survival of donor red cells is almost certainly shortened to the same degree as that of the patient's own cells.

Blood grouping tests

ABO grouping is usually straightforward but the antibody coating on red cells can cause false positive Rh D typing results by albumin, enzyme or antiglobulin methods. This should be unmasked by the finding of unexpected positive results with the appropriate Rh control reagent. Saline-reacting D typing sera, chemically modified and monoclonal D typing reagents usually provide reliable results although controls are necessary with the latter. Autoantibody removal (see above) may enable more reliable genotyping.

2.5 Drug-induced Immune Haemolysis

This probably accounts for a high proportion of *positive direct antiglobulin tests* in patients and a much smaller number of cases of *overt haemolysis*. Specialized laboratory facilities are required for their investigation. Various mechanisms have been shown to result in red cell destruction:

(1) α-*Methyldopa* as a cause of haemolytic anaemia resembling autoimmune hae-molytic anaemia is referred to above.
(2) Penicillin therapy induces a mild haemolytic anaemia in occasional patients. Penicillin (and the chemically similar cephalosporins) both bind to red cells and also provoke anti-penicillin/cephalosporin antibodies which then attack the penicillin- or cephalosporin-coated erythrocytes.
(3) Other drugs (e.g. quinine, quinidine, phenacetin, chlorpropamide, sulpha drugs) form immune complexes with their corresponding antibodies. These then become passively bound to red cells, accelerating their destruction by the reticuloendothelial system; sometimes complement fixation and severe acute intravascular haemolysis follow drug therapy in sensitized patients.

3 IDIOPATHIC THROMBOCYTOPENIC PURPURA

This condition shows some serological, clinical and therapeutic parallels to warm autoimmune haemolytic anaemia, and the principles on which the diagnosis is determined have been described earlier (section 1). Platelet concentrate therapy is not likely to be helpful and is rarely used except for dangerous bleeding episodes and in attempts to reduce blood loss during surgery. The survival of transfused platelets is so short that effective increases in platelet count cannot be obtained. Steroids and/or splenectomy are the well-known and conventional forms of therapy for persistent care but intravenous immunoglobulin (chapter 9, section 3), in certain circumstances, has a valuable role in this condition.

REFERENCES

1   Laine, M.L. and Beattie, K.M. (1985) Frequency of alloantibodies accompanying auto-antibodies. *Transfusion*, 25: 545–546.
2   Wallhermfechtel, M.A., Polh, B.A. and Chaplain, H. (1984) Alloimmunization in patients with warm autoantibodies: a retrospective study employing three donor alloabsorptions to aid antibody detection. *Transfusion*, 24: 482–485.
3   Edwards, J.M., Moulds, J.J. and Judd, W.J. (1982) Chloroquine dissociation of antigen–antibody complexes: a new technique for typing red blood cells with a positive direct antiglobulin test. *Transfusion*, 22: 59–61.

4   Branch, D.R. and Petz, L.D. (1982) A new reagent (ZZAP) having multiple applications in immunohaematology. *Am. J. Clin. Pathol.*, **78**: 161–167.

5   Walker, R.H., Kuban, D.J., Polesky, H.F. and Van Der Hoeven, L.H. (1982) The 1980 Comprehensive Blood Bank Survey of the College of American Pathologists. *Am. J. Clin. Pathol.*, **78**: 610–614.

18

Special Transfusion Problems in General Medicine

1 RENAL FAILURE

1.1 The Anaemia of Renal Failure

Anaemia is usual in chronic renal failure and results from a variety of factors including defective erythropoietin production, reduced erythrocyte survival and accumulation of toxic products impairing bone marrow function. Transfusions have often been given for the treatment of symptomatic severe anaemia but it was recognized they were *not* necessary just because of low haemoglobin levels. Patients with chronic renal failure tolerate blood haemoglobin concentrations, even as low as 5.0 g/dl, surprisingly well. This is partly because the haemoglobin oxygen affinity is reduced as a result of acidosis and high plasma inorganic phosphate levels, both of which enhance 2,3-diphosphoglycerate (DPG) synthesis (chapter 3, section 2.1). Plasma volume expansion occurs in renal failure and this causes the peripheral blood count to underestimate the size of the red cell mass. This is especially true in the presence of hypersplenism, and splenectomy has been found to result in increased haemoglobin levels and decreased transfusion needs.

Despite the ability to tolerate low haemoglobin levels, patients do benefit greatly from improved haemoglobin levels. The management of anaemia in renal failure has now been transformed with the availability of recombinant human erythropoietin (rHuEPO) in therapeutic form.[1] Erythropoietin administered subcutaneously (despite its greater efficacy the intravenous route is impractical for regular use in most dialysis patients) at starting doses of around 300–450 IU/kg per week is given to raise haemoglobin values to 11.0–11.5 g per day. Maintenance therapy can be achieved with substantially lower doses (37.5–150 IU/kg per week). Provision of adequate iron supplies is necessary to ensure optimum response. Despite the usually high storage iron levels limitations in the rate of release necessitate the use of supplementary iron.

Replacement of blood loss

Although patients with chronic renal failure and anaemia compensate well in a stable state, there will be diminished capacity to tolerate further blood losses and these should, therefore, be replaced promptly. Needless to say, in severely anaemic patients, particularly careful attention to oxygenation and maintenance of blood pressure is required. There seems to be agreement that 'top-up' transfusions, raising haemoglobin values above those to which the patients are accustomed, are unnecessary during preparation for surgery. This policy may, however, require reassessment with the recent realization that a low haematocrit appears to lengthen the bleeding time (see section 1.4).

1.2 Blood Transfusion and Renal Transplantation

Blood transfusion before transplantation has, during recent years, been clearly shown to have a beneficial effect on graft survival. As a result blood transfusion prior to transplantation is, under certain circumstances, now regarded as acceptable. This represents a volte-face from the earlier position in which transfusion was believed to induce a high incidence of alloimmunization to HLA antigens, thereby reducing the chances of successful engraftment. Because of these anxieties, a minimum transfusion policy, often utilizing only leucocyte-free products, was espoused by many transplantation centres. The subject is discussed more fully in chapter 22, section 2.3.

1.3 Transfusion and Renal Function

The homeostatic control of plasma volume depends on efficient renal salt and water excretion. These responses will be slower in renal failure; transfusions carry a greater risk of blood volume overload and should therefore be given more slowly.

Hyperkalaemia might be expected to be a particular risk to patients with renal failure. For this reason, where several units are to be given, or if transfusion is required during surgery, it has been suggested that reasonably fresh blood (e.g. 3–5 days of age) should be selected. In practice, the problem appears infrequently for the same reasons as discussed in chapter 12, section 4.6. It has clearly been shown that the practice of using blood of less than 5 days of age is unnecessary for transfusion of chronic dialysis patients.[2] Red cells up to 2 weeks of age were shown to be satisfactory; neither potassium nor post-transfusion haemolysis presented problems.

1.4 Haemostatic Problems in Renal Failure

Uraemia causes a platelet functional defect which may result in bleeding symptoms. The presence of the defect may be indicated by prolonged bleeding times or by reduced performance in platelet adhesiveness tests. Transfused platelets will acquire the same functional impairment and will therefore be of little value in treating haemorrhage. Dialysis improves platelet function and in this respect peritoneal dialysis appears to be more effective than haemodialysis. This seems likely to be due to more efficient loss of the lower molecular weight substances which damage platelet function. The bleeding time appears to be prolonged when the haematocrit is low in patients with uraemia, in the same way that it is in thrombocytopenic disorders. Increasing the haematocrit to above 0.26 has been reported to normalize the bleeding time despite unchanged blood urea values.[3] Arginine vasopressin (DDAVP), with or without cryoprecipitate, has been reported as being helpful in transiently reducing the bleeding time in uraemia;[4,5] this effect appears to be related to the increased blood levels of high molecular weight multimers of von Willebrand factor.

2 CARDIAC DISEASE

Increased cardiac output is an obligatory response to anaemia in otherwise healthy subjects. It follows, therefore, that correction of anaemia in patients with cardiac failure reduces myocardial workload and may improve symptoms. Correction of anaemia also alleviates the myocardial hypoxia that in turn contributes to the cardiac failure.

The transfusion problems of patients with cardiac disease depend of the cardiac lesion, the physiological consequences of cardiac failure (e.g. pulmonary oedema, hypervolaemia) and the presence of other predisposing conditions. Those with angina who are not in cardiac failure will be essentially normovolaemic or only slightly hypervolaemic and will require relief from any anaemia that may have aggravated anginal symptoms. Whether total correction of their haemoglobin deficit is required or whether, alternatively, a moderate degree of haemodilution (chapter 15, section 2) is beneficial remains an area of controversy. Severe anaemia in patients with cardiac failure can be corrected by means of small-volume exchange transfusion (chapter 4, section 1.4) replacing 'anaemic' blood with lower volumes of red cell concentrates. For critically ill patients with severe anaemia blood of near normal DPG content (e.g. that within the first few days of collection) is advisable.

The presence of hypertension or valvular disease may be associated with congestive failure, pulmonary or hepatic congestion, splenomegaly and renal functional impairment. There is also likely to be hypervolaemia due to an expanded plasma volume. In such circumstances it is necessary to use low-volume products such as red cell concentrates and to restrict the use of albumin or plasma products which could contribute to further increases in the plasma volume. Transfusions given overnight, at times when patients are less easily observed, are best avoided. Warming the patient induces peripheral dilation, expands the potential vascular volume and reduces the risk of precipitating left ventricular failure.

Use of albumin concentrates (chapter 10, section 4) to treat oedema and hypo-proteinaemia will cause dangerous plasma volume expansion in the presence of cardiac failure unless effective diuretic therapy is in progress. Pre-existing left ventricular failure in surgical or traumatized subjects seems likely to be an important factor in the genesis of adult respiratory distress syndrome (ARDS). For these patients it may be particularly important to reduce the other risk factors for ARDS. In particular, volume overload should be avoided and microaggregate filters should be used during transfusions of conventional red cell components.

3 PULMONARY DISEASE

Hypoxaemia arising from pulmonary disease normally tends to result in erythrocytosis. However, in the presence of chronic infections, the bone marrow response to hypoxia may be impaired as it is in anaemias associated with chronic inflammatory disease. The resulting haemoglobin level may therefore be inappropriately low for the oxygen transport needs. Where large transfusions are required, for example during surgery in hypoxaemic patients with chronic obstructive pulmonary disease, an attempt should be made to maintain normal blood haemoglobin levels. Provided the alveolar pO_2 exceeds 60 mmHg, use of fresh blood with a right-shifted oxygen dissociation curve is desirable. If alveolar oxygen tensions fall below this value, use of blood with a right-shifted oxygen dissociation curve could theoretically become a disadvantage, as alveolar pO_2 values then fall on the steep descending part of the curve and oxygen uptake might be impaired. It is theoretically possible, although unproven, that high-affinity left 'shifted' blood such as that resulting from storage should allow higher arterial blood oxygen saturation values and permit a greater difference in arteriovenous oxygen content. In contrast, for many pulmonary and cardiac conditions, in which right-to-left shunting from the 'venous' to the 'arterial' circulation occurs, it has been shown that oxygen transport is improved following transfusion of blood of low oxygen affinity.

In general, therefore, selection of reasonably fresh blood where large transfusions are given rapidly to patients with pulmonary disease is probably advantageous. This may not be so helpful for patients in whom alveolar pO_2 values are too low to permit high levels of haemoglobin saturation with a right-shifted oxygen dissociation curve. In this situation the optimum choice of blood is debatable.

4 LIVER DISEASE

Anaemia can occur in liver disease from blood loss, haematinic factor (B_{12}, folate) deficiency, haemolysis or marrow depression. The haemoglobin concentration is sometimes inappropriately low for the size of the red cell mass because of plasma volume expansion. The metabolic problems of liver failure may be compounded by coexisting renal failure (hepatorenal syndrome), making acidosis and hyperkalaemia added transfusion risks. Patients with liver disease may present several problems during blood replacement:

(1) There may be pre-existing deficiencies of vitamin K-dependent clotting factors (II, VII, IX and X and also Factor V). Fresh frozen plasma may be required for preoperative correction of disordered coagulation function at an earlier stage than is usual during extensive blood replacement. Where time permits preoperative correction of coagulation status with vitamin K should be attempted (see chapter 8, section 4).
(2) Patients with portal hypertension and splenomegaly may have thrombocytopenia, in which case platelets may be needed during surgery.
(3) Reduced albumin synthesis, and impaired aldosterone metabolism, may lead to hypoproteinaemia and retention of sodium and water. These eventually cause oedema and an expanded plasma volume. There is, therefore, an increased risk of circulatory overload from inadequately supervised transfusion and fluid balance. Combined use of diuretics and albumin concentrates (chapter 10, section 4) may be required to gain control over hypoproteinaemic oedema.

REFERENCES

1 Macdougall, I.C., Hutton, R.D., Coles, G.A. and Williams, J.D. (1991) The use of erythropoietin in renal failure. *Post. Grad. Med. J.*, **67**: 9–15.
2 Fogh-Andersen, N. and Mogensen, F. (1984) On the safety of using stored blood for chronic haemodialysis patients. *Transfusion*, **24**: 505–507.
3 Fenandez, F., Goudable, C., Sie, P. *et al.* (1985) Low haematocrit and prolonged bleeding time in uraemic patients: effect of red cell transfusions. *Br. J. Haematol.*, **59**: 139–148.
4 Janson, P.A., Jubelirer, S.J., Weinstein, M.J. and Deykin, D. (1980) Treatment of the bleeding tendency in uraemia with cryoprecipitate. *N. Engl. J. Med.*, **303**: 1318–1322.
5 Canavese, C., Salomone, M., Pacitti, A., Mangiarotti, G. and Calitri, V. (1985) Reduced response of uraemic bleeding time to repeated doses of desmopressin. *Lancet*, **i**: 867–868.

19

Therapeutic Apheresis

1 DEFINITIONS

Therapeutic apheresis procedures involve the physical removal of abnormal blood constituents for the purpose of alleviating or controlling disease symptoms. The treatment is palliative rather than curative; it buys time thereby allowing conventional therapy to regain control over the disease process or natural remission to occur. During the procedure an equivalent volume of suitably selected intravenous fluid is replaced so that physiological disturbances are minimized. *Apheresis* is a generic term embracing various types of procedure. *Haemapheresis, cytapheresis* and *plasmapheresis* denote removal of blood, blood cells or plasma respectively; the latter is sometimes referred to as *plasma exchange*. The procedures are developments of the technique of exchange transfusion, which still has a place, particularly in neonatal medicine. Manual exchange of large volumes of plasma or red cells is cumbersome and time consuming. The modern application of therapeutic apheresis followed the development of automated cell separators.

1.1 Automated Apheresis

Therapeutic apheresis machines (cell separators) are similar to those used for blood component collection and mainly utilize the principles of either *continuous* or *discontinuous centrifugation*. Separation of plasma components can also be achieved using *membrane* filtration systems analogous to those used for renal dialysis. The technical field is one of continuous development and manufacturers will readily demonstrate the principles and particular advantages of their own machines. Technical aspects which should be considered include:

(1) The extracorporeal volume: this may vary from 150 to 400 ml over and above the volume of plasma collected. Hypotensive episodes are more likely with larger extracorporeal blood volumes.
(2) Discontinuous centrifugal systems require only a single intravenous needle which suffices for both collection and return. Two needles, one in each arm, are usually required for continuous centrifugal machines.
(3) Simplicity of use, flow rate indicators, air-bubble warning devices, automatic operation, visual display of operating instructions or problem diagnosis are features incorporated into the latest models.
(4) Reliability, service and back-up arrangements, operator training and, of course, costs of the machine and disposable materials.

2 PHYSIOLOGICAL PRINCIPLES

The apheresis principle entails the removal or exchange of unwanted blood constituents which may include:

(1) Red cells, granulocytes, lymphocytes and platelets.
(2) Plasma constituents such as auto- or alloantibodies, immune complexes.
(3) Toxic metabolites such as bilirubin, and protein-bound poisons.

Three main variations are possible:

(1) An *abnormal substance* is removed. Examples include removal of paraprotein in hyperviscosity states, Factor VIII antibodies in treatment-resistant haemophilia patients, or immune complexes which cause tissue damage in systemic lupus erythematosus. Autoimmune disorders form the largest group of diseases for which apheresis is currently used, and in these conditions the procedure is usually designed to remove autoantibodies or immune complexes.
(2) The reduction of an *excessive amount* of otherwise *normal cells* or *plasma constituents* may be required. An instance of this is the removal of red cells to enable rapid correction of the haematocrit and blood viscosity in severe polycythaemia.
(3) Exchange of large volumes of plasma which may be deficient in certain components, e.g. thrombotic thrombocytopenic purpura, in which a natural inhibitor to the pathological platelet aggregation may be lacking from the plasma. Normal plasma is then replaced.

2.1 Arithmetic and Physiological Considerations

In some conditions the clinical response to apheresis is, to a degree, arithmetically predictable. For this to be true:

(1) There must be a clear relationship between the *concentration* of the unwanted material and the *severity* of the disease. This certainly holds true for erythrocytosis and for hyperviscosity syndrome due to IgM paraprotein. The relationship, is however, much less clear with regard to removal of immune complexes in conditions such as systemic lupus erythematosus.

(2) The *distribution* of the substance to be removed between *intravascular* and *extravascular spaces* must be known. IgM immunoglobulins are predominantly intravascular and are therefore removed efficiently by apheresis. IgG immunoglobulins are only about 40% intravascular and removal from the plasma is therefore followed over the next few hours by replenishment from the extravascular fluid.

(3) The rate of *synthesis* and of *degradation* and also how these might be influenced by the apheresis procedure must be considered. The natural half-life is around 3 weeks for IgG and 5 days for IgM. These rates, slow for IgG and more rapid for IgM, proportionally influence the time for plasma levels to recover following apheresis. Whether plasma exchange itself influences turnover rates is not well understood. Natural degradation rates for some materials may be concentration dependent; reduction of blood levels by apheresis might, as a result, slow catabolism. It is also possible that the reduction of immunoglobulin levels during apheresis may, by mechanisms which remain speculative, stimulate further syntheses. This phenomenon has certainly been postulated to account for unexpected difficulties in reducing pathological antibody levels to the extent desired. On occasions plasmapheresis treatment appears to be rather more effective than might be anticipated; the endogenous clearance rate of immune complexes in patients with systemic lupus erythematosus is, for example, thought to be improved following plasmapheresis. It has been proposed that this may be due to the recovery of reticuloendothelial cell function following removal of a 'log-jam' effect caused by accumulation of very high plasma immune complex levels.

2.2 Volume and Frequency of Apheresis

Apheresis procedures principally remove *intravascular* materials, and it is largely during the post-exchange period that the proportion held in the extravascular compartment is returned to the circulation. For this reason repeated small volume exchanges, in which high plasma concentrations are replaced, are more efficient than larger and less frequent exchanges. During large volume exchanges the removed plasma, on a volume-for-volume basis, contains progressively lower concentrations of the abnormal constituent and increasing proportions of exchange fluid.

A convenient approximation for prediction of the plasma levels remaining immediately after exchange is that:

- A one-volume exchange removes 66%.
- A two-volume exchange removes 85%.
- A three-volume exchange removes 95% of intravascular constituents.

The plasma volume can be calculated approximately by assuming the blood volume to be 75 ml/kg body weight and multiplying this value by (1 − haematocrit).

Typical plasma exchange schedules entail removal of 2 l of plasma three times weekly. More aggressive regimens aim to remove 3–4 l on each occasion and nine or more litres per week. These programmes may have to be continued for several weeks, in some conditions, until it is clear whether control of the disease is possible.

2.3 Recovery of Normal Plasma Composition Following Plasma Exchange: Choice of Exchange Fluid[1-5]

Although it would be ultimately desirable, plasmapheresis is not yet a selective process that would allow removal of only the unwanted component from the plasma. (This qualification will not apply if experimental immunoabsorbent systems become practicably feasible—see section 6.) Whole plasma must be removed but the fluids available for return to the patient will differ in composition from normal plasma. An assessment must therefore be made as to the likelihood of physiologically dangerous alterations in the patient's own plasma composition following the exchange procedure. The plasma volume-expanding materials that are available for replacement are described in chapter 10.

The principal concerns surround reductions in:

- Coagulation activity.
- Plasma proteins and oncotic pressure.
- Immunoglobulin concentrations.

The behaviour of the various components of these physiological systems depends on the same factors that relate to removal of pathological materials described above. In assessing the risks of apheresis it is important to recognize those categories of patients least able to tolerate particular disturbances. The following observations relate to patients having sequential exchanges of the order of 0.7–1.0 plasma volumes (approximately 2–3 l) every 48 hours.

Haemostatic changes

Many coagulation factors have relatively rapid turnover rates (half-life less than 24 hours) and are as a consequence not affected to a clinically significant degree during most exchange programmes. *Fibrinogen*, with a half-life of around 4 days, is an exception and it is this protein which appears to be the limiting factor with regard to the intensity of plasma exchange. Levels may be 50% reduced at 24 hours and 30% reduced at 3 days following exchange. Clinically hazardous fibrinogen levels (below 0.5 g/l) have occasionally (in approximately 6% of patients) been reported to occur with repeated exchanges approaching 1.5 plasma volumes. Measurement of pre-exchange fibrinogen levels has been recommended for the identification of patients who might need corrective action. Post-exchange fibrinogen levels can then be predicted from the plasma volume exchanged (see section 2.1).

Prothrombin times and *partial thromboplastin times* are prolonged immediately following exchange (by approximately 15% and 25% respectively following 0.7–1.0 plasma volume and by 60% and 70% following 1.5 plasma volume exchange) but show substantial recovery between 4 and 24 hours later. These tests, however, are poor predictors of a bleeding risk; *it has, in fact, proved to be very difficult to induce significant coagulation abnormalities as a result of plasmapheresis.*

Intensive (1.5 plasma volume) repeated plasma exchanges can result in depletion of Factors II, V, X and antithrombin III by as much as 60–70% from initial levels but these have not proved clinically dangerous. This degree of reduction in antithrombin III levels might be expected to predispose to thrombotic problems (chapter 8, section 6) but the simultaneous reduction in coagulation proteins presumably has a protective effect.[6] Factors VII, VIII and IX appear to be removed less effectively and never fall to clinically dangerous levels.

Platelets will be lost during plasmapheresis particularly during continuous-flow procedures but this may be less than expected since not all will be removed from the plasma that is collected. A 10–15% depletion is usual after single exchanges but no further deteriorations are seen with further courses unless repeated large-volume exchanges are undertaken. Large volume continuous-flow (1.5 plasma volume) exchanges can reduce platelet counts by 50%[5] and when repeated daily have produced counts below $30 \times 90^9/l$ in around 20% of patients. Bleeding symptoms become more likely at this level. Platelet counts should therefore be monitored particularly in those patients in whom for various reasons thrombopoiesis might be defective. These include patients with *haematological malignancies*, those undergoing *cytotoxic therapy* and those with *poor nutritional status.*

Plasma albumin and oncotic pressure[4]

It is generally accepted that *sustained* reduction of plasma oncotic pressures below 10–12 mmHg (corresponding approximately to albumin levels of 20–25 g/l, total protein 35–40 g/l) are necessary before a risk of oedema becomes apparent. The degree of depletion in the patient's plasma albumin during plasmapheresis depends on the albumin content of the returned fluid. A mixture of 5% albumin and normal saline in a 1:1 ratio is commonly used during large volume exchanges. This combination can be used for exchanges of as much as 1.5 plasma volumes on alternate days without more than very transient depressions below 10–12 mmHg oncotic pressure. Colloid oncotic pressures can in any case be expected to return to normal values within 24–48 hours following exchange because of the re-entry into the plasma of extravascular albumin. It is also important to appreciate that low plasma colloid oncotic pressures will not on their own lead to pulmonary oedema in patients with normal cardiopulmonary function.

Albumin solutions should not, therefore, be used too readily. Some plasmapheresis regimens begin by using saline alone and conclude by replacing albumin as a 5% or 25% solution, aiming at a 2–3% overall albumin concentration in the return fluid. This practice allows more efficient use of albumin but there is a risk of more profound though transient depression of colloid oncotic pressure.

Saline or gelatin solutions alone can be safely used in many patients for plasma exchanges not exceeding the total plasma volume. Since crystalloid solutions eventually diffuse throughout the entire extravascular compartment three volumes should in theory be required for each volume of plasma removed. In practice much less than this is needed, probably because the loss of fluid into the extravascular spaces is relatively slow compared to the duration of the plasmapheresis procedure.

Use of 4.5% albumin alone as replacement fluid will not cause appreciable changes in plasma oncotic pressure and either this material or plasma should best be used for patients such as those in congestive cardiac failure at high risk of pulmonary oedema.

Immunoglobulin concentrations

Both IgG and IgM appear to fall by around 65% following single-volume plasma exchange. Both recover to round 35% below normal by 48 hours. Repeated intensive exchanges can cause progressive reduction of immunoglobulin concentrations even to as low as 20% of normal[1] but this has not caused problems except in those already immunosuppressed. An increased incidence of infections has, for example, been reported in patients with renal failure. Under these and similar circumstances use of plasma to supplement the replacement fluid so that IgG does not remain below 0.45 g/l may be helpful. *Complement components* C3 and C4 fall during exchange but recover to close to normal by 48 hours. Repeated exchanges lead to a reduction of around 20% below normal levels but no clinical problems appear to be associated.

Pathological immunoglobulins are reduced by plasmapheresis in the same manner as their normal counterparts but, if substantial reductions are sought, immunoglobulin replacement may need to be given in order to maintain acceptable levels of *normal immunoglobulins*. It has been suggested that the clinical outcome may be better when normal immunoglobulins are replaced and it may be that keeping plasma immunoglobulins at normal levels reduces *de novo* synthesis of the pathological auto- or alloantibodies by some form of feedback mechanism. There are some similarities in this situation with the use of intravenous immunoglobulin for autoimmune disorders discussed in chapter 9, section 3.1.

It is important to ensure that any concurrent immunosuppressive therapy is continued throughout plasma exchange in order to prevent what appear to be rebound increases in unwanted antibody levels following completion of the procedure.

Immune complexes, being large and mainly intravascular, are removed efficiently during plasma exchange.[1] It is unlikely, however, that those already deposited in tissues can be removed.

Red cells

Around 30 ml of red cells may be lost during each procedure. This volume of red cells may, however, include a preponderance of reticulocytes (because of their reduced density compared to mature red cells) and their loss may contribute disproportionately to the risk of producing anaemia in repeatedly treated patients.

Table 1 Haematological and biochemical monitoring during plasma exchange

Haemoglobin concentration	Before first exchange and weekly thereafter
Platelet count	Weekly; more frequently if abnormal
Plasma proteins	Weekly and before exchange if albumin below 30 g/l
Fibrinogen concentration[a]	Before first exchange and before each subsequent exchange if below 1.5 g/l
Prothrombin time,[a] partial thromboplastin time	Before final exchange. Repeat more frequently if more than 1.5 times prolonged

[a]Repeated tests are not required unless there is a history of abnormal bleeding or frequent large volume exchanges are undertaken.

2.4 Choice of Anticoagulant

Citrate anticoagulants are almost universally used. The ratio of anticoagulant to blood may vary in different machines. ACD-A with a high citrate content is used in some machines: the alternative ACD-B has a lower citrate content and a greater volume is therefore required. Citrate solutions anticoagulate only the extracorporeal circulation. Heparin, in contrast, anticoagulates the patient's circulation;[7] this carries a risk of bleeding. Heparin may occasionally produce side-effects such as thrombocytopenia. The response to heparin is also variable, which makes optimum anticoagulation difficult. Heparin is sometimes used as a supplement to ACD-B, particularly if clotting becomes troublesome in the extracorporeal circulation.

Table 2 Selection of replacement fluid

Consider *normal saline* or *gelatin* solution for exchanges below one plasma volume when these are not more than twice weekly
Use equal parts of *albumin 5%* and *normal saline* for repeated intensive regimens
Replace with *5% albumin* alone only for patients at high risk of pulmonary oedema or other problems predisposing to oedema or accumulation of fluid in serous cavities
Give *fresh frozen plasma* as supplement only if there are already coagulation abnormalities at the start of the procedure. Substitute for equal volumes of the 5% albumin up to 30% total replacement volume

3 CLINICAL COMPLICATIONS DURING APHERESIS[8-10]

Complications have been variously reported as occurring in between 2% to 12% of all procedures. In a Canadian series of over 5000 procedures[11] severe reactions were encountered in 0.56% treatment episodes. Approximations from worldwide data suggest a fatality rate of around 3/10 000; both these are severe, but non-fatal reactions, being associated with the use of fresh frozen plasma (FFP) as a replacement fluid.[12-14]

Many of these problems are, however, of a minor nature and easily rectified. Adverse reactions should, of course, be anticipated most frequently in those patients who are already seriously ill. Circulatory instability has caused symptoms related to recurrence of underlying problems, such as *myocardial* or *cerebral ischaemia*, and *pulmonary embolization*. Apheresis procedures on patients with these problems should only be performed where facilities for appropriate emergency treatment are available. In the UK guidelines and codes of practice have been prepared governing apheresis procedures[15] and it is advisable to ascertain whether similar guidelines are available in other areas. Those with *cardiopulmonary disease* require particular attention to the choice and volume of replacement fluid according to the principles discussed above.

Episodes of *hypotension* generally respond to postural change, administration of more replacement fluid or temporary discontinuation of the procedure. Hypotensive episodes are more common in the elderly, and in children as well as smaller adult patients. They are far more liable to occur with discontinuous systems rather than continuous-flow procedures during which the plasma volume is being continually replenished.

Adverse reactions can occur which are side-effects of the plasma volume materials used as exchange fluid. These problems are discussed elsewhere (chapter 10). *Citrate toxicity*, e.g. circumoral numbness, lightheadedness and abdominal discomfort, can result from too rapid reinfusion of citrated blood. Citrate toxicity has also caused dangerous and sometimes fatal cardiac arrhythmias; this risk seems to be greatest when the central veins have had to be used for vascular access. Smaller patients are more at risk, and particularly liable are those with hepatic dysfunction in whom citrate metabolism is impaired. These symptoms are, in practice, uncommon because during plasma exchange most of the citrate is removed with the plasma. A greater risk occurs if FFP is used as the replacement fluid. The problems can usually be ameliorated by temporarily stopping or

---

Table 3 Complications encountered during apheresis procedures

Vasovagal attack
Hypovolaemia
Fluid overload
Difficulties with maintaining venous access
Citrate toxicity
Anaphylactoid reactions if fresh frozen plasma is used
Acute exacerbations of symptoms due to drug removal

slowing the procedure. Supplemental calcium has been used for management of recurrent hypocalcaemia, but there is some doubt as to its value.[11,16]

Removal of drugs during plasma exchange

It is important to recognize that therapeutic drugs, particularly those bound to protein, may also be removed during apheresis. Blood levels of antibiotics, anticonvulsants and cardiac glycosides may all be reduced, resulting in withdrawal effects.

Technical difficulties may arise during the procedures. These include:

(1) Leaks in the apparatus.
(2) Clots appearing in the system.
(3) Loss of venous access, resulting in the inability to return red cells or replacement fluid.

4 CLINICAL MONITORING DURING APHERESIS

Records should be made of:

• Pulse, every half-hour.
• Blood pressure.
• Abnormal symptoms or signs.
• Volumes of fluid removed and returned.

These are most conveniently recorded on specially designed therapeutic plasma exchange sheets (pro forma).

It is most important that *operational procedures* should be laid down in each apheresis unit detailing the measures to be taken in response to any problems that may arise.

5 CLINICAL APPLICATIONS OF APHERESIS[17]

The necessary controlled trials that could firmly establish the value of apheresis are sadly lacking in most of the diseases for which this expensive and labour-intensive treatment is often used. In many instances anecdotal experiences, belief in the theoretical benefits of apheresis and realization of the ineffectiveness of alternative remedies are all combined to justify apheresis therapy. Despite this somewhat illogical background it is sometimes considered unethical to institute controlled trials and, indeed, the clinical variability of some conditions and sometimes their rarity makes this more logical approach difficult.

In all the conditions listed particular indications define those patients for whom treatment may be justified. A much larger list can be drawn up of other conditions in which apheresis may at times be of value, but in which considerably less agreement exists. Some of these are discussed below.

Table 4 Established indications for therapeutic apheresis

Apheresis seems to be a well-founded remedy for:
  Goodpasture's syndrome
  Myasthenic crises
  Thrombotic thrombocytopenic purpura
  Poisoning with protein-bound poisons
  Hyperviscosity syndrome
  Sickle cell disease crisis
  Circulatory problems in severe erythrocytosis
  Guillain–Barré syndrome

Apheresis is also an accepted measure for intractable cases of
  Rheumatoid vasculitis
  Cholestatic pruritis
  Glomerulonephritis with GBM antibodies
  Chronic relapsing polyneuropathy
  Life-threatening scleroderma
  Polymyositis
  Systemic lupus erythematosus

5.1 Haematological Conditions

Erythrocytosis[18,19]

The haematocrit and blood viscosity can be lowered rapidly by this means. Removal of red cells (erythropheresis) may be indicated:

(1) During preparation for emergency surgery.
(2) For treatment of thrombotic episodes or where risks of these seem likely. Only one or two exchanges will usually be necessary and these can be accomplished perfectly well by manual procedures. After this venesection combined with other appropriate therapy should be used.

Erythrocyte exchange has also been utilized for severe *falciparum malaria*,[20,21] *lassa fever*,[22] *babesiosis*,[23] and *legionellosis*.[24]

Sickle cell disease[25,26]

This is also discussed in chapter 4, section 3.6. Exchange of haemoglobin A red cells in place of those containing haemoglobin S may be valuable in severe acute sickling crises although, of course, these will in most cases eventually improve spontaneously. Particular indications include severe pain, acute pulmonary syndrome, priapism, cerebral thrombosis and retinal artery occlusion. Exchanges should aim to reduce the haemoglobin S concentration to below 20%.

Maintenance of low haemoglobin S concentrations appears to minimize the likelihood of complications during surgery and pregnancy, reduce the risk of recurrence of strokes and, in younger patients, preserve renal and splenic function.

Leucocyte removal[27]

Apheresis may be of value in reducing very high leucocyte counts (e.g. greater than 100×10^9/l) in patients with leukaemia (usually acute non-lymphocytic leukaemia and chronic myeloid leukaemia in blast cell crisis) where these may be causing hyperviscosity symptoms. These circulatory problems occur particularly in the cerebral and pulmonary circulations; sometimes they may be so severe as to necessitate emergency leukapheresis. Reduction of high cell counts may also be indicated prior to the initiation of chemotherapy so as to reduce the hyperkalaemia and hyperuricaemia that follow destruction of a large tumour mass. The procedure has, of course, no curative value. Regular leukapheresis has also been used to assist control of the very high peripheral lymphocyte count and massive splenomegaly characteristic of prolymphocytic leukaemia.

Thrombocythaemia

Thrombopheresis has been used for the initial treatment of those patients with platelet counts exceeding 1000×10^9/l who also have associated bleeding or thrombosis. Again treatment is not curative and must be combined with chemotherapy.

Rh haemolytic disease

Plasmapheresis was formerly used by a number of centres to treat very severe Rh D haemolytic disease. This treatment has largely been abandoned in favour of intrauterine transfusion with Rh D-negative red cells. This is discussed in chapter 21, section 5.6.

Hyperviscosity syndrome

Malignant paraproteinaemias with hyperviscosity syndrome are almost certainly improved by plasma exchange. The paraproteins are usually IgM, less commonly polymers of IgA; sometimes the hyperviscosity is due to high levels of IgG. The progress of treatment can be monitored by measurement of plasma viscosity and protein levels.[28] It should be appreciated that plasma viscosity rises exponentially with increasing protein concentration; the exact relationship can be determined for individual patients by laboratory investigation.[29]

Because of this exponential relationship quite modest plasma exchanges can produce clinical improvement. Plasmapheresis is used in combination with chemotherapy as long as the hyperviscosity state persists. Normal saline is regarded as an adequate replacement fluid for individual exchange volumes of up to 1.5 l; for larger and more intensive regimens, dextran 40, which maintains plasma colloid osmotic pressure in the post-exchange period, has been shown to be satisfactory.[30]

Factor VIII inhibitors (see chapter 8, section 1.2)

Plasmapheresis is sometimes used for dangerous bleeds where inhibitor levels prevent high-dose Factor VIII infusions from having any chance of effect. The value of this is not universally agreed.

Protein A immunoabsorbents have also been used experimentally and found effective at reducing Factor VIII inhibitor levels.[31]

Thrombotic thrombocytopenic purpura[32,33]

There seems to be good evidence that plasma exchange can play an important part in the successful treatment of this formerly fatal condition. Although the pathological mechanism in thrombotic thrombocytopenic purpura (TTP) is still uncertain, the combination of endothelial damage and activated platelets which lead to thrombosis is related in some way to the appearance of abnormal polymers of von Willebrand factor (vWF) multimers. These may be the result of depletion of a normal plasma constituent whose role is the reduction of ultra-large vWF to the smaller normal forms. It is speculated that plasma exchange removes the ultra-large abnormal vWF, restores the missing component and provides a natural break to the platelet-aggregating and thrombotic process. The use of cryo-supernatant plasma[34] has been claimed to be even better than plasma since it is largely depleted of vWF multimers. Alternative measures, including steroids, aspirin and dipyridamole, should be continued, and daily haemoglobin, platelet counts and serum lactate dehydrogenase activity are used to monitor progress. Plasmapheresis may also be effective in the closely related *haemolytic uraemic syndrome*.

Plasmapheresis for other haematological conditions

Plasmapheresis has been used for *post-transfusion purpura*,[35] also severe *acute idiopathic thrombocytopenia*[36] and for *severe autoimmune haemolytic anaemia*. In these latter two conditions plasmapheresis probably only has a role in the most desperate of cases refractory to other treatments.

5.2 Rheumatological Disorders

(1) Plasmapheresis is generally believed to benefit selected patients with *systemic lupus erythematosus*. It has been used to treat patients with life-threatening disease which can no longer be managed by more conventional measures.

Such patients are usually distinguished by having high levels of circulating immune complexes and these appear to be instrumental in causing the tissue damage. Indications for plasmapheresis include progressive glomerulone-phritis, systemic vasculitis, multiple organ failure and cerebral symptoms. These patients are usually treated with intensive plasmapheresis regimens lasting several weeks; conventional treatment is given concurrently. The value of plasmapheresis for this condition has been recently challenged by results from a large multi-centre collaborative study which failed to show any advantage from addition of plasmapheresis to the therapeutic regimen.[37]

(2) Occasional very severely affected and treatment-resistant patients with rheumatoid arthritis appear to be improved by intensive plasma exchange.

(3) Plasmapheresis, together sometimes with lymphocyte removal, has also been used for a variety of other related disorders, including systemic necrotizing vasculitis and polymositis, but without convincing benefit.

5.3 Renal Disorders

Goodpasture's syndrome, which comprises pulmonary haemorrhage and glomerular nephritis, appears to be conspicuously improved following plasma exchange. The aetiological agent removed by the procedure is an autoantibody against glomerular basement membrane. It seems to be important to begin plasma exchange before severe renal damage has occurred if the high mortality rate of this disease is to be reduced. Once oliguria has supervened there appears to be little hope of recovery.

Plasmapheresis is being evaluated for a possible role in controlling renal allograft rejection. Results so far are not encouraging.

5.4 Neurological Disease

Probably more than half of all therapeutic plasma exchanges are now performed for patients with *neurological diseases*. For this category of patients evidence for benefit seems to have become more convincing with experience. The prevailing attitude to plasma exchange in neurological diseases has been recently summarized in a consensus conference.[38]

There is increasing suspicion that many neurological disorders are the result of an autoimmune process. *Myasthenia gravis* is known to be due to an autoantibody against the acetylcholine receptor on the post-synaptic membrane. Patients with severe widespread muscle weakness who cannot be controlled by anti-cholinesterase and steroid therapy are candidates for plasmapheresis and this appears to be conspicuously beneficial.

Plasmapheresis has been used for *Guillain–Barré syndrome*.[39–41] When plasma exchange is used it should probably be performed early and be restricted to those more severe cases likely to require pulmonary ventilation. Similarly *Eaton–Lambert syndrome*, a supposedly autoimmune-mediated disorder of the neuromuscular junction, is also accepted as a probable indication for plasma exchange.

There is no satisfactory evidence that plasma exchange has any value in other neurological conditions for which it has been attempted. These include multiple sclerosis, amyotrophic lateral sclerosis and motor neurone disease.

6 SELECTIVE REMOVAL OF PLASMA CONSTITUENTS USING IMMUNOABSORBENTS[42,43]

Exchange of whole plasma as a means of removing an unwanted constituent comprising in many cases less than 1% of the total plasma solutes is clearly a wasteful and inefficient approach. Where the offending pathological material can be identified, there are logical attractions in seeking its removal in a more selective fashion, thereby avoiding unnecessary disturbance of the normal plasma composition. Ligands such as *staphylococcal protein A* with specific affinity for certain IgG subclasses (predominantly IgG1, IgG2 and IgG4) can be coupled to an insoluble supporting matrix and used for removal of pathological IgG.[31] The immunoabsorbent can be packed into a column or filter configuration and incorporated into the plasma return line of an apheresis circulation system. Protein A absorption columns, which are now commercially available, have been used for IgG removal in various autoimmune conditions as well as other clinical problems in which pathological antibody production prevents effective treatment. It has been shown that with plasma perfusion volumes exceeding 7.5 l IgG levels can be reduced to below 20% of starting levels. Albumin and other plasma proteins, including coagulation factors, are not affected.

Protein A immunoabsorption therapy is currently under investigation in a variety of autoimmune states in which plasma exchange has been investigated. The technique has also been applied to coagulation factor VIII inhibitor removal prior to the institution of replacement therapy. As might be anticipated, antibody rebound would be expected to undermine any initial success with this approach, to which the answer might be the pulsed administration of cytotoxic agents, e.g. cyclophosphamide. Protein A immunoabsorption clearly has limitations. IgG3 is not specifically bound; however, it is possible that the alternative protein G can be incorporated into an immunoabsorbent for this purpose. The immobilization of specific monoclonal antibodies would enable an even more highly selective immunoabsorbent procedure. As an example, the low-density lipoprotein removal in patients with homozygous hypercholesterolaemia by means of sepharose-bound apoprotein B appears to be an efficient means of treatment. This can be done without the high-density lipoprotein removal that will occur during conventional apheresis.[43]

Immunoabsorbent techniques are still highly experimental and expensive. Toxic reactions are not uncommon, e.g. those possibly related to the leakage of protein A into the patient's circulation. Selective extraction of plasma constituents seems a promising technique for the future. Its successful implementation will depend upon advances on several fronts:

(1) Precise knowledge of the nature of the pathological entity that must be removed.

(2) Development of specific Ligands for the immunoabsorbent material.
(3) Improvements in biocompatibility of the matrix supporting material so that complement activation 'by-products', a known cause of adverse clinical reactions, are minimized.

REFERENCES

1 Volkin, R.L., Starz, T.W., Windelstein, A. *et al.* (1982) Changes in coagulation factors, immunoglobulins, and immune complex concentrations with plasma exchange. *Transfusion*, **22**: 54–58.
2 Nilsson, T., Rudolphi, O. and Cedergren, B. (1983) Effects of intensive plasmapheresis on the haemostatic system. *Scand. J. Haematol.*, **30**: 201–206.
3 Domen, R.E., Kennedy, M.S., Jones, L.L. and Senhauser, D.A. (1984) Haemostatic imbalances produced by plasma exchange. *Transfusion*, **24**: 336–339.
4 Lasky, L.C., Finnerty, E.P., Genis, L. and Polesky, H.F. (1984) Protein and colloid osmotic pressure changes with albumin and/or saline replacement during plasma exchange. *Transfusion*, **24**: 256–259.
5 Urbaniak, S.J. (1982) Intensive plasma exchange: effects on haemostasis. In: *Massive Transfusion in Surgery and Trauma*, pp. 191–212. New York: Alan R. Liss.
6 Sultan, Y., Bussel, A., Maisonneuve, P., Poupeney, M., Sitty, X. and Gajdos, P. (1979) Potential danger of thrombosis after plasma exchange in the treatment of patients with immune disease. *Transfusion, 19*: 588.
7 Morales, M., Pizzutol, J., Reyna, M. *et al.* (1982) Use of heparin for cytapheresis and plasmapheresis in a continuous flow centrifuge. *Transfusion*, **22**: 384–387.
8 Ziselman, E.M., Bongiovanni, M.B. and Wurzel, H.A. (1984) The complications of therapeutic plasma exchange. *Vox Sang.*, **46**: 270–276.
9 Huestis, D.W. (1983) Mortality in therapeutic haemapheresis. *Lancet*, **ii**: 1025–1026.
10 Das, P.C. and Smit Sibinga, C.Th. (1983) Complications of therapeutic plasma exchange. *Lancet*, **ii**: 455–456.
11 Sutton, D.M.C., Nair, R.C., Rock, G. and the Canadian Apheresis Study Group (1989) Complications of plasma exchange. *Transfusion*, **29**: 124–127.
12 Shumak, K.H. and Rock, G.A. (1984) Therapeutic plasma exchange. *N. Engl. J. Med.*, **310**: 762–771.
13 Bouget, J., Chevret, S., Chastang, C., Raphael, J.C. and the French Co-operative Group (1993) Plasma exchange morbidity in Guillain–Barré syndrome: results from the French prospective, double-blind, randomized, multicenter study. *Crit. Care Med.*, **21**: 651–658.
14 Rosenkvist, J., Berkowicz, A., Holsoe, E., Sorensen, H. and Taaning, E. (1984) Plasma exchange in myasthenia gravis complicated with complement activation and urticarial reactions using fresh-frozen plasma as replacement solution. *Vox Sang.*, **46**: 13–18.
15 British Committee for Standards in Haematology (1991), Code of practice for the clinical use of blood cell separators. In: Roberts, B. (ed.), *Standard Haematology Practice*. Oxford: Blackwell Scientific.
16 Silberstein, L.E., Naryshkin, S., Haddad, J.J. and Strauss, J.F. (1986) Calcium homeostasis during therapeutic plasma exchange. *Transfusion*, **26**: 151–155.
17 Campion, E.W. (1992) Desperate diseases and plasmapheresis. *N. Engl. J. Med.*, **326**: 1425–1427.
18 Newland, A.C. and Wedzicha, J.A. (1984) Isovolaemic haemodilution (erythrapheresis) in polycythaemia. *Apheresis Bull.*, **2**: 24–33.
19 Wedzicha, J.A., Rudd, R.M., Apps, M.C.P., Cotter, F.E., Newlands, A.C. and Empey, D.W. (1983) Erythrapheresis in patients with polycythaemia secondary to hypoxic lung disease. *Br. Med. J.*, **286**: 511–514.
20 Malin, A.S., Cass, P.L. and Hudson, C.N. (1990) Exchange transfusion for severe falciparum malaria in pregnancy. *Br. Med. J.*, **300**: 1240–1241.

21 Govoni, M. and Graldi, G. (1993) Erythrocyte exchange in cerebral malaria. *Vox Sang.*, **64**: 56.

22 Cummins, D., Bennett, D. and Machin, S.J. (1991) Exchange transfusion of a patient with fulminant lassa fever. *Postgrad. Med. J.*, **67**: 193–194.

23 Cahill, E.M., Benach, J.L., Reich, L.M. *et al.* (1981) Red cell exchange: treatment of babesiosis in a splenectomized patient. *Transfusion*, **21**: 193–194.

24 Denning, D., Thomas, P., Harries, M. and Wall, R. (1987) Whole blood exchange as a treatment for legionellosis. *Lancet*, **i**: 227.

25 Nagey, D.A., Alawode, N.A., Pupkin, M.J. and Crenshaw, C. (1983) Isovolumetric partial exchange transfusion in the management of sickle cell disease in pregnancy. *Am. J. Obstet. Gynecol.*, **147**: 693–696.

26 Morrison, J.C., Douvas, S.G., Martin, J.N. *et al.* (1984) Erythrocytapheresis in pregnant patients with sickle haemoglobinopathies. *Am. J. Gynecol.*, **149**: 912–914.

27 Mehta, A.B., Goldman, J.M. and Kohner, E. (1984) Hyperleucocytic retinopathy in chronic granulocytic leukaemia: the role of intensive leucapheresis. *Br. J. Haematol.*, **56**: 661–667.

28 Wahlin, A., Grubb, A., Holm, J. and Marklund, S.L. (1988) Effects of plasmapheresis on the plasma concentration of proteins used to monitor the disease process in multiple myeloma. *Acta Med. Scand.*, **223**: 263–267.

29 Beck, J.R., Quinn, B.M., Meier, R.A. and Rawnsley, H.M. (1982) Hyperviscosity syndrome in paraproteinemia. *Transfusion*, **22**: 51–53.

30 Fujii, H. (1988) Plasma exchange using dextran 40-electrolyte solution as the sole replacement fluid in malignant paraproteinemia. *Transfusion*, **28**: 42–45.

31 Gjrstrup, P. and Watt, R.M. (1990) Therapeutic protein A immunoadsorption: a review. *Transfusion Sci.*, **11**: 281–302.

32 Moake, J.L. (1992) von Willebrand Factor (vWF) abnormalities in thrombotic thrombocytopenic purpura (TTP) and the hemolytic uremic syndrome (HUS). *Transfusion Sci.*, **13**: 27–31.

33 Rock, G., Shumak, K., Kelton, J. *et al.* and the Canadian Apheresis Study Group (1992) Thrombotic thrombocytopenic purpura: outcome in 24 patients with renal impairment treated with plasma exchange. *Transfusion*, **32**: 710–714.

34 Byrnes, J.J., Moake, J.L., Hirsch, R. *et al.* (1990) Effectiveness of the cryosupernatant fraction of plasma in the treatment of refractory thrombotic thrombocytopenic purpura. *Am. J. Hematol.*, **34**: 169.

35 Laursen, B., Morling, N., Rosenkvist, J., Sorensen, H. and Thyme, S. (1978) Post transfusion purpura treated with plasma exchange by Haemonetics cell separator: a case report. *Acta Med. Scand.*, **203**: 539–543.

36 Blanchette, V.S., Hogan, V.A., McCombie, N.E. *et al.* (1984) Intensive plasma exchange therapy in ten patients with idiopathic thrombocytopenic purpura. *Transfusion*, **24**: 388–393.

37 Lewis, E.J., Hunsicker, L.G., Lan, S.P., Rhode, R.D. and Lachin, J.M., for the Lupus Nephritis Study Group (1992) A controlled trial of plasmapheresis therapy in severe lupus nephritis. *N. Engl. J. Med.*, **326**: 1373–1379.

38 Consensus Conference (1986) The utility of therapeutic plasmapheresis for neurological disorders. *JAMA*, **256**: 1333–1337.

39 Greenwood, R.J., Newsom-Davis, J., Hughes, R.A.C. *et al.* (1984) Controlled trial of plasma exchange in acute inflammatory polyradiculoneuropathy. *Lancet*, **i**: 877–879.

40 Guillain–Barré Syndrome Study Group (1985) Plasmapheresis and acute Guillain–Barré syndrome. *Neurology*, **35**: 1096–1104.

41 Dyck, P.J. and Kurtzke, J.F. (1985) Plasmapheresis in Guillain–Barré syndrome. *Neurology*, **35**: 1105–1107.

42 Pineda, A.A. (1989) Editorial: selective extraction of plasma constituents. *Transfusion*, **29**: 283–284.

43 Leitman, S.F., Smith, J.W. and Gregg, R.E. (1989) Homozygous familial hypercholesterolemia: selective removal of low-density lipoproteins by secondary membrane filtration. *Transfusion*, **29**: 341–346.

Part E
PAEDIATRIC TRANSFUSION

20
Neonatal Transfusion Problems

The dramatic advances that have taken place in recent years in the care of sick and premature babies have also been matched by a similar increase in the use of blood transfusion therapy. Transfusion specialists, who were formerly almost entirely preoccupied with growth areas of adult medicine, must now turn their attention to the rather special requirements of their paediatric colleagues. The uncertainties regarding the proper use of transfusion therapy and the associated opportunities for inappropriate practices[1] have stimulated production of a number of guidelines for blood component use.[2–4]

Neonatal medicine poses various blood transfusion-related problems that do not have exact counterparts in adult medicine. Many of the problems affecting the newborn may influence or be influenced by transfusion therapy; these include:

(1) Problems associated with *prematurity* such as anaemia, respiratory distress syndrome (RDS), intraventricular haemorrhage, sepsis and disseminated intravascular coagulation.

(2) *Haemolytic disease of the newborn* and hyperbilirubinaemia.
(3) Anaemia resulting from blood losses during collection of samples for investigational purposes.
(4) Consequences of the relative *immaturity of the haematological system*. The high
oxygen affinity of haemoglobin F, the deficiency of vitamin K-dependent
coagulation factors as well as the poor marrow reserves and the relative unresponsiveness of neutrophil polymorphs towards infective episodes may all
complicate the management of illnesses encountered in neonates.

1   HAEMATOLOGICAL FEATURES OF THE NEONATAL PERIOD

There are significant differences between the haematological systems of neonates
and adults which must be borne in mind during diagnosis and management of
peri-natal transfusion problems.

Haemoglobin, haematocrit, blood volume

The haemoglobin concentration, haematocrit and blood volume of neonates
depend on the volume of placental blood that is allowed to return to the infant's
circulation prior to clamping the cord. The 'normal' blood volume may vary, e.g.
from 85 ml up to 125 ml (mean 95 ml) per kilogram; the highest blood volumes
follow from delayed cord clamping, especially when the infant has been held
below the placental level to facilitate drainage. A controlled amount of placento-
fetal transfusion can reduce the likelihood of post-natal anaemia;[5] if carried to
excess polycythaemia can result. In such instances the excess blood volume
becomes reduced by absorption of the superfluous plasma over the first day of
life. Red cells cannot be disposed of so easily; the haematocrit therefore rises and
values as high as 0.75 may be seen. Generally blood volume values of 85–100 ml/
kg are assumed to be typical for full-term infants in the first week or so. Premature infants tend to have higher initial blood volumes, but an anaemia, the
precise mechanism of which is uncertain, frequently supervenes over the next
2–3 months. Haemoglobin values may fall as low 8–9 g/dl compared with the
10–11 g/dl found in normal full-term infants at a corresponding post-gestational
age. Blood-sampling losses compound this anaemia in intensively managed pre-
term babies.

Fetal haemoglobin

Fetal haemoglobin predominates at birth in full-term infants (60–85% of total
haemoglobin) and to an even greater extent in the premature (>90%). The high
oxygen affinity of fetal haemoglobin is optimal for oxygen uptake at the lower
pO_2 of the placental interface between the fetal and maternal circulations. It is,
however, less suitable for extrauterine life and may even be a handicap in the
presence of respiratory disease. For this reason exchange transfusions have

been given in attempts to improve oxygen transport and tissue oxygenation in the respiratory distress syndrome. However, because of the hazards of the procedure in sick babies, exchange transfusions are now rarely used in these circumstances.

For various biochemical reasons, the *in vivo* P_{50} can vary widely (and hence also the degree of oxygen saturation at any given pO_2); haemoglobin values alone, therefore, do not give an accurate indication of the oxygen transport capabilities of blood, especially during this early period of life. For this reason calculation of 'available oxygen'[6] derived from both the *in vivo* P_{50} and the haemoglobin concentration have been used to assess whether a functional state of 'anaemia' exists and thus provide a better indication for transfusion than the haemoglobin alone.

The diagnostic problem is further complicated by the fact that plasma volumes are sometimes reduced to such an extent that the haemoglobin concentration becomes a poor indicator of the true deficit of red cell mass.[7]

Disordered granulopoiesis

There is evidence that the septic problems to which newborn infants are particularly prone are, in part, a consequence of a defective ability to mount and maintain an adequate neutrophil response to bacterial infection. This is considered in more detail in section 4.

Immaturity of immune functions

Immaturity of immune functions is characteristic of premature infants. As a consequence premature babies have been thought to be susceptible to colonization by donor blood lymphocytes resulting in *graft-versus-host disease* (GVHD) and also to infections by agents such as *cytomegalovirus* that can be transmitted through blood transfusion.

Transplacental passage of maternal IgG does not become fully effective until the third trimester of pregnancy. Very low birth weight (e.g. < 1500 g) babies are characteristically profoundly hypogammaglobulinaemic and hence particularly vulnerable to bacterial infection. These infections are typically acquired around the time of birth and are either from organisms of maternal origin or nosocomial infections acquired later over the next few weeks. The value of immunoglobulin therapy for infection prophylaxis is under investigation[8] (see chapter 9, section 2.2). Intravenous immunoglobulin is also under study for the treatment of established sepsis in premature infants, but again no clear benefit in overall survival has so far been shown.[9]

Bleeding problems

Deficient synthesis of vitamin K-dependent factors may cause bleeding problems arising in the first few days of life in otherwise healthy infants. These arise after birth, when maternal supplies of vitamin K cease and before there has been a chance for replenishment by vitamin K absorbed from the gut.

Coagulation factor deficiencies

Coagulation factor profiles of plasma from newborns differ from those of adults, and interpretation of results of laboratory investigation requires understanding of the normal post-natal development of the coagulation system. Typically, vitamin K-dependent factors, contact factors, plasminogen and many of the coagulation inhibitors are reduced, some to the order of 50% of adult normal values. Factors V, and VIII and von Willebrand factor (vWF) concentrations are, in contrast, similar to adult mean values. It seems likely that a balanced state of equilibrium exists to protect the fetus against abnormal bleeding.

2 RED CELL TRANSFUSIONS

Red cell transfusion may be categorized according to the amount of blood to be transfused. For example:

(1) Small *top-up transfusions* generally to replenish investigational losses and correct mild degrees of anaemia (normally of the order of 5–15 ml/kg). These account for over 90% of all transfusions during the neonatal period. Low birth weight premature babies in special care units are amongst the most intensively transfused of all the hospital patient population. Means of around 9–10 transfusion episodes are not unusual, with some babies transfused even more frequently.[10]

(2) *Partial exchange transfusions* to correct anaemias (or polycythaemias) where blood volume changes must be minimized.

(3) *Full exchange transfusions* for treatment of severe anaemias, hyperbilirubin-aemia, metabolic and toxaemic problems.

(4) *Acute blood loss* must be treated using similar principles to those described for adults. Massive blood loss at birth may be due to fetomaternal haemorrhage, haemorrhages from the circulation of one twin to that of another, or to umbilical cord accidents. These infants usually show pallor or tachycardia and dyspnoea and may need instant resuscitation; 4.5% albumin (20 ml/kg immediately, and repeated as necessary) should be used to correct hypovolaemia until blood transfusion can be started.

2.1 Blood Grouping and Compatibility Testing for Neonates

Blood grouping

Two important considerations must be borne in mind:

(1) Only the *red cells* are required for blood grouping purposes. Any antibodies present in the serum will have been derived solely from the mother and only

those of IgG1 and IgG3 subclasses are likely to be present. The detection even of these antibodies may be difficult since, in the presence of the corresponding alloantigens on the fetal cells, absorption from the serum may result in very little free antibody.

(2) Newborn infants' red cells may show *weak expression of ABO antigens*, thus particular care is required during grouping. P_1, Lewis and I antigens may also be temporarily lacking on neonatal red cells. If *intrauterine transfusion* has been given it must be remembered that the apparent ABO group is that of the donor and not that of the baby. When the antiglobulin test is strongly positive due to immune haemolytic disease there may be such heavy coating with antibody that Rh typing may be difficult even when using saline-reacting or monoclonal reagents. Typing may be possible after unwanted antibodies have been removed by elution. Alternatively, the Rh group can be inferred from the specificity of the eluate.

Compatibility testing

Blood of the infants ABO group can be selected but it must be compatible with the maternal ABO group. For practical convenience, however, *group O blood of low anti-A,B titre* is commonly used. Traditionally, maternal serum has been used for compatibility tests until the infant is 6 months old. Recently, however, this requirement has been abandoned. The maternal serum should certainly be screened for antibodies and this can be done following the routine procedures described in chapter 25, section 2.4. It is now accepted that if the *maternal antibody screen* and the infant's *direct antiglobulin test* are *negative*, transfusions of group O blood may be given *directly*, without further testing, during the first 4 months (subject to the confirmation of the ABO and Rh group on the donor units). Neonates do not form alloantibodies in response to transfusion within this period.[11,12]

This arrangement allows top-up transfusions to be given without the delay and inconvenience of obtaining further maternal samples for the compatibility test. For the much less frequent circumstances in which repeated massive transfusions are given it may be prudent to re-examine the neonatal serum for evidence of previous passively transfused antibodies or the very rare occurrence of alloantibody stimulation.[12,13]

2.2 Rates and Volumes for Transfusion

Great care is essential in controlling and recording the rates and volumes of blood transfused to neonates. Volumes of 2–5 ml/kg per hour are regarded as safe in the absence of active haemorrhage; the lower rate should be selected where there is risk of congestive cardiac failure. All transfusions should be carefully *monitored* for signs of impending *circulatory overloading*. In order to avoid this problem, it is usual to give diuretics mid transfusion, and also to avoid feeding until an hour or so following completion of the transfusion.

Small-volume transfusions, for example up to 25 ml, can be administered via pre-filled syringes. Blood can be drawn into a syringe through a filter and then loaded into a syringe pump (which must incorporate a pressure warning device). Larger volumes of blood are more conveniently administered via specially manufactured burette assemblies which will also incorporate inbuilt 170 μm filters. Provided transfusions are given at the recommended rate, and that the blood is within 5 days post collection, infusion needles as narrow as 23–25 G can be used without excessive haemolysis. Blood warming is only required for exchange transfusions or for rapid transfusions during acute haemorrhage.

2.3   Small-volume 'Top-up' Transfusions[14,15]

Newer developments in neonatal medicine have greatly improved the survival rate of premature and very low birth weight (<1500 g) infants. Anaemia of prematurity is a well-recognized problem (see section 1) but the repeated blood sampling usually required for investigational purposes frequently compounds the problem and may necessitate transfusion. As an alternative, recombinant human erythropoietin is under study for its effectiveness at improving haemoglobin levels. Erythropoietin appears to be effective in some circumstances, the evidence being most conclusive in babies without infections, and blood transfusion requirements are lessened. The importance of other factors affecting erythropoiesis, e.g. iron and nutritional status, needs to be clarified before the proper role of erythropoietin can be agreed.[63,64]

Indications for red cell Transfusion

The indications for transfusion in the neonatal period remain poorly defined, controversial and often subjective. Clinical problems such as lethargy, cardio-respiratory difficulties during feeding and poor weight gain[16] are widely regarded as justifying transfusion particularly when they are unresponsive to other measures. Transfusions are also frequently given to correct anaemia when this is present in infants with respiratory failure. The *haemoglobin* concentration remains the most readily available indication but its interpretation must take into account the following:

(1) The change in normal range according to age: the haemoglobin concentration of healthy infants falls to around 11.0 g/dl 2–3 weeks after birth and for pre-term babies values of 9.0 g/dl are usual at this time. It is customary, however, to consider transfusion for symptomatic babies at haemoglobin levels of 8–10 g/dl over the first few weeks (typically 4–5 weeks) of life, especially if there are other coexisting clinical problems. For pre-term babies with respiratory failure in the immediate neonatal period transfusion might be considered at haemoglobin and haematocrit levels as high as 12.0 g/dl and 0.36. Higher transfusion thresholds are considered appropriate (e.g. Hb 12.0–13.0 g/dl) in the presence of severe pulmonary disease, cyanotic cardiac disease or heart failure.

(2) Without knowledge of *in vivo* oxygen affinity the haemoglobin concentration provides an imperfect indication of the capacity for tissue oxygen delivery. A better indicator, where investigations permit, might be assessment of available oxygen.[6] Haemoglobin concentration does not reliably correlate with the red cell mass. For this reason, the true severity of anaemia may often be masked when there are unsuspected reductions in plasma volume and blood volume.[7]

Walking donor programmes

The need to replenish iatrogenic losses by means of repeated small-volume (e.g. 10–30 ml) transfusions was not, at first, readily or easily met by established transfusion services. As a result, some neonatologists began to collect the small volumes of blood required either from hospital staff or from relatives, for immediate transfusion purposes. These programmes became popularized as 'walking donor programmes' and seemed, for a while, to be a convenient solution to the transfusion needs of such sick infants until the risks became evident.

Such donations, usually collected with heparin, provided 'fresh' blood rapidly and avoided the perceived disadvantages of citrate or low pH associated with bank blood. These concerns have now been shown to be without foundation and confidence has now been gained in the routine issue of designated routine blood bank donations.

Walking donor programmes have been found vulnerable to both serological mishaps and a greater risk of virological transmitted infection, since the quality-assurance disciplines mandated for transfusion services cannot easily be replicated under the usual circumstances of walking donor programmes. It is, therefore, now generally accepted that these collection arrangements have no place in modern transfusion practice.

Selection of blood

Many blood banks now provide special blood packs for neonatal use containing whole blood or red cell concentrate derived as satellites from the main blood pack assembly. The highly important objective of reducing donor exposures and the risk of infection can be achieved by dedication of a single donation per infant and using successive satellite pack aliquots for each transfusion.

Group O Rh D-negative blood with low titres of anti-A,B will be most suitable. The unit may need to be CMV antibody negative (see chapter 24, section 6.1) in addition to meeting normal criteria for acceptability. Although some blood services provide leucocyte-depleted red cells for neonatal use, no proven advantage of leucocyte depletion has yet been demonstrated.

It is important to recognize that red cell replacement is the primary objective during these transfusion programmes. Blood for 'top-ups' can be used up to the accepted normal expiry age. The oxygen affinity of stored donor blood even at its worst would not be very different from the p50 of the infant with its high HbF content but the transfused cells do have the advantage that they will regenerate DPG and regain normal oxygen affinity. Potassium concentrations of supernatant plasma may seem alarming (up to 80 mol/l in bank blood plasma) but at the rates and quantities administered present no risk.[17] In fact, at the amount transfused, potassium provides only a small fraction of the daily K^+ needs. Very fresh blood is sometimes requested for top-up transfusions because of anxieties over the possibilities of haemostatic failure. This suspicion requires confirmatory investigation and therapy in its own right (see sections 3 and 5); in any event the amount of platelets or plasma present in the conventional size of top-up transfusion is too small to provide effective haemostatic therapy. The suitability of red cells preserved in optimal additives for neonatal transfusion has frequently been raised as a concern. Experience matches theoretical expectations that these materials are completely safe for modest red-cell replacement needs.[18] There is little evidence so far to support their safety for massive transfusions, particularly when hepatic or renal failure are present, and in these situations caution is warranted.

Relatives as donors

The place of directed donations is considered in chapter 15. Family pressures are often high to use relatives, particularly the mother, as a source for transfusion support. In this context it should be remembered that the mother is likely to have been immunized to antigens of paternal origin.[19]

Although some maternal antibodies will already have been passively transfused, a proportion will have been retained by the placental barrier. The significance of HLA antibodies in neonatal transfusions is unknown, although uncommon but severe reactions due to leucocyte antibodies are well recognized in adult transfusion. Disease transmission is also possible; HCV for example is not normally transmitted vertically, but could be via maternofetal transfusion. First-degree relative donations are a well-recognized cause of GVHD and should therefore be irradiated (see chapter 23, section 4.1).[20]

2.4 Partial Exchange Transfusions

Symptomatic anaemia, in which haemoglobin values would normally be expected to be less than 10 g/dl, can be rapidly corrected by partial exchange transfusion with concentrated red cells. Exchange transfusion minimizes blood volume changes and can be useful in the presence of congestive cardiac failure or other conditions in which there may be intolerance of circulatory overloading. The procedure can also be useful for correction of neonatal polycythaemia (haematocrit > 0.65)[21] in which case 4.5% albumin solutions or fresh plasma are used. A suitable formula for calculation of the net amounts of blood or plasma to be given is:

$$\frac{\text{Volume to be}}{\text{exchanged}} = \frac{\text{Blood volume} \times (\text{Observed haematocrit} - \text{Desired haematocrit})}{\text{Observed haematocrit}}$$

The blood volume is usually assumed to be 85 ml/kg in full-term infants or 100 ml/kg in very low birth weight newborn infants.

2.5 Exchange Transfusion

This procedure was originally devised for the treatment of haemolytic disease of the newborn (see chapter 21, section 5.4). In this condition treatment has a well-proven role in the *correction of anaemia, removal of bilirubin, removal of antibodies and replacement of red cells* by those compatible with the offending antibodies. A similar approach is sometimes necessary for other forms of severe neonatal haemolysis, e.g. glucose 6-phosphate dehydrogenase deficiency. Exchange transfusion has been used for the treatment of respiratory distress syndrome with the intention of replacing fetal red cells containing HbF with those containing more physiologically appropriate HbA. The treatment has been used for other conditions, including severe neonatal sepsis, disseminated intravascular coagulation and neonatal alloimmune thrombocytopenia. In most such circumstances exchange transfusion would not now be considered if more specific and appropriate therapy, e.g. granulocytes or serologically compatible platelets, could be provided.

Selection of blood for exchange transfusion

Plasma-reduced red cells (haematocrit 0.5–0.6) that are *not older than 5 days of age* are the normally preferred products. These are produced by removal of around 120 ml of plasma from a standard whole blood donation. Use of blood within a few days of collection avoids the risk of *hyperkalaemia*, ensures *good post-transfusion red cell survival* and *acceptable red cell oxygen affinity*. Very premature neonates are at increased risk of *cytomegalovirus* infections and *GVHD*. These risks are admittedly small but prophylactic measures should be considered where facilities exist (see below). Blood for exchange transfusion should be screened for *sickle cell haemoglobin* and also glucose 6-phosphate dehydrogenase deficiency[22] if there is a risk that blood from donors with these abnormalities could be supplied from the transfusion service. If the blood pack label shows both the net weight of blood and the haematocrit, the volume of plasma to be removed to secure any desired haematocrit can be readily calculated. The date of collection and, if designated specifically for neonatal exchange transfusion use, the recommended date of expiry should be shown.

If blood of a suitable age is unavailable then it is acceptable to use hard-packed red cells resuspended in 4–5% albumin. Although fresh frozen plasma (FFP) is sometimes used as a resuspension agent this practice is justified only where there is a coexisting need to restore coagulation factors. In common with all labile blood components, red cells should be transfused through a conventional blood administration filter—there is no strictly justified indication for use of a microaggregate filter although these are sometimes found to be, in practice, a convenient means of enabling filtration. The higher oxygen affinity of stored blood is in fact not a major problem; it may not be substantially different from the fetal blood it replaces and will in any case improve with time. The more serious risk of hyper-kalaemia will, of course, be avoided as a result of the plasma removal. If the infant shows signs of haemostatic problems then fresh components (e.g. FFP and/or platelets) may also be required.

The following additional problems must be considered:

(1) The risks of *over-* or *under-transfusion* necessitate very careful recording of volumes replaced.

(2) *Perforation* of major vessels, *thrombosis* or *embolization* from the catheter site can occur.

(3) *Hypocalcaemia* (e.g. serum-ionized calcium below 0.8 mmol/l): the rate of citrate infusion can be sufficient to cause hypocalcaemia. Blood for exchange should be warmed before use and the baby monitored for evidence of hypo-calcaemia (see chapter 12, section 4.5). Calcium gluconate at a dose of 0.5–1 ml/kg of a 10% solution may be given but only on the basis of proven need. Neonates are more prone to hypocalcaemia than adults because their imma-ture liver is less able to metabolize citrate. In addition, parathyroid function is not well developed and this results in delayed mobilization of skeletal calcium.

(4) *Citrate toxicity*: This manifests as an alkalosis with increased plasma bicarbo-nate and has been a reported problem for premature infants. It now seems to be only a rare occurrence with use of CPD plasma-reduced blood and better control of plasma infusion rate and hypothermia.

(5) *Hypothermia*: blood warming[23] is advised for rapid transfusion rates (e.g. >0.5 ml/kg per minute); for this, in-line warmers equipped with thermometer and audible error warning system are advised. Although the need for warming of small-volume transfusions is doubtful, it is accomplished readily by keeping the syringe within the incubator chamber. Overheating and dangerous haemolysis have occurred from exposure to phototherapy sources.

(6) *Rebound hypoglycaemia*: the commonly used CPDA-1 solutions have an unphy-siologically high glucose content (26 mmol/l). This stimulates increased insulin secretion, which persists after transfusion, and may lead to hypogly-caemia. Babies with haemolytic disease may be particularly prone because of the associated islet cell hyperplasia. Blood glucose levels should therefore be monitored during and following exchange transfusion.

(7) *Thrombocytopenia* is a common problem following exchange transfusion and may partly be due to a dilution effect resulting from the stored blood replace-ment. Platelet counts may fall by 50–70% of initial values. More serious hae-mostatic disturbances may be due to an underlying state of disseminated intravascular coagulation.

(8) *Necrotizing enterocolitis* is probably one of the commonest serious complica-tions of exchange transfusion, particularly in association with erythrocytosis. If necrotizing enterocolitis is suspected on clinical grounds the laboratory should be notified so that the necessary serological examinations or T activa-tion can be performed (see section 4.1).

(9) *GVHD* (see chapter 23, section 4.1) is a rare and poorly quantified risk in neonatal transfusion.[20] Although premature infants of very low birth weight (e.g. below 1500 g) have been considered to be vulnerable, there is insufficient

evidence to justify routine use of irradiated products. The risk is more certain for those with any suggestion of congenital *immune deficiency*; blood components for those babies, for intrauterine transfusions and any subsequent exchanges should be irradiated. Blood from donors sharing an HLA haplotype with the recipient is liable to lead to GVHD. For this reason blood components from first-degree relatives should be irradiated and the possibility clearly also exists where other blood relative donors are considered. Because of the risks of hyperkalaemia red cells for exchange transfusions and other massive transfusions should be irradiated within 4 days of collection and administered within 48 hours.[24]

(10) *Bacterial* or *viral infections*: CMV infection is a particular problem[25] (see chapter 24, section 7).

Blood transfusion during extracorporeal membrane oxygenation[26]

Extracorporeal membrane oxygen (ECMO) has become increasingly used to provide effective support for babies with severe respiratory failure. In transfusion terms the procedure has similarities with cardiopulmonary bypass involving massive blood replacement. Usually, the ECMO circuit will accommodate around 1.5 times the neonatal blood volume and the transfusion problems associated with massive blood replacement (see chapter 12), e.g. colloid osmotic pressure maintenance, haemostatic impairment and metabolic complications, are to be anticipated. Microaggregate blood filters would have a logical role for transfusion during ECMO as with cardiopulmonary bypass and other circumstances in which the pulmonary vascular bed is bypassed.[27]

3 PLATELET TRANSFUSION: NEONATAL THROMBOCYTOPENIA

Clinically significant thrombocytopenia can be observed in around 20% of babies in special care units. Despite the multiplicity of causes, a pattern involving a fall in count over the first post-natal days followed by recovery within 10 days is typical.[28] Falling counts generally coincide with increased mean platelet volumes suggesting that peripheral destruction is responsible.

Thrombocytopenia may be due to *sepsis* and *disseminated intravascular coagulation* following infection by common *bacterial pathogens*. Various other neonatal infections may cause thrombocytopenia; these principally include *cytomegalovirus, toxoplasmosis, rubella, herpes simplex* and *syphilis*. Thrombocytopenia may also occur in circumstances such as *pre-eclampsia, intrauterine death of a twin, abruptio placenta, brain injuries, severe hypoxia* and any state of *shock*. In the absence of these conditions *maternal ITP* or *neonatal alloimmune thrombocytopenia* should be considered. Effective management of the underlying condition, where possible, is probably of more importance than the use of platelet transfusions. Bleeding is believed to be more likely in thrombocytopenic infants who also have infections or other metabolic problems than it is in those who are otherwise fit.

Platelet concentrates are administered using broadly the same criteria as those for adult therapy. On occasions, the difficulties of ensuring adequate samples for diagnosis may result in requests for use of platelets or fresh plasma for sick babies on the basis of rather less rigorous criteria than may be acceptable in adult medicine. The need for treatment should be determined by taking symptoms into account rather than relying absolutely on the platelet count alone. However, at a given platelet count bleeding is believed to be more likely in neonates, premature infants being particularly vulnerable.[29] For term infants prophylactic treatment is regarded as justified at counts of below $30 \times 10^9/l$, a figure well in excess of the adult therapeutic figure, and the threshold for the use of platelets during active bleeding is also correspondingly higher. Again for low birth weight pre-term babies, prophylactic treatment is considered with counts in the region of $50 \times 10^9/l$ or sometimes at even higher levels for the most severely ill. These recommendations are based largely on the basis of observations suggesting an increased risk of intraventricular haemorrhage even with mild thrombocytopenia.[30]

Administration of platelets

(1) One random donor equivalent ($\sim 55 \times 10^9$) pack per 2.5 kg should be sufficient as a single dose.
(2) Fresh platelets, certainly those less than 24 hours old, *also contribute fresh plasma*. This should be remembered during treatment of disseminated intra-vascular coagulation where both platelets and coagulation factors are required.
(3) It may be necessary to reduce the volume administered to avoid circulatory overload. Platelets can be concentrated further, from 50 ml down to 15 ml, by gentle centrifugation and removal of unwanted plasma.[31] The platelet packs must then stand for about 1 hour without disturbance to allow resuspension. The platelets should be administered within 12 hours; prolonged storage in this reduced volume of plasma is not possible.
(4) Platelet concentrates usually contain considerable numbers of leucocytes; CMV transmission is therefore a risk (chapter 21, section 6.2) and also in some circumstances GVHD (see chapter 23, section 4.1).

3.1   Alloimmune (Isoimmune) Neonatal Thrombocytopenia

This condition is the counterpart of haemolytic disease of the newborn. It arises as a result of the maternal sensitization to platelet-specific antigens which may follow an earlier transfusion or the transplacental passage of fetal platelets. It usually presents as an unexpected neonatal thrombocytopenia in otherwise healthy babies with healthy mothers.

Serology

There are several known platelet-specific antigen systems (now designated as human platelet antigens (HPA))[32] but it appears that *anti-HPA-1a* (formerly Zw[a], PL[A]) formed in HPA-1a-negative mothers carrying HPA-1a-positive infants is the commonest cause of this condition. About 98% of the population are HPA-1a positive and those mothers are therefore not at risk. The remaining 2% of mothers who are HPA-1a negative will virtually always have partners who are HPA-1a positive and therefore liable to have babies affected by this condition. In practice, however, clinical thrombocytopenia is rare. First-born babies are involved on about 50% of occasions. The problem of HPA-1a alloimmune thrombocytopenia seems to be more frequent in mothers with HLA-B8 and -DRw52 antigens. Immunization to HPA-5b (formerly Brᵃ) and to a variety of other platelet antigens has also been observed as a cause of thombocytopenia. Many mothers also have coincidental HLA antibodies which are not usually of pathological significance. In approximately 50% of a large series of presumed alloimmune thrombocytopenia no serological diagnosis could be made.[33]

Incidence of alloimmune thrombocytopenia

This condition appears in around one in 10 000 births, but may carry a mortality risk of around 10%. Alloimmune thrombocytopenia is therefore a serious condition; *central nervous system bleeding*, either spontaneous or caused by the trauma of delivery, is responsible for a major part of the morbidity and mortality.

Diagnosis

The condition is diagnosed by an *exclusion* of other forms of neonatal thrombocytopenia, e.g. *maternal ITP, disseminated intravascular coagulation and neonatal infection either of bacterial or viral origin*. The mother should therefore have a normal platelet count and no platelet autoantibodies; the infant should not have any coagulation factor abnormalities indicative of a consumptive state. The diagnosis is confirmed by the demonstration that *maternal serum contains HPA-1a antibodies* (usually by means of immunofluorescence, enzyme-linked immunoassay or the more recently developed monoclonal antibody immobilized platelet protein assay (MAIPA)) when tested against a panel of HPA-1a-positive and -negative platelets. Her own platelets must, of course, be shown to be HPA-1a negative. Future pregnancies of immunized women will also be affected if the fetus is incompatible. Because of the risks and uncertainty of managing affected pregnancies, early knowledge of the fetal phenotype is valuable. Fortunately it has now become possible to identify HPA-1 alleles by PCR-amplified RFLP analysis using DNA from chorionic villus biopsy, and possibly also amniotic fluid fetal cells early in pregnancy.[34,35]

This investigation will generally only be available at the few reference centres which have access to the appropriate laboratory expertise.

Management of thrombocytopenic babies

For the reasons discussed above, rapid serological diagnosis, which should serve as the basis for specific treatment, is difficult. *Washed maternal platelets*, resuspended in compatible plasma, will reliably correct the thrombocytopenia but random donor platelets will not. HPA-1a-negative platelets can be used but it should be remembered that these will only be effective when anti-HPA-1a is the culprit (probably 95% of cases). There is increasing evidence that intravenous immunoglobulin (e.g. at 0.4 g/kg for 5 days)[36] (see chapter 9, section 3.2) is effective in raising the platelet count.

Management of future pregnancies[36–39]

Where mothers are known to be HPA immunized any succeeding pregnancies must be monitored carefully. Where available, fetal blood sampling permits platelet antigen typing and platelet counting. Where there is severe thrombocytopenia compatible platelets can be transfused *in utero*, although the timing, frequency, effectiveness and safety of such interventions has not been fully established. Maternal therapy with IVIg is a less hazardous measure which is sometimes, but not reliably, effective. One approach is to begin treatment at high doses (1 g/kg weekly) after percutaneous umbilical blood sampling (PUBS) at 20 weeks to confirm the diagnosis of an incompatible and affected (e.g. platelet counts $< 100 \times 10^9$/l) fetus. Steroids are sometimes also given with IVIg in the belief that they have a potentiating effect. Depending on the severity of thrombocytopenia, fetal sampling is repeated around 1–4-weekly intervals, particularly as term approaches, to establish the potential risk at delivery. Platelet transfusions can be given when platelet counts are low and where no response to IVIg has occurred. The aim should be to obtain post-transfusion platelet counts $> 500 \times 10^9$/l.[37] Certainly pre-delivery transfusions appear to be a practicable measure to improve safety at the time of greatest danger. Caesarian section is usually chosen as the mode of delivery when the fetal platelet count cannot be raised above 50×10^9/l. After 20 weeks' gestation ultrasound monitoring can be used to detect whether intracranial haemorrhage has already occurred.

3.2 Neonatal Thrombocytopenia due to Maternal Autoimmune Thrombocytopenia

Mothers with autoimmune thrombocytopenia may have affected infants—the likelihood of significant morbidity is, however, far less than with alloimmune thrombocytopenia, and serious thrombocytopenia and intracranial haemorrhage are rare.[40,41] Platelet counts typically reach their nadir a few days post-natally, in contrast to the early thrombocytopenia of alloimmune origin. Prognosis of the infant's condition correlates poorly with maternal platelet counts (they may still be thrombocytopenic even when maternal counts are near normal) and only slightly better with platelet-associated IgG or free antibody levels.[42,43]

Pre-natal platelet counting, which carries some risk, is not generally indicated. Maternal therapy with IVIg or corticosteroids are also not indicated for protection of the fetus since no form of treatment for the mother's thrombocytopenia has been shown to have any effect on the fetus. Vaginal delivery rather than Caesarean section is advised if the maternal platelet count is above $50 \times 10^9/l$.[44]

Significant neonatal thrombocytopenia (e.g. counts below $50 \times 10^9/l$) should be treated with IVIg. Doses of $0.4\,g/kg$ per day for 5 days have been used; 80% of infants appear to show a response within a few days—the value of corticosteroids as an adjunctive measure has not been confirmed. It is generally considered that those rare infants with serious symptoms should receive random donor platelets even though they will not be compatible with the maternal autoantibodies. Even if platelet counts in the immediate post-natal period are satisfactory they should continue to be monitored for a few days as thrombocytopenia may be delayed.

4 GRANULOCYTE THERAPY

4.1 Neonatal Sepsis[45]

Severe *neonatal sepsis* is a potentially devastating illness which contributes significantly to overall neonatal morbidity and mortality. It has been estimated that 0.1–1% of full-term infants and an even greater proportion of premature babies may have septicaemia with an expected mortality of approximately 40%. This vulnerability may in part be related to impaired humoral immunity but it is also a consequence of immaturity and relative unresponsiveness of the neutrophil granulocyte system in response to infection. Several defects have been recognized:

- Reduction of the size of the bone marrow neutrophil storage pool.
- Low rate of replenishment from myelopoietic precursors.
- Suboptimal release of mature granulocytes from the marrow.
- Defective granulocyte migration.
- Impairment of phagocytosis and bacterial killing.

Several controlled trials have been performed which appear to demonstrate the efficacy of *granulocyte therapy* in this category of septic neonates.[46-48] However, an increasing body of opinion regards the benefit of granulocyte therapy as unproven.

Modern alternatives, for example growth factors G-CSF and GM-CSF which are known to stimulate bone marrow production, offer an alternative approach that is currently under study. Advocates of granulocyte therapy have identified the most deserving candidates for therapy as those who are premature, have bacterial sepsis, either proven or presumed highly likely on clinical grounds, and who have *low neutrophil counts* (below $3.0 \times 10^9/l$). These counts do not seem unduly low in comparison with adult neutropenia but must be judged in the context of the expected neutrophilia of healthy neonates. Bone marrow examination is not a feasible routine diagnostic procedure but, if performed, there should be reduced numbers of post-mitotic bone marrow granulocyte precursors (bone marrow storage pool below 7% of total marrow cells) and this depletion will be reflected by a corresponding increase in the proportion of immature cells in the peripheral blood (greater than 70% metamyelocytes or less mature cells).

Treatments used have included:

(1) Granulocytes procured by leukapheresis procedures. A dose of $0.5-1.0 \times 10^9$ granulocytes/15 ml per kilogram is probably adequate. Firm data are not yet available. A typical adult single donor leukapheresis harvest will require to be concentrated into a smaller volume.[49] The dose should probably be repeated in 12–24 hours until there is significant clinical improvement.

(2) Buffy coats prepared from fresh donor blood can be used.[50] These may often be the most readily available materials providing the dose and volume required, although evidence for their benefit is less supportive, possibly because the doses achieved have been lower than the leukapheresis collections. If necessary, the large volumes of granulocyte concentrate can be administered by partial exchange transfusion. Four to five days' consecutive treatment are usually given. CMV transmission and GVHD are particular risks of granulocyte transfusion unless appropriate precautions are taken.

(3) Exchange transfusion with fresh blood[51] is hazardous and probably least effective at improving the supply of granulocytes.

Necrotizing enterocolitis[52,53]

Necrotizing enterocolitis is now a common gastrointestinal emergency of unknown aetiology in neonates. It presents with obstruction, abdominal distension and rectal bleeding usually, in association with clostridial or other bacterial bowel infection. The problem sometimes appears as a complication of exchange transfusion, in which instance hypovolaemic hypotension and mucosal ischaemia are postulated causative factors. Shock and disseminated intravascular coagulation (DIC) are commonly present and require therapy. In clostridial infection damage to red cells, due to the release of the bacterial neuraminidase, exposes reactive antigenic (T antigen) groups that render them prone to lysis by the anti-T antibody naturally present in all donor plasma. Blood transfusion is such cases results in a haemolytic transfusion reaction, but this time of *recipient* and not of donor red cells. This condition used to be disclosed by the finding of polyagglutinability during routine grouping with human serum reagents. Monoclonal reagents do not show this property and their use may result in T activation being overlooked. The diagnosis is confirmed in the laboratory by demonstrating that the T antigen has been exposed on the infant's red cells. This is accomplished by testing the red cells with an anti-T lectin obtained from peanuts (*Arachis hypogaea*), a precaution which may be advisable during pre-transfusion testing of all infants with necrotizing enterocolitis.[54]

If peanut lectin is unavailable incubation of infants' red cells in group AB plasma will disclose the problem. If T activation is confirmed, washed red cells must be used for further transfusions and all products containing plasma avoided.[55]

4.2　Alloimmune (Isoimmune) Neonatal Neutropenia

Although maternal sensitization to HLA antigens of the fetus is common, this appears to have little clinical affect and does not appear to cause either lymphopenia or neutropenia. Possibly, HLA antibodies reaching the fetus are neutralized by the corresponding antigens which are widely distributed throughout the placenta and fetal tissues. Sensitization to neutrophil-specific antigens (e.g. NB1, NA1, NA2, NC1) is rare. The diagnosis can be confirmed by detecting antibodies in the maternal serum against paternal neutrophil specific antigens. The comparative rarity of the condition is difficult to explain. It seems possible that the relatively small number of granulocytes and their shorter life-span compared to red cells renders them less immunogenic when fetal blood is introduced into the maternal circulation. It is also likely that the active marrow and high blood turnover rate characteristic of normal granulopoiesis renders this system less vulnerable to immune damage. The approach to diagnosis of this rare condition follows the lines of neonatal thrombocytopenia. Intravenous immunoglobulin appears to be an effective treatment.

5 COAGULATION FACTOR REPLACEMENT[56-59]

Coagulation factor profiles of the newborn

Levels of contact activation and vitamin K-dependent procoagulant proteins are relatively reduced (approximately 40–60%) in newborns compared to adults. In contrast, Factor VIII and vWF are usually within the adult normal range. Moderate deficiencies are also seen in coagulation inhibitors antithrombin III and protein C. The significance of these differences as a background to the pathological perturbations of the newborn period is unclear. However, both thrombotic problems and intraventricular haemorrhages are risks complicating the newborn period which may at least in part be due to these relative imbalances.

5.1 Neonatal Prothrombin Deficiency

Before the widespread use of prophylactic vitamin K, bleeding during the first few days of life, due to reduced levels of vitamin K-dependent factors, was a frequent occurrence in the newborn. This is attributed to a decline in vitamin K levels after maternal supplies are withdrawn and before that absorbed from the neonatal bowel becomes available. Vitamin K_1 (0.5–1.0 mg i.m. or 2 mg orally) allows hepatic synthesis of coagulation factors to be maintained. FFP (10–12 ml/kg) can be given if there is evidence of bleeding and if waiting for the response to vitamin K_1 seems risky.

5.2 Disseminated Intravascular Coagulation

DIC is the commonest coagulation problem encountered and is particularly associated with *sepsis, respiratory distress syndrome, shock* and sometimes *haemolytic disease of the newborn*. DIC requires broad-spectrum coagulation factor therapy and usually there will be a need for platelets in addition. Diagnosis and treatment on the basis of laboratory findings are more difficult than in adults (see chapter 8); blood-sampling difficulties and difficulties in interpretation of test results are common. When platelets and coagulation factor disturbances coexist, a single fresh platelet concentrate per 2.5 kg body weight provides the most suitable form of therapy. If platelets are not required then either FFP or cryoprecipitate is given. FFP is best made available in a small-volume pack to minimize waste and facilitate rapid thawing. A stock of group AB Rh-negative plasma can be held available for infants of any blood group. Cryoprecipitate, which contains all the plasma coagulation factors but is enriched for fibrinogen and Factor VIII, may be preferred for severe states of consumptive coagulopathy when the coagulation test results are very abnormal.

5.3 Congenital Factor Deficiencies

Symptoms due to deficiencies of specific coagulation factors do not usually cause problems in the neonatal period. Factor XIII deficiency, rare in its own right, is an exception and can cause serious bleeding, as occasionally may also occur with Factor IX deficiency (haemophilia B, Christmas disease). In the former case, FFP (10–12 ml/kg) should be given twice daily, after diagnostic samples have been obtained. Because of their greater predisposition to thrombotic events, high-purity Factor VIII or Factor IX are the preferred products for the respective haemophiliac conditions. The diagnosis of haemophilia should certainly be considered in all instances of otherwise unexplained visceral or intracranial haemorrhage.[60]

FFP was formerly preferred for Factor IX replacement because of concerns over the viral risk and thrombotic vulnerability associated with conventionally available products. This is probably no longer true for the newer preparation of Factor IX concentrates (see chapter 8). Similarly high-purity Factor VIII is now preferred as substitution therapy for haemophilia A.

Neonatal thrombotic problems

The newborn period is characterized by increased vulnerability to major vessel thrombotic episodes. In part, this may reflect suboptimal levels of the anti-thrombotic and fibrinolytic systems as well as increased whole-blood viscosity. The very rare protein C deficiency is characterized by widespread multi-vessel thrombosis and end organ infarction. Early diagnostic suspicion and prompt treatment with FFP is required. Microcirculatory thrombosis in sick neonates has been ascribed in part to pre-maturity-associated antithrombin III deficiencies. The place of antithrombin III replacement in these circumstances has not yet been established. Serious, sometimes life-threatening thromboses occur in around 1% of infants with umbilical catheters. No clear consensus yet exists regarding a management of these problems. Surgical thrombectomy, heparin or thrombolytic therapy have been used.[61]

6 PLASMA VOLUME EXPANSION: USE OF ALBUMIN

The precise clinical role for albumin products is no more firmly agreed for neonates that it is in adult medicine (see chapter 10). Hypoalbuminaemia ($< 30\,g/$ dl) is usual in low birth weight pre-term infants and may, although this is debatable, be an aggravating factor in respiratory distress syndrome. Albumin infusion in this situation has been claimed to be beneficial. Albumin at 4–5% concentration is probably most valuable for treatment of non-haemorrhagic shock states where the haematocrit is above 0.55 and administration of red cells would therefore be harmful. Albumin is preferred when hypoalbuminaemia is a likely consequence of the use of other volume expansion agents or for acute management of the clinical consequences of plasma albumin deficiency. Intraventricular haemorrhage is well known as a frequent neurological complication of pre-term babies which may be related to haemodynamic instability. FFP has been claimed to confirm a protective effect[62] but the topic requires further study, and there is no evidence yet to support the need for coagulation factor replacement therapy. Prophylactic benefit, if confirmed, may equally depend on plasma volume expansion leading to improved cardiovascular stability.

Newborn infants, particularly the most premature and sick, are frequently believed to be at risk from a variety of haemostatic problems and the use of FFP is customarily advocated either as a prophylactic measure or as a resuspending agent when red cell transfusions or exchange transfusions are given. There is no conclusive modern evidence to support the use of FFP under these circumstances and it would seem prudent to reserve its use for patients in whom use could be justified on the basis of clinical and laboratory evidence of coagulation disorder.

REFERENCES

1 Sacher, R.A., Strauss, R.G., Luban, N.L.C. *et al.* (1990) Blood component therapy during the neonatal period: a national survey of red cell transfusion practice, 1985. *Transfusion*, **30**: 271–276.

2 Strauss, R.G., Blanchette, V.S., Hume, H. *et al.* (1993) National acceptability of American association of Blood Banks Pediatric Hemotherapy Committee guidelines for auditing pediatric transfusion practices. *Transfusion*, **33**: 168–171.

3 British Committee for Standards in Haematology Blood Transfusion Task Force (1993) Guidelines for administration of blood products: transfusion of infants and neonates. *Transfusion Med.*, **4**: 63–69.

4 Hume, H.A., Ali, A.M., Dcary, F. and Blajchman, M.A. (1991) Evaluation of pediatric transfusion practice using criteria maps. *Transfusion*, **31**: 52–58.

5 Kimmond, S., Aitchison, T.C., Holland, B.M., Jones, J.G., Turner, T.L. and Wardrop, C.A.J. (1993) Umbilical cord clamping and the preterm infant: a randomized trial. *Br. Med. J.*, **306**: 172.

6 Jones, J.G., Holland, B.M., Veale, K.E.A. and Wardrop, C.A.J. (1979) 'Available oxygen': a realistic expression of the ability of the blood to supply oxygen to tissues. *Scand. J. Haematol.*, **22**: 77–82.

7 Phillips, H.M., Holland, B.M., Abdel-Moiz, A. *et al.* (1986) Determination of red-cell mass in assessment and managment of anaemia in babies needing blood transfusion. *Lancet*, **i**: 882–884.

8 Hill, H.R. (1991) The role of intravenous immunoglobulin in the treatment and prevention of neonatal bacterial infection. *Semin. Perinatol.*, **15**: 41–46.
9 Weisman, L.E., Stoll, B.J., Kueser, T.J. *et al.* (1992) Intravenous immune globulin therapy for early-onset sepsis in premature neonates. *J. Pediatr.*, **121**: 434–443.
10 Strauss, R.G. (1991) Transfusion therapy in neonates. *Am. J. Dis. Child.*, **145**: 904–911.
11 Floss, A.M., Strauss, R.G., Goeken, N. and Knox, L. (1986) Multiple transfusions fail to provoke antibodies against blood cell antigens in human infants. *Transfusion*, **26**: 419–422.
12 DePalma, L. (1992) Review: red cell alloantibody formation in the neonate and infant. Considerations for current immunohematologic practice. *Immunohematology*, **8**: 33–37.
13 Maniatis, A., Theodoris, H. and Aravani, K. (1993) Neonatal immune response to red cell antigens. *Transfusion*, **33**: 90–91.
14 Strauss, R.G., Sacher, R.A., Blazina, J.F. *et al.* (1990) Commentary on small-volume red cell transfusions for neonatal patients. *Transfusion*, **30**: 565–570.
15 Meyer, J., Sive, A. and Jacobs, P. (1993) Empiric red cell transfusion in asymptomatic preterm infants. *Acta Paediatr.*, **82**: 30–34.
16 Stockman, J.A. and Clark, D.A. (1984) Weight gain: a response to transfusion in selected preterm infants. *Am. J. Dis. Child.*, **138**: 828–830.
17 Batton, D.G., Maisels, M.J. and Shulman, G. (1983) Serum potassium changes following packed red cell transfusions in newborn infants. *Transfusion*, **23**: 163–164.
18 Luban, N.L.C., Strauss, R.G. and Hume, H.A. (1991) Commentary on the safety of red cells preserved in extended storage media for neonatal transfusions. *Transfusion*, **31**: 229–235.
19 Elbert, C., Strauss, R.G., Barrett, F., Goeken, N.E., Pittner, B. and Cordle, D. (1991) Biological mothers may be dangerous blood donors for their neonates. *Acta Haematol.*, **85**: 189–191.
20 Sanders, M.R. and Graever, J.E. (1990) Post-transfusion graft-versus-host disease in infancy. *J. Pediatr.*, **117**: 159–163.
21 Letsky, E.A. (1991) Polycythaemia in the newborn infant. In: Hann, I.M., Gibson, B.E.S. and Letsky, E.A. (eds), *Fetal and Neonatal Haematology*, pp. 95–121. London: Baillière Tindall.
22 Shalev, O., Manny, N. and Sharon, R. (1993) Post-transfusion hemolysis in recipients of glucose-6-phosphate dehydrogenase-deficient erythrocytes. *Vox Sang.*, **64**: 94–98.
23 Iserson, K.V. and Huestis, D.W. (1991) Blood warming: current applications and techniques. *Transfusion*, **31**: 558–571.
24 *Guidelines for the Blood Transfusion Service* (UK) (1993) London: HMSO.
25 Tegtmeier, G.E. (1988) The use of cytomegalovirus-screened blood in neonates. *Transfusion*, **28**: 201–203.
26 Bjerke, H.S., Kelly, R.E., Jr, Foglia, R.P., Barcliff, L. and Petz, L. (1992) Decreasing transfusion exposure risk during extracorporeal membrane oxygenation (ECMO). *Transfusion Med.*, **2**: 43–49.
27 DePalma, L. and Luban, N.L.C. (1990) Blood component therapy in the perinatal period: guidelines and recommendations. *Semin. Perinatol.*, **14**: 403–415.
28 Castle, V., Andrew, M., Kelton, J. *et al.* (1986) Frequency and mechanism of neonatal thrombocytopenia. *J. Pediatr.*, **108**: 749–755.
29 Gibson, B. (1989) Neonatal haemostasis. *Arch. Dis. Child.*, **64**: 503–506.
30 Lupton, B.A., Hill, A., Whitfield, M.R. et al. (1988) Reduced platelet count as a risk factor for intraventricular hemorrhage. *Am. J. Dis. Child.*, **142**: 1222–1224.
31 Moroff, G., Friedman, A., Robkin-Kline, L., Gautier, G. and Luban, N.L.C. (1984) Reduction of the volume of stored platelet concentrates for use in neonatal patients. *Transfusion*, **24**: 144–146.
32 von dem Borne, A.E.G. and Decary, F. (1990) ICSH/ISBT Working Party on Platelet Serology. *Vox Sang.*, **58**: 176.
33 Meuller-Eckhardt, C., Kiefel, V., Grubert, A. *et al.* (1989) 348 cases of suspected neonatal alloimmune thrombocytopenia. *Lancet*, i: 363–366.

34 Williamson, L.M., Bruce, D., Lubenko, A., Chana, H.J. and Ouwehand, W.H. (1992) Molecular biology for platelet alloantigen typing. *Transfusion Med.*, **2**: 255–264.
35 Andersen, B.R., Georgsen, J., Madsen, H.O., Taaning, E., Grunnet, N. and Sveijgaard, A. (1993) Human platelet antigen-1(Zw) typing using PCR-RFLP. *Transfusion Med.*, **3**: 153–156.
36 Levine, A.B. and Berkowitz., R.L. (1991) Neonatal alloimmune thrombocytopenia. *Semin. Perinatol.*, **15**: 35–40.
37 Murphy, M.F., Waters, A.H., Doughty, H.A. *et al.* (1994) Antenatal management of feto-maternal thrombocytopenia: report of 15 affected pregnancies. *Transfusion Med.*, **4**: 281–292.
38 Lynch, L., Bussel, J.B., McFarland, J.G., Chitkara, U. and Berkowitz, R.L. (1992) Antenatal treatment of alloimmune thrombocytopenia. *Obstet. Gynecol.*, **80**: 67–71.
39 Marzusch, K., Schnaidt, M., Dietl, J., Wiest, E., Hofstaetter, C. and Golz, R. (1992) High dose immunoglobulin in the antenatal treatment of neonatal alloimmune thrombocytopenia: case report and review. *Br. J. Obstet. Gynaecol.*, **99**: 260–262.
40 Cook, R.L., Miller, R.C., Katz, V.L. and Cefalo, R.C. (1991) Immune thrombocytopenic purpura in pregnancy: a reappraisal of management. *Obstet. Gynecol.*, **78**: 578–583.
41 Pillai, M. (1993) Platelets and pregnancy. *Br. J. Obstet. Gynaecol.*, **100**: 201–204.
42 Kelton, J.G., Inwood, M.J., Barr, R.M. *et al.* (1982) The prenatal prediction of thrombocytopenia in infants of mothers with clinically diagnosed immune thrombocytopenia. *Am. J. Obstet. Gynecol.*, **144**: 449–454.
43 Scott, J.R., Rote, N.S. and Cruikshank, D.P. (1983) Antiplatelet antibodies and platelet counts in pregnancies complicated by autoimmune thrombocytopenic purpura. *Am. J. Obstet. Gynecol.*, **145**: 932–936.
44 Janes, S.L. (1992) Thrombocytopenia in pregnancy. *Postgrad. Med. J.*, **68**: 321–326.
45 Yoder, M.C. and Polin, R.A. (1986) Immunotherapy of neonatal septicemia. *Pediatr. Clin. North Am.*, **33**: 481–501.
46 Laurenti, F., Ferro, R., Isacchi, G. *et al.* (1981) Polymorphonuclear leukocyte transfusion for the treatment of sepsis in the newborn infant. *J. Pediatr.*, **98**: 118–123.
47 Christensen, R.D., Rothstein, G., Anstall, H.B. and Bybee, B. (1982) Granulocyte transfusions in neonates with bacterial infection, neutropenia, and depletion of mature marrow neutrophils. *Pediatrics*, **70**: 1–6.
48 Cairo, M.S. (1991) The role of granulocyte transfusions as adjuvant therapy in the treatment of neonatal sepsis. *Transfusion Sci.*, **12**: 247–256.
49 Kalmin, N.D. and Liles, B.A. (1984) Preparation of granulocyte concentrates for neonatal patient transfusion. *Transfusion*, **24**: 240–242.
50 Rock, G., Zurakowski, S., Baxter, A. and Adams, G. (1984) Simple and rapid preparation of granulocytes for the treatment of neonatal septicemia. *Transfusion*, **24**: 510–512.
51 Christensen, R.D., Anstall, H.B. and Rothestein, G. (1982) Use of whole blood exchange transfusion to supply neutrophils to septic, neutropenic neonates. *Transfusion*, **22**: 504–506.
52 Placzer, M.M. and Gorst, D.W. (1987) T activation haemolysis and death after blood transfusion. *Arch. Dis. Child.*, **62**: 743–744.
53 Wiswell, T.E. and Cornish, J.D. (1986) Fresh frozen plasma partial exchange transfusion and necrotizing enterocolitis. *Pediatrics*, **77**: 786–787.
54 Seger, R., Joller, P., Kenny, A., Hitzig, W., Metaxas, M. and Metaxas-Bühler, M. (1979) Potential hazards of blood-transfusion in clostridia-associated necrotising enterocolitis. *Lancet*, **i**: 48–49.
55 Levene, C., Sela, R., Blat, J., Friedlaender, M. and Manny, N. (1986) Intracellular hemolysis and renal failure in a patient with T polyagglutination. *Transfusion*, **26**: 243–245.
56 Andrew, M., Paes, B., Milner, R. *et al.* (1988) Development of the human coagulation system in the healthy premature. *Blood*, **72**: 1651–1657.
57 Andrew, M., Paes, B., Milner, R., Johnston, M., Mitchell, L., Tollefsen, D.M. and Powers, P. (1987) Development of the human coagulation system in the full-term infant. *Blood*, **70**: 165–172.

58 Smith, P.S. (1990) Congenital coagulation protein deficiencies in the perinatal period. *Semin. Perinatol.*, **14**: 384–392.
59 Beardsley, D.S. (1991) Hemostasis in the perinatal period: approach to the diagnosis of coagulation disorders. *Semin. Perinatol.*, **15**: 25–34.
60 Bray, G.L. and Luban, N.L.C. (1987) Hemophilia presenting with intracranial hemorrhage. *Am. J. Dis. Child.*, **141**: 1215–1217.
61 Bray, G.L. (1991) Normal and disordered coagulation in the neonate. *Transfusion Sci.*, **12**: 231–245.
62 Beverley, D.W., Pitts-Tucker, T.J., Congdon, P.J., Arthur, R.J. and Tate, G. (1985) Prevention of intraventricular haemorrhage by fresh frozen plasma. *Arch. Dis. Child.*, **60**: 710–713.
63 Strauss, R.G. (1994) Erythropoietin and neonatal anemia. *N. Engl. J Med.*, **330**: 1227–1228.
64 Maier, R.F., Obladen, M., Scigalla, P. *et al.* (1994) The effect of epoetin beta (recombinant human erythropoietin) on the need for transfusion in very-low-birth-weight infants. *N. Engl. J. Med.*, **330**: 1173–1178.

21

Haemolytic Disease of the Newborn

1 NATURAL HISTORY OF HAEMOLYTIC DISEASE

The term *haemolytic disease of the newborn (HDNB)* refers to the haemolytic anaemia that affects fetuses or neonates caused by the transplacental passage of maternal alloantibodies directed against fetal red cell antigens. These antibodies are not naturally occurring but will have been stimulated either by leakage of fetal red cells into the maternal circulation or by blood transfusion.

The haemolytic process varies greatly in severity and the differences in the criteria used for definition can cause confusion when statistics concerning risks and incidences are quoted. In its mildest form haemolytic disease of the newborn is shown only by the combination of *alloantibodies in maternal blood and a positive direct antiglobulin test* result on the infant's red cells due to coating by the offending antibody. The only action necessary in such mild cases is clinical observation coupled with a complete laboratory investigation.

More severe degrees of HDNB involve red cell haemolysis which shows as *anaemia* at birth together with *jaundice* due to increasing post-natal levels of unconjugated bilirubin. After birth there is continued *haemolysis* of antibody-coated cells which can continue for weeks as newly formed red cells become damaged by the passively acquired maternal antibody. *Anaemia* and *congestive cardiac failure* are dangers, but the most serious hazard is that of damage to the central nervous system caused by high levels of unconjugated bilirubin. This can be seen at autopsy as yellow staining of the brain, particularly in structures such as the corpus striatum, the thalamus and the nuclei in the floor of the fourth ventricle. The condition, known as *kernicterus*, shows clinically as severe brain damage with high-tone deafness, athetoid cerebral palsy and sometimes mental retardation. Jaundice and kernicterus occur only as post-natal problems; prior to delivery fetal bilirubin crosses the placenta to be removed by the maternal circulation and metabolized. The neonatal liver is functionally too immature to conjugate the large amounts of bilirubin derived from the haemolysed red cells. Furthermore liver function may also be impaired by gross erythroid hyperplasia.

Kernicterus was a tragic sequel to many cases of haemolytic disease of the newborn before modern management of this condition became available (see below). Its cause and the means for its prevention are now so well known that new cases should not occur.

At its worst the haemolytic process causes *severe anaemia, cardiac failure and fetal death*, sometimes as early as 20 weeks' gestation. There is gross erythroid hyperplasia of the spleen and liver and in consequence abdominal distension. Disturbed liver function and cardiac failure produce *oedema, ascites and serous effusions* to complete the clinical picture known as *hydrops fetalis*. Infants born with hydrops require immediate exchange transfusion to have any hope of recovery. Respiratory distress syndrome, haemorrhagic problems due to disseminated intravascular coagulation or reduced hepatic synthesis of coagulation factors and episodes of cardiovascular instability during exchange are common causes of death.

The anaemia of HDNB may persist for some weeks after delivery. This appears to be a result of continued haemolysis due to the residual antibody both in the plasma and also throughout the extravascular fluid. It appears particularly frequently in premature infants in whom the erythroid marrow shows hyporesponsiveness to anaemia.

Over 95% of all cases of clinically significant HDNB of the newborn affect Rh D-positive infants born to Rh D-negative mothers. Typically mothers become sensitized to D-positive fetal cells at delivery of the first Rh-positive infant and subsequent Rh D-positive infants are progressively more severely affected. It is important to appreciate that this pattern does not always hold true; sometimes severe disease is seen even in the first recorded pregnancy. Clinical HDNB due to anti-D should, under ideal circumstances, be a disease of the past. The remainder of this chapter is concerned with ways in which HDNB can be prevented or established cases recognized and treated to prevent severe illness.

2 ANTENATAL TESTING OF MATERNAL BLOOD

Serological examination of maternal blood samples represents the cornerstone of any system for management of HDNB. Testing has two principal aims:

(1) To detect the presence of irregular alloantibodies and thereby identify and allow assessment of mothers at risk of HDNB.
(2) Additionally to ensure that any maternal and neonatal transfusion problems can be anticipated in advance.

When very unusual antibodies are found it may be necessary to:

(1) Examine the blood of other members of the family in case they may be suitable as blood donors should the mother or baby require transfusion.
(2) Collect autologous maternal blood.
(3) Seek the assistance of the national rare-donor panels.

It may also be expeditious to arrange induced delivery so that the procurement of blood and its likely need can be coordinated. Maternal serum samples must therefore be screened for the presence of *irregular alloantibodies*. When these are found their *specificity* must be determined and their *potency* estimated. This should be followed by demonstration that the maternal red cells lack the corresponding antigen—an observation which serves to confirm the accuracy of the previous results. Where clinically significant antibodies are found that could necessitate intervention before the natural end of pregnancy, the paternal red cells should be typed for the antigen concerned and where possible homozygosity or heterozygosity determined.

2.1 Routine Grouping

This usually comprises *ABO and Rh D grouping*. Rh genotyping and determination of other groups become necessary only if alloantibodies are found. Accuracy in Rh D grouping of antenatal samples is particularly important[1] and it is a wise precaution to assign Rh D groups only after:

(1) testing on two separate occasions; or
(2) use of two independent reagents or techniques together with appropriate controls (see chapter 25, section 2.2).

Rh-negative women erroneously grouped as Rh positive carry the risk of:

(1) Transfusion with Rh-positive blood and in consequence sensitization to the Rh D antigen and severe haemolytic disease of succeeding pregnancies.
(2) Not receiving prophylactic anti-D immunoglobulin, with the same potential consequences (see section 6.2).
(3) Delayed detection of significant antibodies (see section 2.2), as a result of the reduced frequency of serological examination selected.

It is not necessary to distinguish the *Rh D^u* mothers from amongst those that appear to be Rh D negative. It seems largely immaterial whether they are treated as Rh positive or negative. However, mothers in whom the Rh D^u status has been recognized are not candidates for anti-D immunoglobulin (see section 6.2) and Rh D-positive blood may be used for transfusion. Very weakly reacting apparent D^u blood samples encountered late in pregnancy may in fact be examples of large fetomaternal leaks of D-positive cells in Rh D-negative mothers and this requires prompt investigation and treatment.

Early gestational diagnosis of fetomaternal blood group incompatibility

Direct confirmation of the presence of fetomaternal incompatibility particularly for D and K antigens may be helpful in mothers with a history of previous severe haemolytic disease who have a heterozygous partner. Fetal blood typing can be performed on chorionic villus samples between 9 and 11 weeks' gestation.[2] Alternatively, the genotype can be determined by using polymerase chain reaction (PCR) amplification of DNA from amniotic cells[3] or from fetal cells in maternal peripheral blood.[4] These investigations are most useful when proceeding with a severely affected pregnancy is not possible and termination is under consideration.

2.2 Examination for Irregular Antibodies

The principles of investigation for irregular alloantibodies need not differ from those applied in routine serological practice. Automated screening systems such as twin-channel autoanalysers comprising low ionic strength Polybrene (hexadimethrine bromide) and bromelin methylcellulose channels have been successfully employed in many laboratories with large workloads.[5] Positive antibody screen results require confirmation by manual techniques followed by determination of specificity and potency.

Cold-reacting antibodies do not cause HDNB. They are best left unreported by the laboratory unless the routine compatibility testing protocols in use involve a room temperature incubation phase, in which case they may cause delay and difficulties at a later stage if transfusion is required. These IgM antibodies, which usually show I, P or Lewis specificity, cannot cross the placenta to damage the fetal erythrocytes. Furthermore the strength of the corresponding antigens on fetal erythrocytes is much reduced. The Lewis system is of particular interest during pregnancy although it is, fortunately, of little practical relevance. Maternal red cells frequently lose their Lewis antigens while Lewis antibodies commonly appear during pregnancy. Provided serological reactions cannot be shown at 37 °C these Lewis antibodies are not important.

Frequency of testing

The frequency at which maternal samples should be examined varies according to the *Rh group, antibody status* and the previous *obstetric history*. Rh-negative women should be tested more frequently than Rh-positive women, and those with anti-

Table 1 Frequency of antenatal testing

Rh-positive mothers (without antibodies)	At booking, 32–34 weeks*
Rh-negative mothers (without antibodies)	At booking, 24–26 weeks
	32–34 weeks
	Delivery
Mothers with anti-D and or past history of HDNB	Test sera monthly until 28 weeks, every 2 weeks thereafter

If antibodies are found which pose a severe risk of HDNB, more frequent testing may be required as advised by the laboratory.

*Particularly for multipara or those previously transfused.

bodies and a previous history of HDNB must be monitored with the greatest vigilance. Care should be taken that over-cautious serological concern does not result in unnecessarily frequent serological testing, causing annoyance to obstetricians as well as anxiety to the women concerned. A satisfactory testing schedule is that shown in Table 1.

Analysis of the samples from RhD-positive women constitute a major part of the workload of the antenatal screening programme as it is in this area that there is greatest scope for economies in testing frequency. In particular the need to repeat testing late in pregnancy (e.g. 34 weeks) has been questioned where the booking sample shows no abnormalities. Although it has been claimed that the *de novo* immunization seen only late in pregnancy can result in potentially pathological levels of antibody[6] this is highly unlikely for women who have not been transfused or who have not had earlier pregnancies.[7]

Specificities of antibodies causing haemolytic disease

Anti-D has been by far the commonest antibody found during serological testing of mothers and it also causes the most destructive haemolysis. However, the success of the *anti-D prophylactic programme* (see section 6.2) has resulted in reduction in the incidence of new cases of sensitized women to around 10% of those formerly found. In parallel with this change other Rh antibodies and also antibodies to non-Rh blood group systems have become more prevalent. This probably reflects the increased frequency of mothers with a previous transfusion history as well as a progressive increase in the sensitivity of serological test procedures. Anti-c, and -K are well-known examples of antibodies that can occasionally cause significant HDNB. A more complete list of antibodies, their frequencies, source of stimulation and clinical significance is shown in Table 2.

Special problems during serological examination. Occasional patients, especially those belonging to ethnic minority groups, may have antibodies to high-frequency antigens (e.g. anti-U), in which case antigen-negative blood is usually best sought in the same ethnic group. These sera will show positive results against all panel cells tested, the mode of the action being the same against each. Their behaviour may differ from that of sera containing *mixtures of antibodies* where some subdivision may be possible by taking advantage of the different serological character-istics of each antigen–antibody system. In contrast, antibodies to *low-frequency antigens* not always carried on screening cells (e.g. C^W) or to antigens largely restricted to certain races (e.g. Js^a in Negroes) can cause difficulties; the latter category should be borne in mind during the examination of sera from ethnic minority women. A similar difficulty obtains when antibodies to *private* or *family* antigens exist. Such cases will generally be first discovered by the finding of a direct positive antiglobulin on the cord cells. Examination of the maternal serum against paternal red cells should confirm the presence of this type of problem.

Paternal blood typing

HDNB cannot occur unless the fetal red cells carry the antigen against which the maternal alloantibody is directed. Since clearly the antigen must be paternal in origin, typing of paternal blood should show whether the fetus could be at risk. There will, for example, be no risk to the infant of a mother with anti-K if the father is K negative. In such a case the antibody is likely to have been stimulated by previous transfusion rather than pregnancy. In contrast, where a mother has anti-c and a R_2R_2 (*cDEcDE*) husband, some degree of risk to the fetus will be unavoidable. There are, of course, dangers in over-reliance on such conclusions! Paternal samples should only be sought where the results are necessary for safe management of the fetus, i.e. for those situations in which some form of active intervention is likely before the natural end of pregnancy. These antibodies include:

- Antiglobulin-reactive antibodies of D, c and K specificities.
- Enzyme anti-D (which may transform during the course of pregnancy).
- Rare or unusual antibodies which have been recognized to cause severe HDNB (e.g. Wr^a, $-Jk3$, $-V$, $-P + P_{1+}P^k$).

Paternal samples should also be examined where the obstetric history or the previous finding of an unexpected positive cord antiglobulin test suggests the occurrence of HDNB due to low frequency or private antigens.

Characteristics of antibodies determining their clinical significance

Anti-D antibodies are always potentially haemolytic and must have a quantitative estimate made of their potency in order to determine future management (see section 4). The situation is much less clear for other antibodies. Their specificity gives some guide (see Table 2). *IgM antibodies*, typically those that are saline reacting and of I, P and Lewis specificities, *cannot cause HDNB*. Antibodies of other specificities, e.g. anti-E, may also be predominantly IgM and in consequence convey no risk. Even anti-D may have a significant IgM component and this may be one of the reasons why quantitation results do not correlate as closely with clinical outcomes as would be desired. *IgG antibodies are assumed to be capable of causing HDNB*. IgG is carried across the placenta by an active transport mechanism, presumably the normal method for transfer of the maternal anti-bodies conveying passive immunity.

Placental tissue is believed to bear Fc receptors which assist the undirectional transfer of maternal immunoglobulin to the fetus. It seems that IgG subclasses IgG_2 and IgG_4 may not be important in this context. Antibodies of *subclass IgG_1,* however, appear to be transported readily throughout pregnancy and can haemolyse fetal cells. IgG_3 crosses most efficiently in late pregnancy and may be of greater clinical significance around the time of delivery. 'Enzyme-only' antibodies, as long as they remain so, are not important and if they coexist with antibodies active by antiglobulin methods need not restrict the choice of blood used for exchange transfusion.

It has been claimed that the haemolytic potential of anti-D sera can be assessed by their ability to promote *in vitro* macrophage destruction of Rh-positive cells (mononuclear cell phagocytosis assay, chapter 2, section 5.4). It seems that sera coating red cells with IgG of subclasses 1 and 3 are most efficient in this respect and this observation is in accord with clinical experience. The results of testing sera by other methods, either based on *in vitro* cellular haemolysis (the antibody-dependent cell-mediated cytotoxicity (ADCC) test)[8] or by chemiluminescent measurement of monocyte phagocytic activity,[76] have also been shown to correlate more closely with the eventual clinical outcome than total anti-D levels measured by conventional techniques.

3 TESTS ON CORD BLOOD AND MATERNAL BLOOD AT DELIVERY

The blood of all Rh D-negative mothers should be examined after delivery for the presence of *fetal cells* arising from episodes of fetomaternal haemorrhage (see section 6). Large fetomaternal leaks require additional anti-D immunoglobulin (see section 6.2).

The opportunity should also be taken to repeat the *maternal antibody screen* on RhD-negative mothers at delivery. A *direct antiglobulin test* should be performed on *cord blood* from all infants born to mothers with antibodies. This will be positive in all cases of HDNB (with the exception of occasional cases of ABO HDNB) and those cases needing treatment will usually show more strongly positive results. This observation is not, however, a reliable guide to severity. Up to 50% of all positive direct antiglobulin tests, even when strongly positive, are associated with mild disease requiring no treatment. It is sometimes suggested that a direct anti-globulin test should be performed on all cord samples. This practice offers:

(1) A chance to detect HDNB due to antibodies against rare or private antigens which may be of greater significance in later pregnancies.
(2) The best chance to detect the presence of ABO HDNB.

Most laboratories do not do this and it seems unlikely that the cost could be justified by the clinical benefits. It is important to appreciate that the cord blood anti-globulin test may very occasionally be positive as a result of ante-natal therapeutic immunoglobulin administration. This is not clinically important but will cause confusion if unsuspected.

Table 2 Antenatal antibodies: causes and characteristics

Antibody	Stimulus for formation	Occurrence of HDNB	Comments
Anti-D	Usually pregnancy	Yes Principal cause of severe HDNB	Prevention: anti-D immuno-globulin after delivery, amnio-centesis or any other manipulation. Always transfuse Rh D-blood to Rh D-women
Anti-c	Pregnancy 75% Transfusion 25%	Yes Can be severe. About 90% of c+ infants affected to some degree.	Only R_1R_1 (*CDe/CDe*) persons form this antibody. Incidence can be reduced if R_1R_1 women are given R_1R_1 blood
Anti-E	Pregnancy 50% Transfusion 20% Remainder unknown	Yes, together with Anti-c. Rarely severe alone	Possibly sometimes stimulated by bacteria or viruses with an E-like antigen. Only 30% babies on average are at risk (i.e. E+)
Anti-C	Pregnancy and transfusion equally No obvious stimulus in 10%	Yes but uncommon Rarely severe	
Anti-e	Usually pregnancy Transfusion less frequently	Unusual for infant to be affected even if e+	Rare
Anti-K	Mostly by transfusion Pregnancy occasionally No obvious stimulus in about 10%	Yes Can be severe	Father is usually K– or heterozygous (*Kk*) so infant is usually K– and not at risk
Anti-k (Cellano)	Mostly transfusion but stimulation by pregnancy reported	Yes Very rare	Finding compatible (*KK*) blood difficult
Anti-Fy^a	Usually by transfusion Pregnancy in the remainder	Rare can be severe	
Anti-Jk^a	Transfusion and pregnancy about equally	Rare	
Anti-Jk^b	Transfusion and pregnancy about equally	Rare	
Anti-S	Transfusion and pregnancy about equally	Yes but unusual	
Anti-s	Transfusion Pregnancy	Yes but unusual	
Anti-M	Usually naturally occurring. Can be immune	Yes, rare	

Table 2 *Continued*

Antibody	Stimulus for formation	Occurrence of HDNB	Comments
Anti-A and anti-B	Naturally occurring Can be immune	Yes Not usually severe	Typically immune antibodies stimulated in group O mothers by group A or B infants
Anti-Le^a	Naturally occurring	No	Commoner during pregnancy but the reason for this is not known
Anti-Le^b		No	
Anti-I	Naturally occurring antibodies	No	Associated with anaemia due to cold autoantibodies
Anti-HI			
Anti-P$_1$	Naturally occurring	No	Very common in pregnant women but no evidence that it is caused by immunization

Serological studies on cord blood can be useful in cases of diagnostic difficulty. The cord blood sample, which should include both EDTA and clotted specimens, provides a larger volume of serum, and also of cells for preparation of eluates, than will be available from later samples from the baby. This sample should be collected using a syringe and needle to avoid contamination with Wharton's jelly—a sticky material from the cord tissue which can cause false positive antiglobulin and blood-grouping results. If the maternal blood contains alloantibodies then:

(1) These can also be confirmed in the cord serum. Free antibody in cord serum may sometimes be undetectable but instead be bound to fetal cells.
(2) *Eluates* from fetal cells confirm the presence of fetomaternal incompatibility and indicate those that are significant out of a combination of maternal antibodies. It will be necessary to examine eluates from cord cells in suspected cases of HDNB where it has not been possible to examine the maternal serum for antibodies or where previous tests have not shown antibodies. Cord eluates from cases of HDNB which do not react with panel cells may indicate HDNB due to a *low frequency antigen*. Alternatively the positive antiglobulin tests may reflect the presence of complement alone on cells. When the cord eluates react with *all panel cells* the presence of antibodies to *high-frequency antigens, multiple alloantibodies or maternal warm autoimmune haemolytic anaemia* must be considered.
(3) During the investigation of HDNB, cord cells should be typed for the appropriate antigen system. When ABO grouping is performed only the baby's cells are used. Reverse grouping using cord serum is unnecessary since any antibodies present must be of maternal origin. If the direct antiglobulin test is positive, extra care is necessary during Rh genotyping (see chapter 25, section 2.2).

Table 3 Haemolytic disease of the newborn: haematological studies at delivery (Rh D-negative mothers)

Determine ABO and Rh D type of cord cells
Perform direct antiglobulin test on cord cells
Cord blood haemoglobin

For babies that are Rh D positive:
Measure serum bilirubin (if direct AGT positive)
Examine maternal blood for fetomaternal leakage (this determines the dose of prophylactic anti-D required)
Examine maternal serum for antibodies (in case RhD sensitization has already occurred)

---

4 QUANTITATION OF THE ANTIBODIES FOUND IN ANTENATAL SERA

Quantitation is performed in order to make a better assessment of the likely effects of the antibody on the outcome of pregnancy. Unfortunately, although the prognostic value of *antibody titres* or titre scores is not very good, antibody titres and in particular *rising titres* are still the best available initial guide as to the need for further investigation or alteration in the management of the pregnancy. This is particularly true with regard to anti-D. Intervention before natural delivery in pregnancies in which other antibodies are concerned is rarely necessary but regrettably antibody titrations are often of limited help in making this decision. There are several theoretical and practical factors to account for the poor correlation between antibody titres and their clinical effect. These include:

(1) The immunoglobulin class of the antibody (see section 2.2).
(2) The avidity of the antibody.
(3) The sensitivity of the technique used for its measurement. Because of their greater sensitivity, low ionic strength saline (LISS) antiglobulin anti-D titres will clearly be higher than those obtained by normal saline antiglobulin or albumin agglutination techniques. The results are therefore not comparable. Even when laboratories use similar techniques, minor variations including differences in the composition of the cell pool and in the titre endpoint recorded by operators prevent valid comparisons.
(4) The haemolytic effect will depend on the efficiency of transplacental antibody passage, the efficiency of the fetal reticuloendothelial phagocytic system for red cell removal and the regenerative capacity of the erythroid tissue for replacing red cell losses.
(5) The antigenicity of fetal red cells will affect their susceptibility to destruction. R_2 (cDE) cells carry more D antigen sites than R_1 (CDe) cells and it appears that any given anti-D concentration has nearly twice the haemolytic potential when an R_2 rather than an R_1 fetal genotype is involved.[9]

Group A and B antigen expression on fetal cells also shows a considerable degree of individual variation and this probably affects the haemolytic consequences of the corresponding immune alloantibodies.

4.1 Quantitation of Anti-D

Manual titration

Despite the limitations discussed above, titration of maternal anti-D levels has played an important part in the assessment of risks to the fetus. Antiglobulin titres (performed in normal saline) of the order of 8–32 have been generally used as threshold levels above which further investigation is necessary. Individual laboratories working with local obstetricians generally establish the clinical significance of their own titration results. Meticulous training of staff is necessary to achieve standardization of procedures and reporting of results. Where significant changes in titre seem to be taking place serial samples can be retested together to avoid between-batch variation. Because a two-fold alteration in antibody concentration must occur before the titre result is affected, titres are relatively insensitive indicators of changing serum antibody levels. This limitation was particularly noticeable when mothers with Rh immunization were treated by plasmapheresis; the antibody titres often remained unchanged despite removal of large amounts of antibody.

Automated antibody quantitation

Generally continuous flow analytical principles have been used to overcome these limitations. Antibody reactivity of test serum dilutions against reagent cells is measured as optical density peaks which can then be compared with those obtained in the same assay by anti-D standard solutions. Serum sample results are then expressed either in terms of micrograms per millilitre or more recently as international units (IU) per millilitre. These methods undoubtedly improve the clinical value of anti-D measurement but unfortunately the expression of results in these quantitative terms suggests a greater degree of analytical precision than may be justified. Inter-laboratory assay comparisons on the same samples have revealed major discrepancies in the results and it has only been as a result of extensive effort in terms of standardization of technical procedures and use of national and international standards that the position has improved.

Clinical significance of anti-D quantitation results

High-risk pregnancies in which severe HDNB is possible before term usually have maternal anti-D levels of over 4–5 IU/ml. At this level around 20% of infants in one study had cord haemoglobins below 10 g/dl and over 75% required exchange transfusion.[10] In contrast, when anti-D levels were 4 IU or less:

- The cord haemoglobin was always above 10.0 g/dl.
- The cord bilirubin was below 80 μmol/l (5.0 mg/dl).
- Only 4% of babies required exchange transfusion.

With anti-D levels >30 IU, 60% of infants will develop severe anaemia, but even at this level 40% will not[8]—a reflection of the frustratingly limited value of prediction from anti-D estimates.

On the basis of these findings amniocentesis is certainly not indicated while anti-D titres remain below 4 IU/ml, irrespective of the previous obstetric history. Any given anti-D level carries a worse prognosis in the presence of an R_2 fetus than it does for an R_1 fetus.[9]

5 MANAGEMENT OF PREGNANCIES AT HIGH RISK FROM HAEMOLYTIC DISEASE[11,12]

The declining incidence of HDNB has in most hospitals led to a loss of expertise in the care of severely affected pregnancies. It is therefore essential that mothers are referred to centres where sufficient numbers are seen to maintain the highest possible standards of management. The intention of further management is to identify pregnancies in which treatment must be given before the natural end of pregnancy to avoid progression to *hydrops fetalis* or death.[13]

Candidates for further investigation comprise those mothers with anti-D levels exceeding 4–5 IU/ml or antibody titres of the order of 1/8 to 1/32. Titration figures for prognosis are most reliable in the first pregnancy. The history of a *previously affected infant* impairs the prognosis as HDNB tends to worsen in severity through succeeding pregnancies. The previous history therefore dictates the choice and timing of invasive procedures for further investigation. Various procedures are available to help in assessment or treatment of high-risk pregnancies.

Traditionally amniocentesis has been used to detect and determine the severity of the fetal haemolytic process. Severely affected infants were, where possible, delivered early, this approach being encouraged by improvements in the management of very pre-term infants. Delivery was followed by exchange transfusion to correct anaemia and control the haemolytic process. Very severely affected infants, i.e. those at imminent risk from hydrops, were given intraperitoneal transfusion to sustain them until delivery was possible.

The very recently developed expertise in gaining direct access to the fetal circulation has profoundly altered the management of haemolytic disease. Amniocentesis is still used to gain the first indication of the presence and degree of fetal haemolysis. Where this seems significant confirmation is sought by direct sampling of fetal blood, followed if necessary by intravascular transfusion, to prevent hydrops development. Programmes of fetal transfusion have become sufficiently successful to reduce the necessity for early delivery and the attendant need for 'rescue' exchange transfusions. *Ultrasonic* examination (see section 5.2) can also provide warning of the appearance of hydrops, particularly in cases where invasive investigations have not yet been undertaken. Plasmapheresis of the mother to remove anti-D has been used as a means of treating high-risk pregnancies but this approach, never universally agreed to be effective, has been superseded now that reliable means of replacing fetal blood with immunologically compatible red cells are available. A number of mothers have apparently been successfully treated with intravenous immunoglobulin (IVIg) and this approach may deserve further investigation.[14,15]

5.1   Amniocentesis

The procedure

Amniocentesis is indicated whenever there is a risk of severe haemolytic disease requiring some form of intervention before delivery at term. To perform amniocentesis the infant and placenta must be localized, usually by ultrasonic examination. A needle is passed through the anterior abdominal wall of the mother and then through the uterine wall to enter and sample amniotic fluid from the amniotic sac. The sample of amniotic fluid should be free from haemolysed cells; it must also be kept dark since bilirubin is light sensitive, and the supernatant should be analysed as soon as possible. After centrifugation to remove debris and red cells, the supernatant is examined in a spectrophotometer scanning over a wavelength range of 350 to 700 nm.

The results of amniotic fluid spectroscopy

A normal trace shows a linear increase in optical density (OD) as the wavelength increases. The presence of bilirubin causes a deflection from this line with a peak at 450 nm (Figure 1). The difference in OD between the peak height at 450 nm and the rising background line is proportional to the bilirubin concentration. This optical density difference (ΔOD) is therefore used as the index of severity of the haemolytic state. The figure cannot be used directly for this purpose, however, because the normal increase in amniotic fluid volume that occurs throughout pregnancy progressively dilutes the bilirubin and lowers the optical density. A stable state of bilirubin production is therefore associated with a linear decline in ΔOD$_{450}$ as gestational age increases. This difficulty in interpretation is most easily overcome by plotting the spectroscopic results graphically. Various charts have been devised for this purpose; a common feature is the use of a semi-logarithmic

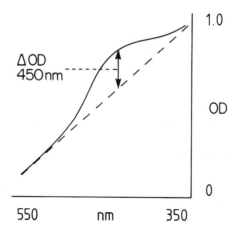

Figure 1   Spectroscopic tracing of amniotic fluid. The trace, typical of a severely affected pregnancy, shows a large optical density deviation (ΔOD) from the normal trend indicated by the inclined dotted line

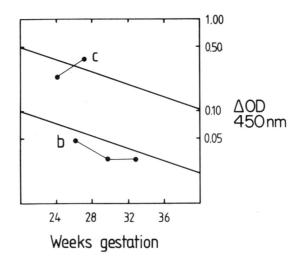

Weeks gestation

Figure 2 Modified Liley chart for prediction of severity of HDNB from amniotic spectro-scopy. ΔOD_{450} readings are plotted according to gestational age. The chart shows upper (severely affected), middle (moderately affected) and lower (mild or unaffected) zones. patient b shows three consecutive readings giving no cause for concern. Patient c shows deterioration between the first and second determinations

vertical axis calibrated according to the scale of optical density values and a hor-izontal axis marked according to gestational age.[16]

One example is shown in Figure 2. Examining Figure 3 it can be seen that diagonal lines falling from left to right (early to late pregnancy) divide the chart into three principal zones:

- Zone 1—the lowest zone. ΔOD_{450} values in this zone indicate unaffected or mildly affected infants which can safely progress to delivery at term.
- Zone 2—sometimes further subdivided into upper and lower portions—reflects intermediate levels of severity. The risks of unaffected, moderate or more severe disease can be expressed in terms of the probability of each event.
- Zone 3—high ΔOD values in this zone denote the presence of very severe fetal disease and a need for immediate treatment or delivery.

It is usual to perform repeated amniocentesis investigations because a better indi-cation of risk is given by the *trend of change*. Action can then be initiated if future results seem likely to approach or enter zone 3. In practice ΔOD_{450} values exceed-ing 0.25 before 30 weeks' gestation and exceeding 0.15 after 30 weeks are usually taken to be indicative of a severely affected fetus.

Timing of amniocentesis

Initial amniocephteses are usually performed after 26 weeks' gestation. When antibody levels are high and particularly when the *previous history* is also bad, amniocentesis has been performed as early as 20 weeks. Unfortunately, interpretive charts cannot be extrapolated to cover the period before 26 weeks and amniocentesis is accordingly less reliable as a prognosticator of haemolysis. Under these circumstances fetal blood sampling is preferred[11]

How the amniocentesis results affect management of the pregnancy

The action to be taken following amniocentesis depends on the gestational age, the fetal maturity, and the ΔOD_{450}. Amniotic fluid can also be used for measurement of the surfactant lipids lecithin and sphingomyelin, which provide an indication of fetal lung maturity. Provided that the fetus is sufficiently mature, OD_{450} values associated with severe haemolysis are an indication for delivery to be followed by exchange transfusion. Immature fetuses in which the amniocentesis results are indicative of severe disease need prompt action. This usually entails cord sampling for confirmatory diagnosis and an opportunity for direct transfusion. Where amniocentesis results are less clear cut, the decision is usually taken to repeat measurements, for example, in 2 weeks time. Because of the imprecision of amniocentesis results the management of mid-trimester-affected fetuses presents particular difficulties. A cautious approach is to proceed to fetal blood sampling where significant haemolytic disease cannot be excluded.[17]

Once intrauterine transfusions have been given, there is usually no point in performing further amniocenteses as the results will be affected by leakage from lysis of the transfused cells.

Risks of amniocentesis

These depend on the skill of the operator and the accuracy of fetal and placental localization. (The improved quality of modern ultrasonic techniques has made determination of the fetal and placental position much easier.) A most important *serological risk* is that of causing a further fetomaternal leak and consequently *boosting anti-D levels*. The procedure has sometimes boosted modest titres to potentially lethal levels.[18] Precipitation of labour and *abruptio placentae* are also risks. For all these reasons the investigation should not be done unless other information (e.g. serology findings, previously affected infants) suggests that intervention may be necessary before full-term delivery.

5.2 Ultrasonic Assessment of the Severity of Haemolytic Disease of the Newborn

Ultrasound techniques, sometimes combined with Doppler waveform analysis, are proving to be helpful in the assessment of patients at risk from HDNB; ultrasound in particular can be helpful where ascites is developing but is less valuable in the absence of ascites as a monitor of severe HDNB.[19-21]

Comparison of the abdominal dimensions with the biparietal diameter can be used to provide warning of hydrops development. Radiologists also look for evidence of generalized fetal oedema, placental thickening, hepatic enlargement and an increase in the diameter of the umbilical vein as evidence of incipient hydrops. This method, particularly when combined with ultrasound waveform analysis of fetal haemodynamics as an indicator of anaemia, holds promise as a relatively safe non-invasive approach to identifying affected fetuses. However, its reliability and sensitivity need to be improved.

Causes of hydrops

From a blood group serologist's perspective, hydrops is usually of immune origin but it should be borne in mind that other causes (e.g. *cardiac malformations, α-thalassaemia and twin-to-twin bleeds, myotonic dystrophy, syphilis and parvovirus infection*) are also possible.[22]

5.3 Early Delivery in Rh Haemolytic Disease of the Newborn

For many years early delivery combined with exchange transfusion was the only approach to management of severe HDNB. Babies with incipient hydrops and at risk of death before 32 weeks could not be treated in any other way until the development of techniques for intrauterine transfusion. However, improvements in neonatal intensive care allowed deliveries to be planned as early as 28 weeks although at that age pulmonary immaturity was a problem.[23]

Policies involving conservative management and early delivery are still appropriate provided that a reasonably mature, non-hydropic fetus can be anticipated. Early delivery must be combined with *prompt exchange transfusion* and it is essential that compatible blood is prearranged for this purpose. Early delivery of a premature, potentially affected infant would not now be regarded as a suitable course of action unless interuterine transfusion was unavailable. Certainly, hydropic fetuses tolerate intravascular transfusion better than post-natal exchange transfusion.

5.4 Exchange Transfusion for Management of Rh Haemolytic Disease

Exchange transfusion for HDNB has the following aims:

(1) Treatment of anaemia and cardiac failure.
(2) Replacement of antibody-coated red cells with compatible red cells.
(3) Removal of plasma containing anti-D immunoglobulin.
(4) Removal of bilirubin.

The initial exchange procedures secure the first two objectives; subsequent transfusions are required to continue the clearance of antibodies and bilirubin. Hydropic infants will require diuretic therapy (e.g. frusemide 1–2 mg/kg) as well as drainage of ascites and of pleural effusions. Severe pulmonary oedema necessitates intubation and ventilation.

Indications for exchange transfusion in Rh HDNB

Policies in different neonatal units vary but the following are typical criteria.

(1) At delivery, cord haemoglobin below 11.0 g/dl and/or cord bilirubin above 80 μmol/l (5 mg/dl).
(2) After delivery, the potential *rise in serum bilirubin* provides the principal reason for performing exchange transfusion. The bilirubin should not be allowed to exceed 450 μmol/l and a lower target such as 250 μmol/l is considered more appropriate for *premature infants* or those with RDS, *sepsis or acidosis*.[24] To play safe, a rate of rise exceeding 10 μmol/l (0.6 mg/dl) per hour can be used to justify exchange transfusion. Four-hourly monitoring may be needed.

Other clinical considerations that reinforce decisions to perform exchange transfusion include the presence of RDS and *prematurity* or a *history of exchanges required for previous children*. The now routine use of phototherapy for these infants can sometimes reduce the frequency at which exchange transfusions are necessary.

Selection of blood

Blood for exchange transfusion should be of the same ABO group as the baby if this is compatible with the mother, otherwise group O Rh D-negative blood (for HDNB due to anti-D) can be used. Compatibility testing should be performed against the maternal serum (see chapter 20, section 2.1).

Blood less than 6 days old anticoagulated with CPD or CPD-A is generally satisfactory (for other aspects of exchange transfusion see chapter 20, section 2.6). The less acid pH of CPD as compared to ACD has rendered unnecessary the former practice of using heparinized blood for exchange as a means of reducing the acid load.

Partial plasma reduction to achieve a haematocrit of 0.50–0.60 is generally preferred. If the haematocrit of conventional red cell concentrates is unacceptably high, 4–5% albumin solution can be used as a resuspension agent. Plasma albumin binds unconjugated bilirubin, making it less available to diffuse into and damage nervous tissue, thereby causing kernicterus. The complications of hypocalcaemia and alkalosis are also less likely when the citrated plasma has been removed.

If there is exceptional difficulty in providing serologically compatible blood (e.g. for antibodies against high-frequency antigens) then washed maternal red cells can be used resuspended in albumin.

Volume of blood to be exchanged

Two units of partially packed red cells (haematocrit ∼0.55) will usually be required for the initial exchange transfusions. In practice an exchange equal to one blood volume ensures that around 75% of an infant's red cells are replaced; this rises to 90% after two blood volumes have been exchanged. Bilirubin levels fall to only 50–60% of pre-exchange values because of the large amount distributed throughout the extravascular fluid which diffuse back into the plasma to replace that removed. Blood is usually exchanged via a catheter inserted into the umbilical vein, then through the ductus venosus as far as the inferior vena cava. Using a syringe and three-way tap, or specially prepared exchange transfusion devices, volumes of 10–15 ml are withdrawn and exchanged for donor blood in repeated cycles. A two-unit exchange requires about two hours for completion. Alternatively blood can be withdrawn from the umbilical artery and transfused blood returned via a peripheral vein. Blood should be warmed before infusion.

Laboratory investigations

Pre- and post-exchange blood samples are collected for:

- Bilirubin estimation.
- Haemoglobin determination and platelet count.
- Urea and electrolytes, calcium and glucose.

The pH and blood gases are usually determined during the procedure. Samples for coagulation screening tests may be required (for babies in whom DIC is suspected).

Complications of exchange transfusion

These are discussed in chapter 20, section 2.6.

5.5   Direct Fetal Blood Sampling

The development of the percutaneous umbilical fetal blood sampling (PUBS) technique and with it the capability of administering red cells directly into the fetal circulation has transformed the management of severe haemolytic disease. Although amniocentesis is usually performed first to give an indication of the severity of an affected fetus, fetal blood sampling for haemoglobin measurement provides a more direct and precise measurement of morbidity and whether corrective action is required. In centres where expertise is available fetal blood sampling is likely to replace amniocentesis for the continued surveillance of severely affected pregnancies.

In addition to haemoglobin measurement, Rh grouping and a direct antiglobulin test can be done. The mean corpuscular volume (MCV) and Kleihauer–Betke blood film examination confirms the sample to be of fetal origin. If the fetus appears to be severely affected a platelet count is also advisable.

Fetal blood-sampling results may indicate the need for immediate treatment (e.g. anaemia where Hb values are >2 SD below mean for gestational age).[11] or a prognosis of poor risk, for example, but with mild anaemia (haematocrit $\geqslant 0.30$) but with strongly positive DCT (3+) and reticulocyte count >97.5 percentile.[25]

Table 4 Analysis of PUBS samples

Haemoglobin concentration
Rh D group
Direct antiglobulin test
MCV and/or Kleihauer–Betke to confirm fetal origin
Reticulocyte count
Platelet count

The sampling needle is introduced using ultrasound guidance to puncture (if possible) the umbilical vein close to its placental origin (see Figure 3). Anterior implantation of the placenta may necessitate access to cord vessels via the placenta rather than the amniotic cavity, and the risk of fetal maternal haemorrhage is greater. If feasible, amniocentesis might be preferred where anterior placentation is present.[26]

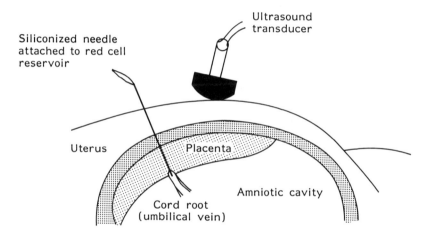

Figure 3 Percutaneous approach to fetal transfusion via maternal abdomen under real-time ultrasound guidance

Selection of cases for PUBS fetal blood sampling will be indicated:

(1) Where a previous fetus has been severely affected. PUBS is considered about 10 weeks prior to the age that the previous pregnancy showed severe HDNB (but not before 18 weeks of fetal age).
(2) On the basis of significantly elevated antibody titres (e.g. > 15 IU/ml).[27]
(3) If amniotic fluid spectroscopy or ultrasonic evidence of haemolytic disease is seen.

The technique is possible from about 18 weeks' gestation onwards. The exact timing will depend upon the presumed severity of the HDNB. The presence of anaemia as judged against available reference values[28,29] dictates the need to proceed to intravascular transfusion.

There is some debate regarding the relative merits of amniocentesis and PUBS for the early assessment of potentially severe haemolytic disease. Points of concern include:

(1) Threshold for investigation. Since both procedures carry risks there should be convincing evidence that the clinical and serological circumstances warrant invasive study.
(2) PUBS can be performed technically, rather earlier (e.g. from 18 weeks' gestation, compared to the 26th week, in which it is conventionally agreed amniocentesis is most reliable.
(3) Amniocentesis is generally safer, requires less expertise and is less liable to provoke fetomaternal haemorrhage and subsequent antibody boosting.
(4) PUBS provides direct assessment of the state of fetal haemolysis and can confirm blood group compatibility as well as providing an opportunity for immediate transfusion.

5.6 Intravascular Transfusion

Intravascular transfusion is now the preferred approach for the treatment of potentially severely affected fetuses, and it is essential that mothers be referred to centres where expertise exists. Transfusions are usually given in conjunction with fetal blood sampling (see section 5.5). Packed red cells are given—the amount can be calculated by use of normograms.[30,31]

Red cells are usually irradiated, CMV antibody negative and infused through a microaggregate filter because no pulmonary filtration is available to shield the cerebral circulation. The preferred haematocrit is usually of the order of 0.70–0.85.

A typical schedule involves repeating the transfusion after 1 week and every 2 weeks thereafter. The falling fetal haematocrit provides a guide—a decline of around 1% per day is to be expected; transfusion policy is generally to maintain the haemoglobin/haematocrit above 10.0 g/dl/0.30. Hydrops becomes increasingly likely if the haemoglobin falls towards 4.0 g/dl.

The intravascular transfusion route has advantages.

(1) Direct transfusion into the fetal circulation.
(2) Measurement of pre- and post-transfusion haemoglobin values.
(3) It can be performed earlier during pregnancy.
(4) The complete replacement of fetal red cell mass enables the infant to be delivered in a relatively mature state (e.g. approx. 37 weeks).
(5) Post-natal exchange transfusions are not usually necessary. Mortality rates for this procedure have now fallen to the order of 1–2% while survival rates, even for fetuses with hydrops, exceed 80%. The fetus, with its large placental circulatory volume, seems surprisingly tolerant of the extra transfused volume. Accordingly, intrauterine exchange transfusion has not been found to be necessary. There is some evidence that too energetic an elevation of the haematocrit (e.g. >4 ×)[32] or volume load (>20% combined fetoplacental blood volume)[33] is associated with higher mortality, possibly because cardiac function is incapable of tolerating the increment of viscosity as the red cell mass is increased. The main complications of intravascular transfusion include

premature labour, infection, chorioamnionitis, bradycardia, feto-maternal hemorrhage and most frequently blood leakage from the cord puncture site. Transfusion may temporarily aggravate pre-existing fetal acidosis, and in such cases blood gas measurements are necessary. Following successful intra-vascular transfusions, post-natal exchange transfusions are rarely necessary, although erythroid suppression persists for some 3–4 months, during which top-up transfusions may be required.[34]

Apart from its recognized value in severe HDNB, intravascular transfusion has been used to correct anaemia due to massive fetomaternal haemorrhage and for hydrops due to anaemia from other causes (e.g. parvoviral infection).

5.7 Intraperitoneal Transfusion

Before the techniques for intravascular transfusion were developed, transfusion was given via the intraperitoneal route. The procedure is still used for less severely affected fetuses, particularly later in pregnancy. The presence of ascites, however, makes the intravenous route essential. Ultrasonic imaging techniques are used to assist placement of a needle into the fetal peritoneal cavity. Contrast medium is usually injected into the peritoneal cavity to confirm that the needle is in the right place. A red cell suspension of high haematocrit (~ 0.90) is then infused into the peritoneal cavity. The infusion pressure must be monitored carefully: too high a pressure causes obstruction of the portal and umbilical veins and reduces the venous return. The fetal heart rate is monitored throughout the procedure to give warning of circulatory embarrassment. Donor blood injected into the peritoneal cavity is largely absorbed into the fetal circulation during the week following transfusion. This takes place via uptake of red cells into the lymphatic system.

Selection of blood and the volume to be given

Group O Rh D-negative blood tested for compatibility against maternal serum is used. This should be cytomegalovirus antibody negative unless the mother has been shown to be seropositive. It should also be irradiated to prevent the risk of graft-versus-host disease. The volume to be infused depends on the capacity of the combined fetal and placental circulation. This can be estimated from the following formula:

$$\text{Volume to be administered (ml)} = (\text{Age in weeks} - 20) \times 10$$

6 FETOMATERNAL LEAKS AND MATERNAL ALLOIMMUNIZATION

6.1 Incidence of the Problem

Maternal sensitization to the Rh D antigen occurs as a result of fetomaternal leaks across the placental barrier which normally separates the two circulatory systems.

There appears to be a slight natural risk of the occurrence throughout pregnancy but they occur with greatest frequency at delivery. The size of the leakage should be measured at each delivery (see section 6.2).

Frequency of fetomaternal leakage

Fetomaternal haemorrhages of some degree probably occur in most pregnancies. Of transplacental leaks 96–98% involve transfer of 1 ml or less of fetal blood, but it has been estimated that 0.3% of pregnancies result in fetomaternal leakage of over 30 ml. Fetomaternal leaks are also liable during *abortions*; the risk is greater for terminations of pregnancy than for spontaneous abortions. Before 12 weeks the risk of sensitization, as a result of spontaneous miscarriage, is probably negligible.[42] Fetomaternal leaks occur with increased frequency later in pregnancy and are particularly associated with procedures such as *amniocentesis* (amniocenteses early in pregnancy, e.g. for chromosome examination, are also risky), *version* or when *premature placental separation* and *accidental haemorrhages* occur.

Frequency of anti-D immunization

The natural incidence of Rh immunization appears to be about 5–15% of all Rh-negative pregnancies. Fetal and neonatal deaths due to Rh HDNB were formerly (1950–1960) of the order of 1.5 per 1000 births in Britain, accounting for over 1000 deaths each year, thus making a considerable contribution to overall perinatal mortality. Early delivery combined with exchange transfusion successfully cut the perinatal loss rate until by the late 1960s it had fallen to around 0.3 per 1000 births. This figure is now acknowledged to underestimate the true significance of Rh immunization as a continuing problem as it does not include fetal deaths through pregnancy termination or spontaneous losses before 28 weeks.[35]

Introduction of the anti-D prophylactic programme has reduced the incidence of maternal sensitization by over 90% and of peri-natal deaths due to HDNB to about 0.08 per 1000 births.

6.2 Anti-D Immunoglobulin Prophylactic Programme

Antibody-mediated clearance of immunogenic cells

The reduced frequency of Rh alloimmunization that was observed in ABO-incompatible pregnancies prompted investigation of the possibility that accelerated antibody-mediated cell clearance (due to naturally occurring anti-A or anti-B iso-antibodies) was the basis for the effect and if so whether this result could be obtained by other means. In the late 1960s it was shown that immunization of male volunteers to the Rh D antigen could be prevented by administration of Rh D antibody prior to injection of Rh-positive cells. Passively transfused antibody was, in these instances, responsible for removal of incompatible cells. These successes led to trials in pregnant women and by 1968–1970 sufficient confidence had been gained to advise the universal use of the anti-Rh D immunoglobulin in a prophylactic programme. This was initially applied to first pregnancies; later, when immunoglobulin became more freely available, it was used for all pregnancies occurring in women who had not already been sensitized.

Despite this successful achievement it is by no means clear exactly how the protective effect of Rh immunoglobulin is achieved.[36] The simple explanation that immunogenic cells are rapidly removed from the circulation seems unlikely to be the sole explanation. Antibody-coated cells may be cleared rapidly but their ultimate fate is to the spleen, an organ rich in antigen recognition sites. The dose of immunoglobulin is also insufficient to cause complete coating of all the antigenic sites and thereby hide them from recognition.

Therapeutic recommendations

In the UK[37] 500 IU of anti-D immunoglobulin (formerly 100 μg) are given within 72 hours after delivery when:

- The mother is Rh D negative.
- No anti-D is detectable in her serum.
- The infant is group Rh D positive.

This dose was calculated to be sufficient to prevent sensitization provided no more than 4 ml of fetal red cell leak had occurred. Different amounts of immunoglobulin were selected as the routine dose in other countries. In the USA, for example, 1500 IU (300 μg) are given which should allow protection against fetomaternal bleeds of the order of 12 ml (red cells). This higher dose level has now been endorsed in Europe by the Committee for Proprietary Medicinal Products and the requirement for a routine post-natal test for fetomaternal is no longer mandated.[75]

Within the UK, it is currently recommended that the size of any fetomaternal leak should be measured on each occasion (see section 6.2). Further doses of immunoglobulin (125 IU/ml of fetal red cells) are required for unusually large fetal cell counts.

Doses of immunoglobulin should also be administered for other potentially sensitizing episodes.[38–40] There is no good evidence to support the necessity of treatment for first-trimester domiciliary miscarriages,[41,42] although a study of women presenting with threatened abortions up to 20 weeks did demonstrate a significant incidence of transplacental haemorrhage.[43]

Rh D^u mothers (chapter 2, section 3.3) should be treated as Rh positive and anti-D should *not* be given.[44] Those rare mothers who are D variants are potentially capable of making anti-D against the portion of the D mosaic they lack. Rare instances of HDNB have been reported[45,46] but most infants have been only mildly affected. Anti-D is probably advisable although it has been claimed that it would be largely autoabsorbed and therefore ineffective at fetal cell clearance.

A suggested protocol is indicated in Table 5.

Table 5   Anti-D administration protocol (UK)

A. *At delivery* all previously unsensitized Rh D-negative women should be given 500 IU of anti-D:
   Re-examine maternal serum for irregular antibodies
   Perform group and antiglobulin test on cord cells
   Assess size of any fetomaternal leak

B. *Amniocentesis, version, APH*: give 500 IU of anti-D, perform Kleihauer and give further anti-D if necessary

C. *Before 20 weeks* (amniocentesis, spontaneous and therapeutic abortions): Rh D-negative women with no detectable antibodies should be given 250 IU of anti-D immunoglobulin

---

Rh D sensitization: a continuing problem

The anti-D prophylactic programme has reduced the incidence of Rh D-sensitized mothers to around 10% of the natural occurrence rate. Recent years have, however, shown a slowing of the rate of this decline and complete abolition of the problem now seems unlikely, judged by present trends.[47]

Mothers currently found to have anti-D fall into the following categories:

(1) Mothers who were sensitized before the prophylactic programme began.
(2) Failure to give anti-D immunoglobulin: this may be due to errors in testing the blood group of either mother or baby,[48,49] early discharge of the mother before anti-D could be given, or simple organizational errors.
(3) Sensitization despite administration of immunoglobulin: this occurs when the fetomaternal leak exceeds the capacity of the standard dose of immunoglobulin. This *should* be recognized if a properly performed test for fetal cells is carried out and a larger dose of immunoglobulin can then be given.
(4) Unrecognized fetomaternal leaks also take place early in pregnancy and sensitize the mother before the standard post-natal dose of immunoglobulin is given. This group comprises most of the remaining immunized women.[50]
(5) Small numbers of women may be sensitized by unrecognized or untreated abortions and, regrettably, a few become sensitized as a result of inadvertent transfusion with Rh-positive blood.

The case for antenatal prophylaxis[51–54]

Administration of anti-D immunoglobulin to Rh-negative primipara *during the antenatal period* has been shown to further reduce the incidence of maternal sensitization by a factor of eight without risk to the fetus.[55]

Successful schedules have involved dosages of 500 IU (100 µg) at 28 and 34 weeks' gestation, followed by further treatment at delivery if the infant is Rh positive. Maternal blood should still be examined for fetomaternal leaks after delivery or any other sensitizing episodes and extra doses given as described above. Antenatal prophylaxis would be expected to reduce sensitization due to accidental failure to give immunoglobulin at delivery and should also protect against that arising from fetomaternal leaks occurring late in pregnancy. The success of the early trials confirmed observations that such leaks are most frequent during the last trimester. It has been estimated that around one-third of the British deaths from Rh haemolytic disease in 1982 and 1983 (7.0 and 5.4 respectively per 100 000 births) could have been prevented by a programme of antenatal therapy.[56]

Antenatal therapy is not without drawbacks. A considerable increase in the supply of anti-D immunoglobulin is required to allow full implementation of such a programme. This is partly because around 40% of all pregnancies in Caucasians will be carrying Rh-negative infants. There is also a risk arising from immunization of increased numbers of male volunteers who, if they require emergency transfusion, must then receive only Rh-negative blood or, worse still, blood that must also be compatible with any other antibodies they may have formed. It is now expected that therapeutic preparations of monoclonal anti-D will eventually become available for the Rh prophylactic programme and this would remove the need for immunization and boosting of volunteer donors.[57] Ante-natally administered anti-D will persist for some weeks in the maternal plasma and may cause confusion during routine serological studies unless the laboratory is notified. A biological half-life of around 3 weeks has been reported;[58] following injections of 125 μg (625 IU) maximum plasma levels were 2.9–11.6 ng/ml falling to 1 ng/ml by around 70 days. It can therefore be reasonably assumed that levels clearly in excess of 0.5 IU/ml represent active immunization rather than residual therapeutic anti-D.

Quantitation of fetomaternal leakage

Sensitization will not be prevented if the transplacental passage of fetal blood exceeds that covered by the dose of immunoglobulin given. For this reason estimation of the proportion of fetal cells present in the maternal circulation must be carried out on each occasion treatment is necessary. Several methods for this have been devised and technical details are readily available in practical manuals. Popular methods include:

(1) *Kleihauer–Betke acid elution method:*[59] a routinely prepared film of maternal blood is dried, incubated in acid buffer and then stained with eosin. The stained film is examined microscopically. Fetal cells stain pink because fetal haemoglobin resists elution in the acid buffer, while adult cells show only as pale red cell outlines leached of haemoglobin. The size of the fetal bleed can be estimated from the proportion of fetal to adult red cells on the film. The Kleihauer–Betke test is sensitive, being capable of detecting of the order of 4 ml (0.1%) fetal cells but it is difficult to standardize and to ensure reproducible and accurate results. This test detects *fetal* haemoglobin-containing cells; the serological tests described below detect *Rh-positive* cells in the maternal blood.

(2) *Enzyme-linked antiglobulin tests*[60] have been claimed to offer equal sensitivity to the Kleihauer–Betke test and be easier to perform and more reproducible. The maternal red cell suspension is incubated with anti-D. The red cell-bound anti-D is then estimated by means of the addition of the enzyme-linked antiglobulin followed finally by enzyme substrate. The absorbance of the coloured product is proportional to the amount of anti-D bound and therefore to the number of Rh-positive red cells in the maternal blood.

(3) Rh-positive fetal cells in maternal blood can also be detected by means of the *antiglobulin anti-D grouping test* if the results are examined microscopically. Although in widespread use, the test is relatively insensitive and a 12% risk of failure to identify bleeds exceeding 30 ml has been reported. The procedure can be a useful means of verifying the accuracy of very high estimates of fetomaternal bleeds obtained using the Kleihauer–Betke method.

(4) A *rosetting technique* which has been reported to be convenient, reproducible and sensitive can be used for visual identification of Rh-positive fetal cells.[61] Enzyme-treated Rh-positive reagent cells are added to a washed suspension of anti-D-treated maternal blood (as in (2) above). The enzyme-treated cells, their D antigen sites exposed by enzyme action, attach to free binding sites of the anti-D antibodies coating Rh-positive fetal cells. The ring of attached cells forms rosettes which can be easily counted.

(5) Where facilities are available flow cytometry is accurate, precise and sensitive.

Anti-D administration for the treatment of large fetomaternal leaks or inadvertent transfusion of Rh-positive blood

Anti-D immunoglobulin is administered on the basis of 125 IU (25 μg) of anti-D for each 1.0 ml of fetal Rh-positive red cells. Large fetomaternal bleeds and Rh-positive transfusions therefore need correspondingly larger doses of immunoglobulin. Large fetomaternal bleeds detected by the Kleihauer–Betke method should be confirmed by serological means such as the microscopic D^u grouping procedure ((3) above). The distribution of HbF-containing cells should also be critically re-examined for the appearance of the heterogeneous F distribution within red cells typical of β-thalassaemia trait.

The infant's Rh group must be determined for the records so that the success of therapy can be assessed at a future date. Clearly, if the baby is Rh negative Rh immunoglobulin is not required. The mother's serum must also be examined to confirm the absence of pre-existing sensitization. After delivery, the infant's haemoglobin result should be obtained: the presence of anaemia will support the diagnosis of a large fetomaternal leak and this may need urgent treatment in its own right.

After immunoglobulin treatment of the mother, daily blood samples will be required until fetal cells have been shown to be cleared. Around 90% of the fetal cells should, if they are Rh positive, be lost within 48 hours. The maternal serum should be examined for the presence of residual passively acquired anti-D. If this is present and cell clearance has been efficient, further doses will be unnecessary. Otherwise give further doses of anti-D as determined by the fetal cell count.

Maternal serum samples should be examined around 3–6 months later to determine whether active anti-D immunization has occurred. It is also important to note the progress of any future pregnancies as a means of assessing the results of therapy. Recommendations for dosage of Rh immunoglobulin following transfusion mishaps have been published.[48,62]

7 ABO HAEMOLYTIC DISEASE OF THE NEWBORN

Fetomaternal ABO incompatibility occurs in around one in six of pregnancies in the UK but fortunately the observed incidence of some degree of HDNB is much lower, probably at the most around 3% of all births. ABO haemolytic disease, albeit mild, is still one of the commonest causes of this condition. In contrast to Rh D HDNB, ABO HDNB rarely needs treatment, although some form of action is most likely to be required when it occurs in *premature infants. Phototherapy or exchange transfusion* following natural delivery is usually sufficient; hydrops is virtually unknown;[63] premature induction or other antenatal intervention is never indicated. This state of affairs is fortunate because the available laboratory tests for diagnosis and prognosis of ABO haemolytic disease have not proved to be reliable.

The condition usually occurs in group A or B infants of group O mothers and is due to the transplacental passage of immune IgG anti-A or anti-B. These titres are typically higher in group O mothers and this phenomenon is particularly pronounced in many black communities, where it corresponds to a conspicuously higher incidence of clinically significant haemolytic disease.[64]

The elevated isoantibody levels have been ascribed to environmental factors; presumably microbial and parasitic infections are the most likely causes. The direct antiglobulin test on cord cells may be weakly positive but this finding may not persist in samples collected later. Anaemia is most unusual at delivery. Jaundice is more typical; this appears in the first 24 hours, to reach a peak during the next 2 weeks. Cord blood films may show spherocytosis, reflecting the presence of antibody-damaged red cells, a phenomenon which for some reason is not typically seen in Rh HDNB. The maternal serum should contain immune IgG antibody, haemolysing at 37 °C and sensitizing group A (or B) cells by the antiglobulin test. These serological changes are unfortunately not confined to clinically affected cases of HDNB and are therefore of little prognostic significance. Anti-A or anti-B can be eluted from cord cells to confirm the diagnosis of ABO HDNB: the potency of the eluate has been claimed to reflect the severity of the haemolytic process.

Treatment follows similar indications as for Rh HDNB. Phototherapy is usually sufficient to control hyperbilirubinaemia. If not, exchange transfusion with group O red cells resuspended in AB plasma will be required. Conclusive diagnosis of significant ABO haemolysis is not straightforward; it is important to recall that prematurity, sepsis and haemorrhage also contribute to the differential diagnosis of neonatal jaundice. Late-onset anaemia can be a problem and the haemoglobin should be monitored for 6–8 weeks.

ABO HDNB frequently affects first pregnancies but does not increase in severity with later pregnancies: in these respects it differs from Rh haemolytic disease.

Once it has occurred later children, if ABO incompatible, will be likely to be affected but only to the same extent as the first.[65]

8 HAEMOLYTIC DISEASE OF THE NEWBORN DUE TO OTHER ANTIBODIES

The anti-D prophylactic programme has been so successful in reducing the incidence of mothers with anti-D that they are now outnumbered by women with antibodies against the other Rh and non-Rh antigens.[66] Fortunately, clinically significant haemolytic disease is unusual and only on exceptional occasions do the serological findings necessitate consideration of early delivery or antenatal assessment or treatment.[67] The serological results do, however, provide warning of the need to search prospectively for compatible blood in case of need by the mother or her baby.

Serological testing of antenatal maternal samples, cord blood and paternal blood is discussed in section 2. A list of the more frequently occurring antibodies capable of causing HDNB is shown in Table 2. All are considerably less frequent as causes of HDNB than anti-D; mortality and serious morbidity from the commonly occurring antibodies are virtually confined to pregnancies affected by c, E and K antibodies. A British survey covering neonatal death due to haemolytic disease showed 5% to be due to anti-c and anti-E antibodies.[68]

Blood should be made available for exchange transfusion of the infant should the need arise, as well as for the mother in case of obstetric mishap requiring transfusion. Where antibodies to *high-frequency antigens* are present it may be necessary to obtain help from panels or banks of rare donor blood (see Appendix A). Maternal blood can also be used for neonatal transfusion; this may be:

(1) Collected well in advance and stored frozen.
(2) Collected in CPD-A1 and accumulated over a short period prior to delivery (see chapter 15, section 3.1). Before use for neonatal exchange transfusion, the cells can be packed and resuspended in 4.5% albumin.

It is obviously easiest to consider using the maternal red cells if they are ABO compatible with the infant. In fact, even ABO compatibility is not essential[69] because the infant will not have antibodies other than those of maternal origin.

It is only rarely necessary to employ invasive management measures for patients with antibodies other than anti-D. Nevertheless, severe erythroblastosis and hydrops, sometimes even requiring IUT, has been described with anti-c, -E and -K and exceptionally rarely with C, Jk^a and Fy^a.

These antibodies should be titrated and the results taken in conjunction with the previous history to decide the time and nature of further interventions. A variety of rare antibodies, some of which are reactive against low-frequency antigens, have been associated with severe HDNB.[67,70]

Anti-K is, after Rh antibodies, the most frequent cause of HDNB. An important but unresolved concern raised by several recently published large series of anti-K-affected pregnancies was whether amniocentesis results are unreliable indicators of the severity of haemolytic disease.[71-73]

Non-invasive techniques such as ultrasonic examination[19,74] (section 5.2) should be helpful in the monitoring of babies at risk. Serological criteria for such interventions are not well defined; for anti-K, titres for eight or greater are commonly taken as a threshold for clinical significance. For other antibodies it seems most reasonable to those titres locally accepted for anti-D HDNB (section 5). For potentially dangerous antibodies (e.g. those with a specificity and potency likely to cause severe HDNB during the pregnancy) it is important to establish whether the father possesses the offending antigen. If he does not then clearly HDNB is impossible. In such instances, the antibody must either be naturally occurring, have been stimulated by an earlier pregnancy with a different father, or may have formed as a result of blood transfusion.

REFERENCES

1 Schmidt, P.J., Pautler, K. and Samia, C.T. (1983) Prenatal Rh typing errors. *Am. J. Obstet. Gynecol.*, **145**: 884–885.
2 Kickler, T.S., Blackemore, K., Shirey, R.S. *et al.* (1992) Chorionic villus sampling for fetal Rh typing: clinical implications. *Am. J. Obstet. Gynecol.*, **166**: 1407–1411.
3 Bennett, P.R., Le Van Kim, C., Colin, Y. *et al.* (1993) Prenatal determination of fetal RhD type by DNA amplification. *N. Engl. J. Med.*, **329**: 607–610.
4 Lo, Y.M.D., Bowell, P.J., Selinger, M. *et al.* (1991) Prenatal determination of fetal Rh D status by analysis of peripheral blood of Rh negative mothers. *Lancet*, **341**: 1147–1148.
5 Powell, S.B., Howell, P. and Renton, P.H. (1981) Automated screening of antenatal samples using a low ionic strength polybrene system. *Clin. Haematol.*, **3**: 343–350.
6 Bowell, P.J., Allen, D.L. and Entwistle, C.C. (1986) Blood group antibody screening tests during pregnancy. *Br. J. Obstet. Gynaecol.*, **93**: 1038–1043.
7 Gottvall, T., Selbing, A. and Hilden, J.-O. (1993) Evaluation of a new Swedish protocol for alloimmunization screening during pregnancy. *Acta Obstet. Gynecol. Scand.*, **72**: 434–438.
8 Garner, S.F., Wiener, E., Contreras, M. *et al.* (1992) Mononuclear phagocyte assays, AutoAnalyzer quantitation and IgG subclasses of maternal anti-RhD in the prediction of the severity of haemolytic disease in the fetus before 32 weeks gestation. *Br. J. Haematol.*, **80**: 97–101.
9 Morley G. (1978) Relationship between maternal anti-D levels, fetal phenotype, and haemolytic disease of the newborn. *Vox Sang.*, **35**: 324–331.
10 Bowell, P., Wainscoat, J.S., Peto, T.E.A. and Gunson, H.H. (1982) Maternal anti-D concentrations and outcome in Rh haemolytic disease of the newborn. *Br. Med. J.*, **285**: 327–329.
11 Tannirandorn, Y. and Rodeck, C.H. (1991) Management of immune haemolytic disease in the fetus. *Blood Rev.*, **5**: 1–14.
12 Whittle, M.J. (1992) Rh haemolytic disease. *Arch. Dis. Child.*, **67**: 65–68.
13 Spinnato, J.A. (1992) Haemolytic disease of the fetus: a plea for restraint. *Obstet. Gynecol.*, **80**: 873–877.
14 Berlin, G., Selbing, A. and Gottvall, T. (1990) Plasma exchange and intravenous immunoglobulin treatment of the mother to diminish fetal Rh haemolytic disease. *Transfusion Sci.*, **11**: 85–90.
15 Berlin, G., Selbing, A. and Ryden, G. (1985) Rh haemolytic disease treated with high-dose intravenous immunoglobulin. *Lancet*, **i**: 1153.
16 Fairweather, D.V.I., Whyley, G.A. and Millar, M.D. (1976) Six years' experience of the prediction of severity in Rh haemolytic disease. *Br. J. Obstet. Gynaecol.*, **83**: 698–706.
17 Parer, J.T. (1988) Severe Rh isoimmunization: current methods of in utero diagnosis and treatment. *Am. J. Obstet. Gynecol.*, **158**: 1323–1329.

18 Dubin, C.F. and Staisch, K.J. (1982) Amniocentesis and fetal–maternal blood transfusion: a review of the literature. *Obstet. Gynecol. Surg.*, **37**: 272.

19 Benacerraf, B.R. and Frigoletto, F.D. (1985) Sonographic sign for the detection of early fetal ascites in the management of severe isoimmune disease without intrauterine transfusion. *Am. J. Obstet. Gynecol.*, **152**: 1039–1041.

20 Chitkara, U., Wilkins, I., Lynch, L., Mehalek, K. and Berkowitz, R.L. (1988) The role of sonography in assessing severity of fetal anemia in Rh- and Kell-isoimmunized pregnancies. *Obstet. Gynecol.*, **71**: 393–398.

21 Nicolaides, K.H., Fontanarosa, M., Gabbe, S.G. and Rodeck, C.H. (1988) Failure of ultrasonographic parameters to predict the severity of fetal anemia in Rh isoimmunization. *Am. J. Obstet. Gynecol.*, **158**: 920–926.

22 Santolaya, J., Alley, D., Jaffe, R. and Warsof, S.L. (1992) Antenatal classification of hydrops fetalis. *Obstet. Gynecol.*, **79**: 256–259.

23 Quinlan, R.W., Buhi, W.C. and Cruz, A.C. (1984) Fetal pulmonary maturity in isoimmunized pregnancies. *Am. J. Obstet. Gynecol. Surg.*, **148**: 787–789.

24 Dodd, K.L. (1993) Neonatal jaundice: a lighter touch. *Arch. Dis. Child.*, **68**: 529–532.

25 Weiner, C.P., Williamson, R.A., Wenstrom, K.D., Sipes, S.L., Grant, S.S. and Widness, J.A. (1991) Management of fetal hemolytic disease by cordocentesis. I Prediction of fetal anemia. *Am. J. Obstet. Gynecol.*, **165**: 546–553.

26 MacGregor, S.N., Silver, R.K. and Sholl, J.S. (1991) Enhanced sensitization after cordocentesis in a Rh-isoimmunized pregnancy. *Am. J. Obstet. Gynecol.*, **165**: 382–383.

27 Nicolaides, K.H. and Rodeck, C.H. (1992) Maternal serum anti-D antibody concentration and asessment of Rh isoimmunisation. *Br. Med. J.*, **304**: 1155–1156.

28 Nicolaides, K.H., Rodeck, C.H., Millar, D.S. and Mibasham, R.S. (1985) Fetal haematology in Rh isoimmunisation. *Br. Med. J.*, **290**: 661–663.

29 Ludomirski, A., Ashmead, G., Weiner, S. *et al.* (1988) Percutaneous umbilical fetal blood sampling procedure: safety and normal hematological indices. *Am. J. Perinatol.* **5**: 264–266.

30 Nicolaides, K.H., Soothill, P.W., Clewell, W.H., Rodeck, C.H., Mibashan, R.S. and Campbell, S. (1988) Fetal haemoglobin measurement in the assessment of red cell isoimmunisation. *Lancet*, **i**: 1073–1075.

31 Ludomirski, A. (1991) The anemic fetus: direct access to the fetal circulation for diagnosis and treatment. In: Kennedy, M.S. and Kelton, J.G. (eds), *Perinatal Transfusion Medicine*, pp. 89–101. Arlington, VA: AABB.

32 Radunovic, N., Lockwood, C.J., Alvarez, M., Plecas, D., Chitkara, U. and Berkowitz, R.L. (1992) The severely anemic and hydropic isoimmune fetus: changes in fetal hematocrit associated with intrauterine death. *Obstet. Gynecol.*, **79**: 390–393.

33 Selbing, A., Stangenberg, M., Westgren, M. and Rahman, F. (1993) Intrauterine intravascular transfusions in fetal erythroblastosis: the influence of net transfusion volume on fetal survival. *Acta Obstet. Gynecol. Scand.*, **72**: 20–23.

34 Thorp, J.A., O'Connor, T., Callenbach, J. *et al.* (1991) Hyporegenerative anemia associated with intrauterine transfusion in Rh hemolytic disease. *Am. J. Obstet. Gynecol.*, **165**: 79–81.

35 Bowell, P.J., Entwistle, C.C. and Mackenzie, I.Z. (1985) Deaths from Rh (D) haemolytic disease of the newborn in England and Wales. *Br. Med. J.*, **291**: 1351–1352.

36 Leading Article (1982) Low-dose Rh immunoprophylaxis. *Lancet*, **ii**: 1028.

37 Wagstaff, W. (1978) Practical aspects of anti-D prophylaxis of haemolytic disease of the newborn. *Association of Clinical Pathologists Broadsheet*, 90.

38 Tabsh, K.M.A., Lebherz, T.B. and Crandall, B.F. (1984) Risks of prophylactic anti-D immunoglobulin after second-trimester amniocentesis. *Am. J. Obstet. Gynecol.*, **149**: 225–226.

39 Brewer, C., Ball, E.W., Beard, R. and Gittins, P. (1981) Comparative risks of Rh autoimmunization in two different methods of mid-trimester abortion. *Br. Med. J.*, **282**: 1929–1930.

40 Hensleigh, P.A. (1983) Preventing Rh isoimmunisation. *Am. J. Obstet. Gynecol.*, **146**: 749–755.

41 Everett, C.B. (1988) Is anti-D immunoglobulin unnecessary in the domiciliary treatment of miscarriages? *Br. Med. J.*, **297**: 732.

42 Contreras, M. (1988) Is anti-D immunoglobulin unnecessary in the domiciliary treatment of miscarriages? *Br. Med. J.*, **297**: 733.

43 von Stein, G.A., Munsick, R.A., Stiver, K. and Ryder, K. (1992) Fetomaternal hemorrhage in threatened abortion. *Obstet. Gynecol.*, **79**: 383–386.

44 Konugres, A.A., Polesky, H.F. and Walker, R.H. (1982) Rh immune globulin and the Rh-positive, Du variant, mother. *Transfusion*, **22**: 76–77.

45 White, C.A., Stedman, C.M. and Frank, S. (1983) Anti-D antibodies in D- and Du positive women: a cause of haemolytic disease of the newborn. *Am. J. Obstet. Gynecol.*, **145**: 1069–1075.

46 Lacey, P.A., Caskey, C.R., Werner, D.J. and Moulds, J.J. (1983) Fatal haemolytic disease of a newborn due to anti-D in an Rh-positive Du variant mother. *Transfusion*, **23**: 91–94.

47 Chavez, G.F., Mulinare, J. and Edmonds, L.D. (1991) Epidemiology of Rh hemolytic disease of the newborn in the United States. *JAMA* **265**: 3270-3274.

48 Pinkerton, P.H., Wood, D.E., Bernie, K.L. *et al.* (1981) Proficiency testing immuno-haematology in Ontario, Canada, 1977–1979. *Clin. Lab. Haematol.*, **3**: 155–164.

49 Schmidt, P.J., Pautler, K. and Samia, C.T. (1983) Prenatal Rh typing errors. *Am. J. Obstet., Gynecol.*, **145**: 884–885.

50 Tovey, L.A.D. and Taverner, J.M. (1981) A case for the antenatal administration of anti-D immunoglobulin to primigravidae. *Lancet*, i: 878–881.

51 Tovey, G.H. (1980) Should anti-D immunoglobulin be given antenatally? *Lancet*, ii: 466–468.

52 Leading Article (1981) Prevention of haemolytic diseases of the newborn due to anti-D. *Br. Med. J.*, **282**: 676–677.

53 Lim, O.W., Fleisher, A.A. and Ziel, H.K. (1982) *Obstet. Gynecol.*, **59**: 477–480.

54 McMaster Conference of Prevention of Rh Isoimmunisation (1979) *Vox Sang.*, **36**: 50–64.

55 Tovey, L.A.D., Stevenson, B.J., Townley, A. and Taverner, J. (1983) The Yorkshire antenatal anti D immunoglobulin trial in primigravidae. *Lancet*, ii: 244–246.

56 Clarke, C.A., Mollison, P.L. and Whitfield, A.G. W. (1985) Deaths from rhesus haemolytic disease in England and Wales in 1982 and 1983. *Br. Med. J.*, **291**: 17–19.

57 Selinger, M. (1991) Immunoprophylaxis for Rh disease: expensive but worth it? *Br. J. Obstet. Gynaecol.*, **98**: 509–512.

58 Eklund, J., Hermann, M., Kjellman, H. and Pohja, P. (1982) Turnover rate of anti-D IgG injected during pregnancy. *Br. Med. J.*, **284**: 854–855.

59 Kleihauer, E., Braun, H. and Betke, K. (1957) Demonstration von fetalem Hamoglobin in den Erythocyten eines Blutausstrichs. *Klin. Wochenschr.*, **35**: 637–638.

60 Riley, J.Z., Ness, P.M., Taddie, S.J., Barrasso, C. and Baldwin, M.L. (1982) Detection and quantitation of fetal maternal hemorrhage utilizing an enzyme-linked antiglobulin test. *Transfusion*, **22**: 472–474.

61 Sebring, E.S. and Polesky, H.F. (1982) Detection of fetal maternal hemorrhage in Rh immune globulin candidates. *Transfusion*, **22**: 468–471.

62 Warebranch, D., Guymon, G. and Scott, J.R. (1985) Failure to prevent Rh immunization with Rh immune globulin after incompatible blood transfusion. *Lancet*, i: 393–394.

63 Sherer, D.M., Abramowicz, J.S., Ryan, R.M., Sheils, L.A., Blumberg, N. and Woods, J.R. (1991) Severe fetal hydrops resulting from ABO incompatibility. *Obstet. Gynecol.*, **78**: 897–899.

64 Vos, G.H. Adhikari, M. and Coovadia, H.M. (1981) A study of ABO incompatibility and neonatal jaundice in Black South African newborn infants. *Transfusion*, **21**: 744–749.

65 Katz, M.A., Kanto, W.P. and Korotkin, J.H. (1982) Recurrence rate of ABO haemolytic disease of the newborn. *Obstet. Gynecol.*, **59**: 611–614.

66 Hardy, J. and Napier, J.A.F. (1981) Red cell antibodies detected in antenatal tests on Rh positive women in South and West Mid Wales, 1948–1978. *Br. J. Obstet. Gynecol.*, **88**: 91–100.

67 Weinstein, L. (1976). Irregular antibodies causing haemolytic disease of the newborn. *Obstet. Gynaecol. Surv.*, **31**: 581–591.

68 Clarke, C. and Whitfield, A.G.W. (1984) Deaths from Rh haemolytic disease in England and Wales during 1980 and 1981 and a comparison with earlier years. *J. Obstet. Gynecol.*, 4: 218–222.
69 Gottschall, J.L. (1981) Letter to the editor: haemolytic disease of the newborn with anti U. *Transfusion*, 21: 230–231.
70 Giblet, E.R. (1964) Blood group antibodies causing haemolytic disease of the newborn. *Clin. Obstet. Gynecol.*, 7: 1044–1055.
71 Caine, M.E. and Mueller-Heubach, E. (1986) Kell sensitization in pregnancy. *Am. J. Obstet. Gynecol.*, 154: 85–90.
72 Leggat, H.M., Gibson, J.M., Barron, S.L. and Reid, M.M. (1991) Anti-Kell in pregnancy. *Br. J. Obstet. Gynecol.*, 98: 162–165.
73 Bowman, J.M., Pollock, J.M., Manning, F.A., Harman, C.R. and Savas Menticoglou (1992) Maternal Kell blood group alloimmunization. *Obstet. Gynecol.*, 79: 239–244.
74 Berkowitz, R.L., Beyth, Y. and Sadovsky, E. (1982) Death in utero due to Kell sensitization without excessive elevation on the delta OD450 value in amniotic fluid. *Obstet. Gynecol.*, 60: 746–749.
75 Committee for Proprietary Medicinal Products, Commission of the European Communities (1994) Note for guidance: core summary of product characteristics for human anti-D immunoglobulin im. Brussels: GEC (111/34463/92EN).
76 Buggins, A.G.S., Thilaganathan, B., Hambley, H. and Nicolaides, K.H. (1994) Predicting the severity of Rh alloimmunization: monocyte-mediated chemiluminescence versus maternal anti-D antibody estimation. *Br. J. Haematol.*, 88: 199–200.

Part F
TISSUE ANTIGENS: TRANSPLANTATION AND TRANSFUSION

22
Organ Transplantation and the Transfusion Laboratory

1 THE MAJOR HISTOCOMPATIBILITY ANTIGEN SYSTEM

The clinical need to replace, by transplantation, organs that are irreversibly diseased has, over the last two decades, led to an extraordinary growth in the knowledge of cellular antigens and the immunological conditions that must be met before foreign tissue can be grafted. The genetic loci coding for the most important tissue antigens (major histocompatibility complex, MHC) are concentrated in one small segment of the short arm of chromosome 6. The gene products of this localized region are expressed on the surfaces of cell membranes, where they play a crucial role in the ability of an individual to distinguish between self and non-self tissues, and also to mount effective immunological defence reactions. These surface structures are recognized during laboratory investigation as cellular antigens, and the study of these and the antibodies they provoke provides the basis of the tissue-typing studies necessary for organ transplantation and for provision of certain HLA-compatible blood components. Successful organ transplantation depends to a considerable extent on the selection of donors whose tissue antigens differ as little as possible from those of the recipient. Transfused platelets and granulocytes, although not retained as transplants, persist long enough to immunologically sensitize the recipient to novel donor tissue antigens. This complication eventually results in premature destruction of transfused platelets known as *refractoriness* and seriously hampers prolonged platelet therapy. Once it has arisen the problem can only be overcome by employing sensitive typing and compatibility testing procedures analogous to those used for red cell transfusions.

HLA (human leucocyte system A) *antigens* are the most important tissue antigens in the context of transfusion and transplantation. These antigens are common to many body tissues and also, fortunately for laboratory purposes, readily detectable on peripheral blood lymphocytes. Individual organ or tissue systems and blood cell lines have their own unique antigenic characteristics not shared uniformly throughout the body. This is certainly true for granulocytes and platelets as well as for various lymphocyte subsets and haemopoietic cells at different stages of maturation.

Poorly matched grafts are likely to be *rejected*, this process being mediated by a variety of immunological mechanisms involving, for example, *cytotoxic lymphocytes, complement-fixing cytotoxic antibodies* and *activated macrophages*. In order to arrest this process, relatively non-specific immunosuppressive drugs are used, and these have side-effects that can complicate recovery following transplantation. *Azothiaprine* and *corticosteroids* have been traditionally used for renal transplants; *antilymphocyte globulin (ALG)*, *monoclonal CD3 lymphocyte antibodies (OKT3)* and *cyclosporin A* are more recent additions to the therapeutic armamentarium; the latter in particular has substantially improved transplant graft survival.

Although transplantation between identical twins establishes the yardstick of success beside which genetically (and antigenically) dissimilar grafts must be judged, there are considerable uncertainties regarding the precise requirements for tissue matching to ensure successful grafting. Evidence is, however, at last emerging to clarify the picture particularly with regard to renal transplantation. Despite the excellent early results from good HLA matches the need for a high standard of HLA matching as a general policy for unrelated transplants was not universally accepted. Evidence from many quarters had been used to refute the claim that the benefits of good matching were worth the logistic difficulties of organ procurement. However, impressive support for the value of HLA matching has now emerged from large studies extending over several years and drawn from large numbers of transplant centres worldwide. These show that grafts that are well matched, particularly if judged in terms of the accuracy and precision attainable by modern typing techniques, can be shown to survive almost as well as phenotypically identical related donations.[1]

Analysis of the effect of HLA matching has been considerably complicated by the influences of other clinical factors, for example the pre-graft *transfusion history* and the nature of the *immunosuppressive regimens*, both of which affect the prognosis. Attention is now being paid to the development of agents capable of controlled attenuation of the rejection process. For many years it has been recognized that blood transfusions may, for ill-understood reasons, improve the survival of renal transplants. On a more refined level monoclonal antibodies suppressing specific T cell subpopulations (helper cells) or natural killer cells or having anti-idiotypic actions are a not too distant possibility. These approaches favour development of a state of tolerance towards the transplanted tissues.[2]

1.1 HLA Antigens

HLA tissue antigens are the products of at least six closely linked gene loci on chromosome 6. The principal loci are designated HLA-A, -B, -C and three D region loci (DR, DP, DQ) and at each locus there are many alternative alleles. Every individual has therefore a total of 12 loci—six of maternal and six of paternal origin—and at each of these numerous allelic alternatives are possible. It is not surprising therefore that the chances of phenotype identity between randomly selected (unrelated) individuals is extremely small.

In addition to the major histocompatibility complex (MHC) antigens, and the recognized tissue-specific antigen systems, there also appear to be various poorly characterized *minor histocompatibility antigens*. Antigenic disparities in these minor systems are postulated to explain the difference in graft survival between, for example, related as compared with unrelated grafts, when both are identically matched for major histocompatibility antigens.

Fortunately, acceptably successful transplantation does not depend on *absolute identity* between donor and recipient tissues. Some degree of mismatch is tolerable in certain situations (e.g. renal transplantation) though it may necessitate a corresponding increase in the amount of immunosuppressive drug therapy in order to reduce the immunological rejection process.

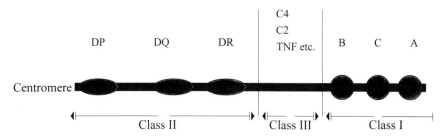

Figure 1 Organization of HLA gene complex on chromosome 6 (C4, B2, complement protein-coding loci, TNF, tumour necrosis factor locus)

1.2   The Development of HLA Matching

Class I (HLA-A, -B, -C) antigens

The first HLA gene products to be recognized were those of the A and B loci. HLA typing for organ transplantation therefore began with A and B locus matching alone. Four antigens are potentially detectable in an individual, unless there is homozygosity at one or two of the loci, in which case only three or two antigens respectively will be found. Antigenic products of an additional locus, the C locus, do not appear to be so important during transplantation, and C locus typing does not, therefore, figure prominently in HLA-matching studies.

HLA-A, -B and -C typing using lymphocytotoxicity tests

Leucocyte antigens are detected by means of specific antisera. Historically leucocyte agglutinating antibodies were used, but now typing is more sensitively and reliably performed using *complement-dependent cytotoxic antibodies*. The standard lymphocytotoxicity test requires *lymphocytes* (bearing HLA antigens), *antiserum* (containing antibodies against specific HLA antigens), *complement* and an *indicator dye* such as eosin. Positive reactions, which entail antigen–antibody reactions and complement-mediated cell death, are revealed because the dead cells become permeable to and stained by the dye (Figure 2). Where no antigen–antibody reaction occurs the lymphocytes remain viable and are able to exclude the dye and remain unstained. As with red cell serological procedures the basic technical method can be used either for cell typing or for antiserum analysis. The basic lymphocytotoxicity test is the cornerstone of HLA serological work.

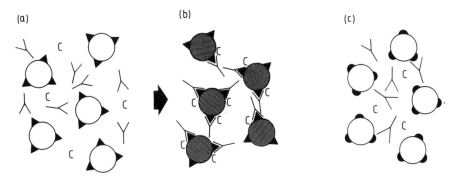

Figure 2 Lymphocytotoxicity test for HLA-A and -B typing or antibody screening. (a) Lymphocytes carrying HLA-A and -B determinants are incubated with serum containing HLA antibodies and complement (C). (b) In the presence of antibodies specific for HLA determinants carried by the test lymphocytes, complement-mediated cell killing occurs and the dead cells become stained by the indicator dye. The principle can be used for HLA typing in the presence of specific antisera or, alternatively, for serum examination where the cellular antigenic constitution is known. (c) Negative reaction obtained when the antiserum is non-reactive with lymphocyte HLA antigens

Where the lymphocytotoxicity test is used for antibody screening, e.g. of pre-transplant patients sera (see section 2.1), maximum sensitivity is required. Sensitivity can be improved, particularly for detection of non-complement-fixing antibodies, by addition of a further complement-fixing antiglobulin phase. However, the most sensitive means of demonstrating recipient lymphocyte–HLA antibody incompatibility is the use of flow cytometry. This has been advocated for renal graft cross-matching, particularly for patients in whom the first graft has failed.

Polymorphism of class I antigens

So far 27 HLA-A and 59 HLA-B specificities have been defined and numbered accordingly.[3] Prior to the 1991 histocompatibility nomenclature workshop, certain antigens carried a prefix 'w' (w = workshop), e.g. Aw33, indicating that their numerical designation was only provisional and awaited full agreement regarding their identity. Biochemical analysis of gene products or DNA genotyping of the corresponding alleles has resolved these uncertainties. Accordingly, use of the 'w' prefix has now been discontinued save for two exceptions. These include the 'supertypic' (see below) antigens Bw4 and Bw6 and also the C locus antigens. In the latter case, use of the prefix differentiates them from gene products of the complement system. Sometimes previously recognized HLA antigens are subdivided (split), e.g. A10 into A25 and A26, when recognizably distinct portions of the original 'broad' antigen are discovered. Under these circumstances, all members of the family of 'splits' will share a common antigenic epitope while each individual member will also be characterized by its own unique epitope. Public antigens (epitopes) are those common to even larger groups of HLA class 1 specificities (e.g. Bw4 and Bw6 denote alternative supertypic epitopes shared amongst the whole series of B locus antigens. Some specificities will be Bw4 associated, while others will carry Bw6). All members of the supertypic group will therefore share a degree of cross-reactivity ascribable to their common ownership of a public epitope. HLA antisera may either react solely against specific private epitopes, or as is often the case be multi-specific, reacting against public antigens shared by the family of cross-reactive antigens.

Cross-reactivity of HLA antigens

Some of the currently defined antigens of the HLA-A and -B loci show a degree of similarity (cross-reactivity) to other antigens of the same locus. Certain antisera react, for example, with both A2 and A28, indicating the presence of structural homology between the two antigens. Some well-recognized cross-reactive antigens showing this behaviour are listed in Table 2. Conversely, A2 may be regarded as less antigenic to an A28 recipient than would, for example non-cross-reactive antigens such as A1 or A9. This phenomenon has considerable practical relevance, both during laboratory work and also for assessing the degree of biological compatibility of various donor-recipient pairs. In the absence of full matching at the A and B loci, knowledge of the cross-reactivity of antigens enables selection of dona-

tions with various degrees of relative compatibility which will be clinically acceptable, e.g. in the provision of HLA-matched platelets. A more discriminating
approach is advantageous for selection of renal and bone marrow donors. For
example, there is evidence that renal and bone marrow grafts typed and matched
for split antigens show better survival than if matched for broad antigens alone.
The interrelationships of HLA antigens are now so complex that computers are
used for selecting the most suitable donor–recipient pairs.

Biochemical analysis of class I antigens

A further level of HLA complexity has been revealed by biochemical analysis of
class I allelic products.[4] Sequencing of PCR-amplified genomic DNA has also
shown that some of what were formerly regarded, on serological evidence, as
discrete specificities actually comprise several variants. The expressed protein
products of these variants generally show conformational differences in the
peptide-binding groove of the MHC molecule. Some of these variant class I allelic
proteins are sufficiently different in size and charge density to be detectable by
isoelectric focusing, and this technique can be used to further resolve class I
specificities. It has been necessary to update HLA nomenclature to include recognition of these newly defined phenotypes (e.g. HLA-3 is now recognized to
comprise two variants, designated A^{*0301}; A^{*0302}—this same alphanumeric
numbering principle is also applied to the newly recognized HLA DR and DQ
specificities (see 'class II typing using DNA analysis', below)).

Role of class I antigens

Class I antigens are believed to constitute individual tissue recognition markers
important for self and non-self recognition. They therefore enable recognition of
foreign antigens by cytotoxic T cells, an important part of defence mechanisms
against invasion by pathogens.

Class II (HLA-D region) antigens

Class II antigens form an additional category of cellular antigens which are
distinct from class I products. Class I and II genes show strong linkage disequilibrium as they are encoded on a closely adjacent part of chromosome 6.
HLA-DR gene products were the first of a series of several class II antigens (principally DR, DP, DQ) to be recognized (see Figure 1). The products of the D region
are mainly expressed on B lymphocytes but not on resting T lymphocytes.

Discovery of D locus antigens: mixed lymphocyte culture studies

D locus antigens were first detected when lymphocytes from antigenically different individuals were cultured together. Under these conditions they both recog-

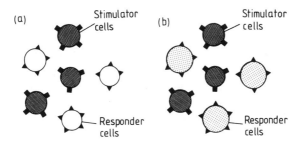

Figure 3 Mixed lymphocyte reaction. (a) Killed B lymphocytes (stimulator cells) are incubated with viable (responder) T lymphocytes, where both stimulator and responder cells bear differing class II D antigens. (b) The responder cells enlarge, undergo DNA synthesis and show blastic transformation. The reaction can be detected by measurement of the uptake of tritiated thymidine.

nize their mutual antigenic differences by undergoing blastic transformation—a process that requires DNA synthesis and can, therefore, be shown by the uptake of radioactive thymidine. This is the principle of the *mixed lymphocyte reaction (MLR)*. The MLR may be regarded as an *in vitro* counterpart of *in vivo* lymphocyte immunological behaviour following transplantation.

D locus compatibility testing using the MLR

For many years the MLR was commonly used for examination of class II antigen disparity as the basis of a *donor–recipient cross-match procedure*. In particular the MLR has been in popular use as the final arbiter during selection of potential bone marrow transplant donors. Pre-treatment of either donor or recipient lymphocytes by the use of cytotoxic drugs or irradiation destroys their ability to undergo blastic transformation in the face of antigenic challenge. In this way the separate capacity of either the potential donor or recipient to recognize antigenic differences in the other party can be established. Despite its conceptual appeal as a compatibility procedure the MLR test is laborious and inaccurate; the results have not provided the desired reliable predictions of transplantation outcome.

The improvements in class II typing by serological methods and more recently by DNA genotyping have led to a reduction in the use of MLR testing for donor recipient matching. The MLR is sometimes still performed during the selection of unrelated bone marrow donors in the expectation that it may detect further class II differences, e.g. at the DP locus, although the clinical significance of these incompatibilities is still uncertain.

Serological analysis of the HLA-D region: DR antigens

At first, D locus typing (known as Dw typing) could only be performed by cellular techniques—basically modification of the MLR in which the stimulator cells were of known phenotype. Fortunately, faster, more reliable serological cyto-toxicity-based methods were devised. Subdivision into at least three loci (DR, DP and DQ) was recognized and currently about 40 serologically defined gene products have been identified. DR typing, performed on purified B cell suspensions, has now become well established and appears to be an important compatibility requirement for both renal and bone marrow transplantation. However, the value of even these advances is being superseded by improvements in the speed and accuracy of DNA genotyping of the DR locus.

Class II typing using DNA analysis[4]

The greatest advance in class II typing and matching has now come from the ability to analyse HLA class II differences at the genomic level. Comparisons of serological and DNA-based techniques have now shown that a substantial proportion (up to 25%) of routinely performed serological DR assignments have been erroneous. This observation has an important bearing on attempts to analyse the relationship between match quality and graft outcome. In particular, for renal transplants, the benefits of good matching can be most clearly shown where the accuracy of DR status is confirmed by DNA genotyping. There are now many methods for HLA-DR typing from genomic DNA, the objectives being to improve speed, accuracy and economy and eventually to enable the immediate matching of, for example, potential cadaveric renal donors. Some popular techniques include the following.

RFLP (restriction fragment length polymorphism) techniques

In these techniques, DNA must be extracted from cells or tissue and digested using a selected restriction enzyme into nucleotide chain fragments. The length of these fragments varies (they are therefore described as polymorphic fragments) according to the position of restriction sites where the enzyme cleaves the nucleotide chain, which relates to the DRB genotype. After separation by electrophoresis, these polymorphic fragments of DNA are identified by the binding of complementary radiolabelled DNA probes (cDNA) chosen to be specific for the locus under study. The DRB alleles can then be identified following autoradiography from the electrophoretic band patterns identified following autoradiography. Unfortunately RFLP analysis is a time-consuming technique and the whole process may take up to 2 weeks to complete. As a consequence, the technique cannot be applied to prospective matching before solid organ transplantation. Although providing a valuable advance RFLP techniques are in turn being superseded by faster PCR-based methods.

Polymerase chain reaction-based methods

Typing using sequence-specific oligonucleotide probes[5]   This approach to HLA class II typing makes use of the ability of sequence-specific oligonucleotide probes (SSOP) to identify and bind to complementary DNA segments. In principle, the PCR reaction is used with group-specific primers first to amplify exon 2 of the DRB genes. The amplified DNA product is applied as dots to an appropriate membrane, which can then be 'stained' by applying biotin-labelled SSOPs. The bound biotin labelled probe is then identified enzymatically, typically by using avidin-labelled peroxidase as an indicator system (see Figure 4).

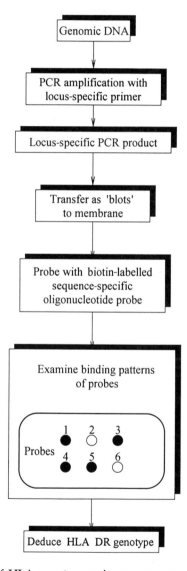

Figure 4 Determination of HLA genotype using sequence-specific oligonucleotide groups. DNA amplified from exon 2 of the DRB locus is applied as dot blots to the membrane. The HLA genotype is then inferred from the binding pattern obtained using a panel of biotin-labelled oligonucleotide probes

Typing using sequence-specific primers for PCR amplification[6]   In this procedure, now well established for DR analysis, typing specificity is obtained from the use of sequence-specific oligonucleotide primers which are selected to amplify alleles corresponding to serological DR specificities.

An amplified product can only be obtained if the primers anneal precisely with the corresponding DRB nucleotide sequence. The amplified gene products are subjected to brief agarose gel electrophoresis and identified under UV illumination. Using this method the DR genotype can be deduced from the presence or absence of PCR products using a series of PCRs with different primer combinations (see Figure 5).

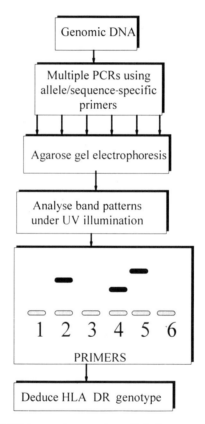

Figure 5 Determination of HLA genotype using allele/sequence-specific primers. In this technique the HLA DR genotype is disclosed by the specificity or specificities of the allele/sequence-specific primers which achieve successful amplification

Function and distribution of class II antigens

In contrast to the ubiquitous appearance of class I antigens throughout body tissues, those of class II loci are confined to cells forming components of the

Table 1 Frequencies of HLA genes

A locus	B locus	DR locus
Over 20% frequency		
A2		
15–20% frequency		
A1	B12	DR5
		DR7
10–15% frequency		
A3	B7	DR2
5–10% frequency		
A24	B5	DR1
A11	B8	DR3
A29	B18	DR4
	B40	DR6
		DR8
1–5% frequency		
A23	B13	
A25	B14	
A26	B27	
A28	B15	
A30	B38	
A31	B39	
	B21	
	B22	
	B37	

immune system. These include macrophages, B lymphocytes, epithelial cells and activated 'blastoid' T lymphocytes but not small T lymphocytes. Class II antigens are necessary for foreign antigen presentation to the immune system and for the various cell-to-cell cooperative functions (e.g. between B lymphocytes, macrophages and T helper cells) that are integral components of the immune response.

1.3 HLA Gene Frequencies

Linkage disequilibrium

Certain HLA-A and -B antigens occur in combination more frequently than would be expected by chance alone based on their individual gene frequencies. This situation resembles that found in the Rh system where certain haplotypes, e.g. *CDe* and *cde*, occur commonly while others, e.g. *cDe*, are unusual. This phenomenon is the result of the continued inheritance of evolutionarily older ancestral haplotypes that have not become altered by crossover during meiosis.

The chances of finding HLA-compatible donors, either of organs or platelets, are considerably improved if the potential recipient possesses one of the more

Table 2 Common HLA haplotypes

Haplotype	Frequency (%)
A1, B8, C7, DR3	5
A3, B7, C7, DR2	2.6
A2, B12, C5, DR4	1.7
A33, B14, C8, DR1	1.7
A2, B7, C7, DR2	1.7
A23, B12, C4, DR7	1.5

Table 3 Common examples of HLA-A and -B antigen cross-reactivity

A locus antigens	B locus antigens
A1, A3, A11	B5, B35, B18
A2, A28	B7, B27, B22
A10, A11	B8, B14, B18
A10, Aw19	B12, B21, B40, B13

common HLA haplotypes. It may, in fact, prove virtually impossible to provide compatible donors for those with rarer antigen combinations.

HLA and disease association

Many associations between HLA phenotypes and disease conditions have been described. Well-accepted examples include those shown in Table 4.

There are several reasons why it may be important to establish HLA–disease associations. Close association can be helpful in supporting the diagnosis of certain disease, in identification of potentially affected family members or, as in the case of HPA-1a negative mothers, highlighting a subpopulation at increased risk of affected pregnancies. It is also possible, though unproven, that certain HLA antigens may actually play a part in pathogenesis of the associated disease.

In routine practical terms HLA associations are, with the exception of B27 and ankylosing spondylitis, generally too weak to provide conclusive diagnosis of individual cases. Widespread testing for this purpose would therefore be very wasteful of effort and reagents. Family studies can be useful for predicting the likely appearance of diseases such as haemochromatosis within succeeding generations of a family. Large-scale population studies, on a research basis, offer at least the prospect that any associations that come to light might eventually help in elucidating the mechanism of the disease concerned.

Table 4   HLA and disease association[7]

Disease	HLA antigens	Relative risk (%)
Narcolepsy	DR2	>100
Ankylosing spondylitis	B27	>50
Goodpasture's syndrome	A3	13.8
Coeliac disease	DR3	11.6
HPA-1a immunization (NAIT)	DR52a	8.4
Idiopathic		
Haemochromatosis	A3	6.7
Rheumatoid arthritis	DR4	3.8

1.4   HLA Antibodies

Origin

Formation of the commonly found polyclonal HLA antibodies of human serum is stimulated by exposure to foreign HLA alloantigens. This occurs:

(1) *During pregnancy*: up to 25% of women develop lymphocytotoxic antibodies directed against paternal antigens by completion of their second pregnancy. Fortunately, these do not appear to have any harmful effects on the fetus. Antibody formation is stimulated by fetal lymphocytes which cross the placenta and reach the maternal circulation.
(2) *Following transfusion*: the incidence of both leucoagglutinating and lymphocytotoxic antibodies increases with increasing donor exposures. Around 15–20% of multi-transfused patients receiving over 20 units have lymphocytotoxic antibodies. The actual risk of occurrence depends on the amount of any concurrent immunosuppression, the types of blood products transfused, the nature of the primary diagnosis and possibly also the degree of innate immune responsiveness of the patient concerned.
(3) As a result of *organ transplantation*: the development of lymphocytotoxic antibodies clearly has a bearing on the success of the transplantation treatment.

Monoclonal antibodies, synthesized by hybridoma cell lines, are useful for revealing the complex nature of the assembly of epitopes which comprise the HLA antigens conventionally defined by polyclonal antibodies. However, only a limited number of specificities have so far been produced and monoclonal antibodies have not been able to supplant human serum-derived polyclonal reagents for routine HLA typing.

Specificity

HLA antibodies found during or following pregnancy are likely to have a specificity largely directed against paternal antigens and may therefore, if monospecific (single antigen specificity), be useful as reagents. This will not be so true for those formed as a result of transfusion when broadly reactive (multispecific) antibodies appear. The specificity of HLA antibodies is determined with cell panels following the principles used for red cell antibodies. Up to 200 panel cells may be required to cover the greater number of antigens and resolve the many possible specificities.

Sera containing mixtures of antibodies may be purified by absorption to produce monospecific reagents. If, however, cross-reactive antibodies predominate in a serum, absorption will remove all the specificities and such sera are therefore of no value as reagents.

Clinical significance of HLA antibodies

HLA antibodies are clinically important as causes of:

(1) Non-haemolytic transfusion reactions: this applies particularly to potent leucoagglutinins (see chapter 23, section 3).
(2) Refractory responses to platelet transfusion (see chapter 5, section 6).
(3) Allograft rejection.

2 RENAL TRANSPLANTATION

Transplantation is now accepted as the treatment of choice for most patients in end-stage renal failure. Overall first-time graft survival rates (from cadaveric donors) are of the order of 80% at 1 year and 50% at 5 years. These are average figures; in fact there are very considerable differences in results from different centres which must be linked in some way to differences in the preparatory regimens as well as to differences in pathological diagnosis and criteria for patient selection.

Immunological factors determining renal allograft survival

Despite the fact that many thousands of kidney transplants have been performed worldwide over the last 20 years, there are still uncertainties about the importance of many common practices with regard to donor selection or management of the recipient. A history of previous *blood transfusion* is, for example, now recognized to *enhance* graft survival for most patients, whereas for many years transfusion was feared for its effect on causing pre-sensitization to HLA antigens and prompt graft rejection. The outlook is, however, worse for those patients who do become sensitized from transfusion or rejection of a previously grafted kidney. The advent of *cyclosporin A* as a powerful new immunosuppressive agent has greatly improved overall graft survival rates. Indeed cyclosporin has been so effective the need for good HLA matching to ensure graft survival has been challenged.[8] The perceived shortcomings of HLA matching may, however, be explained by the newly recognized limitations of HLA analysis by conventional serological means. The variable quality of typing sera, and differences in techniques and proficiency within typing laboratories have been shown to result in typing inaccuracies. These have helped to confound attempts to correlate patient outcomes with match grade.[9] As a further complication, DNA genotype analysis is now revealing the diversity of epitope variability that may be hidden within what had hitherto been recognized as single serological specificities. Proponents of HLA matching now claim that these advances have paved the way towards improvements in typing accuracy that will minimize chronic graft rejection and the need for potent immunosuppressive therapy, and ensure long-term graft survival. Greater resolution of HLA at the biochemical level, if combined with effective national organ-sharing schemes, should therefore improve the long-term outcome for transplanted patients. From the largest and most comprehensive studies[10,11] it has been shown that cyclosporin improves survival rates and first-year graft retention rates are greater, but thereafter the survival half-life of grafts remains unaffected.[12] Cyclosporin alone does not prevent the chronic rejection process. Data from the US nation-wide organ-sharing scheme has shown graft survival half-lives of 17.3 years for full 6 (HLA-A, B, DR) antigen matching, compared with only 7.8 years for mismatched grafts.[11] Matching for antigen splits (see section 1.2), as a further refinement over and above ensuring broad antigen matches, was also shown to be beneficial in the European collaborative transplant study.[10] At 3 years, HLA -A and -B matches had 18% better survival and this improved to 31% when DR split mismatches were avoided. Proponents argue that the extra costs and logistic difficulties of improving match quality can be offset by savings from a reduction of immunosuppression and the need to replace grafts that have failed.

2.1 Graft Selection: HLA Typing

In contrast to bone marrow transplants, in which donors and recipients are usually related, and selected according to strict histocompatibility criteria, most kidneys for grafting are obtained from cadaver donors and match quality may be subservient to clinical expediency. These donors are largely victims of traumatic injury or acute illnesses unassociated with renal pathology. A minority of grafts are, however, obtained from close relatives; these usually share at least

Table 5 Immunological factors determining renal graft survival (in order of probable importance)

T cell cross-match compatibility
Cyclosporin A immunosuppression
HLA-DR matching
HLA-A and -B matching
History of previous blood transfusion

one haplotype with the recipient. Lymphocyte-borne HLA-A, -B, and -DR antigens reflect the nature of tissue antigens within renal parenchyma and vascular endothelium. The search for maximum histocompatibility is therefore designed to minimize the likelihood of immune-mediated damage against renal tissues.

Prospective recipients are patients in chronic renal failure maintained on a dialysis programme. These patients are often anaemic, due mainly to the effects of uraemia, and the inevitable blood losses occurring during each haemodialysis episode. Patients in whom the anaemia is not adequately correctable by ery-thropoietin and haematinic therapy require blood transfusion.

Studies on potential graft recipients

Routine studies on prospective recipients include:

(1) HLA-A and -B typing.
(2) HLA-DR typing.
(3) Serum screening for lymphocytotoxic antibodies.

Sera from pre-transplant patients are usually examined on a 3-monthly basis. Reactivity against cell panels can change over time; samples showing the highest level of activity are identified for later use in cross-match testing.

The results of these studies are usually gathered centrally in computer-based files (e.g. those organized by the UK Transplant Service or the United Network for Organ Sharing in the USA) so that when a donor becomes available the most compatible and geographically convenient recipients can be efficiently selected. This procedure depends on the cooperation of the participating centre notifying the results of HLA-A, -B and -DR typing on the *kidney donor* to the computer registry. In many instances there will be local patients who are suitable recipients for the available donor kidneys and the facilities of the computer registry may not be required. Kidney donors must additionally be compatible for the ABO blood groups.

Group O kidneys are well accepted by non-O recipients, but in a very small number of cases immunocompetent B lymphocytes of donor origin have synthe-sized sufficient anti-A or anti-B to induce a transient haemolytic episode bearing all the hallmarks of an *in vivo* ABO haemolytic reaction.[13]

2.2 Cross-match Studies[14]

Cross-matching is undertaken in order to identify potentially incompatible grafts. Incompatibility can take various forms; in its most dramatic manifestation the transplanted kidney shows immediate immune-mediated damage known as *hyperacute rejection*. At the other end of the spectrum, *chronic rejection*, character-istically makes its appearance from 8 to 10 months following transplantation.

Cross-matching is performed to elicit evidence of pre-formed HLA sensitization with the aim of avoiding early graft loss.

Table 6 Causes of graft rejection[14]

Type of rejection	Time of appearance	Immune mediators	Outcome
Hyperacute	Minutes to hours	ABO alloantibodies Pre-formed cytotoxic HLA antibodies	Graft loss
Accelerated	3–4 days	Cytotoxic T cells Secondary cytotoxic antibody response therapy	Poor even with anti-rejection therapy
Acute rejection	3–5 weeks	Primary immune response Cytotoxic T cells?	May be controlled by anti-rejection therapy
Chronic rejection	> 8–10 months	Alloantibody to donor antigens	Unresponsive to therapy

Donor selection

Donors are selected from amongst those who appear to be the most HLA compatible and who lack antigens reactive with antibodies identified in the recipient serum (they should also lack antigens that were incompatible on any previous graft).

Donor lymphocytes (usually obtained from lymph nodes or splenic fragments) are cross-matched against the latest and the previous most highly reactive serum sample from the recipient.

Antibody characteristics

Initially, it appeared that rapid immunological rejection of grafted kidneys (hyperacute rejection) was due to the presence of any lymphocytotoxic antibodies reacting against donor cells. Accordingly, transplantation of grafts incompatible with lymphocytotoxic antibodies was avoided. It now seems that various forms of lymphocytotoxic antibody may be present, not all of which have such destructive effects, and their full clinical significance has yet to be fully understood.

The different categories of antibodies recognized so far include:

(1) Antibodies reacting against T lymphocytes: 'warm' 37 °C reactive cytotoxic anti-T cell antibodies seem to be most strongly associated with acute rejection.
(2) Antibodies against B cells: these include antibodies recognizing HLA-A, -B or -C determinants. Reactivity can sometimes also be demonstrated against surface-bound immunoglobulin as well as against DR antigens. Most of these antibodies do not appear to be clinically significant, with the exception of DR antibodies which are believed to be associated with chronic rejection.
(3) Autoantibodies: these are usually non-specific and react against most panel cells. They do not, for some reason, react against lymphocytes from patients

with chronic lymphocytic leukaemia and this characteristic assists their laboratory identification.

(4) Immunoglobulin class: whereas IgG alloantibodies are usually assumed to be significant, IgM antibodies, which may be either auto- or alloreactive, are not. Reducing agents such as Dithiothreitol (DTT) disrupt the pentameric structure of IgM and remove antibody reactivity. Use of DTT permits the distinction between IgM and IgG antibodies.

These analyses are accomplished by testing sera against purified B or T lymphocytes, sometimes at various temperatures, e.g. 4 °C, 22 °C and 37 °C. Auto-antibodies can be distinguished by their optimal reactivity at lower temperatures or more usually by their susceptibility to DTT treatment. They do not appear to be clinically important other than presenting as a positive cross-match which requires resolution.

After renal transplantation the recipient serum can be examined for the emergence of lymphocytotoxic antibodies that might signal the onset of a rejection episode. Attempts are made to suppress these rejection episodes with agents such as heterologous anti-lymphocyte globulin (ALG) or monoclonal T cell antibodies (e.g. OKT3). Use of ALG serum for treatment of rejection episodes has sometimes led to red cell cross-matching difficulties.[15,16] Some heterologous antisera, e.g. ALG of equine origin, may have residual anti-human red cell activity causing positive direct antiglobulin test results and their presence in the patient's serum may therefore be confused with autoantibodies.

Cross-match techniques

Cross-matches are conventionally performed using the standard NIH microlymphocytotoxicity test (see section 1.2). In order to distinguish between T cell reactivity (clinically significant) and B cell reactions (of which the importance is less certain) cross-matches can be performed on separated T cells and B cells. Because of concerns that these might not detect all potentially significant alloantibodies, some laboratories increase the test sensitivity by use of an extra antiglobulin phase the (AHG cross-match). Cross-match procedures using flow cytometry provide even greater sensitivity.[93] This test procedure utilizes reagents such as fluorescein isothiocynate-labelled anti-human IgG to demonstrate reactivity between alloantibodies in patients' serum and donor cells.

Interpretation of cross-match results

Cross-matches performed in the work-up prior to renal transplantation do not provide absolute certainty about the likely success of the graft. Clinical interpretation of cross-match results will depend upon a variety of factors, e.g:

(1) The stringency of cross-match compatibility requirements: these are greater for replacement grafts than for first time grafts.

(2) Intensity of immunosuppression and anti-rejection therapy: certain categories

of cross-match incompatibility may be tolerable now that increasingly effective measures for countering early graft rejection are available (e.g. cyclosporin, monoclonal T cell antibodies (OKT3)).
(3) Sensitivity of methods used for antibody detection (e.g. flow cytometry as opposed to lymphocytotoxicity testing), nature of target cell reactivity (e.g. T or B cell).

Highly sensitized patients

Most transplant centres have a waiting list of patients who, as a result of previous blood transfusion or failed grafts, have become sensitized to the majority (e.g. >85%) of random donor cells. For these patients most cross-matches will be incompatible and graft selection is accordingly more difficult. Management approaches include:

(1) Consideration as to whether the antibodies revealed during cross-matching are clinically significant (see above).
(2) Selection of well-matched donors (e.g. DR-matched or matches involving no more than one A or B locus mismatch, provided that the mismatched antigens are not cross-match incompatible) using the offices of the national organ sharing schemes.[17,18]
(3) Some success has been claimed using antibody removal techniques, e.g. staphylococcal A immunoabsorbants (see chapter 19), either alone or coupled with cytotoxic immunosuppression.[19]

2.3   Blood Transfusion and Kidney Transplantation[20,21]

In the early years of kidney transplantation, the practice of transfusing potential recipients was identified as jeopardizing the chance of successful engraftment. *Hyperacute rejection* of the kidney was seen to be due to the presence of lymphocytotoxic antibodies in the recipient's serum which had arisen as a direct consequence of previous blood transfusions. Multi-transfused patients develop even more antibodies, and these typically show a wide spectrum of reactivity; the chances of selection of compatible grafts therefore becomes correspondingly reduced. Most transplant centres have accumulated 'difficult-to-match' patients who required longer maintenance on dialysis and in consequence more transfusions. The patients eventually developed broadly reactive antibodies which diminished further their chances of obtaining a successfully matched kidney. The presence of this hard core of ungraftable patients emphasized the undesirable link between transfusion and development of lymphocytotoxic antibodies. It seemed logical, therefore, to limit, as far as possible, transfusions to prospective graft recipients and, when transfusion was unavoidable, to use only leucocyte-free red cell preparations.

These policies were pursued to a variable extent in transplant centres until it became clearly apparent from retrospective analysis that *transfused patients actually had better graft survival rates* than those not transfused.

So overwhelming was this evidence that, prior to the introduction of cyclo-sporin, policies of *deliberate transfusion* were then adopted in order to take advantage of what obviously seemed to be a protective effect. It clearly then became necessary to reconcile the two apparently opposing influences resulting from blood transfusion.

The effect of transfusion on development of lymphocytotoxic antibodies

Around 10–15% of transfused patients develop lymphocytotoxic antibodies. The risk is enhanced by previous pregnancies but not to a serious extent. For most patients, therefore, blood transfusion does not prejudice the chances of successful transplantation[22] although a small but unpredictable proportion do become highly sensitized and liable to hyperacute rejection.

Donor-specific transfusion

The practice of transfusing blood from the prospective donor (donor-specific transfusions—a procedure only applicable in the case of related donors) has also been shown to benefit graft survival. Such donors will, of course, not necessarily be very well matched. About 30% of recipients become sensitized to donor antigens, thus prohibiting transplantation from the donor concerned, but graft survival seems to be improved for the remainder. There is evidence to suggest that transfusions of blood in which one HLA haplotype is matched with the recipient[23] and possibly also class II disparity on the unshared haplotype[24] appear to abrogate cytotoxic T cell responsiveness to the donor. This tolerance has been ascribed to the induction of a low level of haemopoietic chimerism.

Transfusions can be combined with immunosuppression in order to obliterate the reactive lymphoid cells that might produce lymphocytotoxic antibodies.

Despite the advantageous graft survival seen for many patients, fear of the significant risk of sensitization for a minority has prevented widespread acceptance of donor-specific transfusion as a means of inducing graft tolerance.

The mechanism of the protective effect

The mechanism by which blood transfusion reduces the risk of graft rejection remains to be elucidated. The following are speculations:

(1) Transfusion selects patients for grafting by excluding those that are most responsive to the HLA antigens of the donor.
(2) Transfusion appears to favour the proliferation of suppressor T cells which then induce graft tolerance. Suppressor/helper T cell ratios are in fact increased in multi-transfused patients, both in those receiving blood products (such as haemophiliacs) and in chronically transfused patients (e.g. those with haemoglobinopathies or aplastic anaemia). Many cell-mediated immune

functions such as phytohaemagglutinin (PHA) or MLR responses appear to be reduced after a week or so following transfusion (see chapter 23, section 4.4).

(3) Transfusions may stimulate the formation of anti-idiotypic antibodies or lymphocytes that specifically suppress HLA antibody responses.[25]

(4) It has been suggested that the destruction of effete red cells of transfused units occupies the reticuloendothelial system so fully that the normal process of antigen recognition and presentation to the lymphoid tissues is impaired.

This intriguing beneficial effect of transfusion on graft survival has now diminished in importance beside the powerful effects of cyclosporin in improving graft retention.[26] Such is the current success of renal graft retention that dissection of the influence of other residual factors such as blood transfusion has become very difficult. The use of erythropoietin has very dramatically reduced the need for blood transfusions as an essential support for pre-transplant patients. It does seem likely, however, that limited exposure to transfusion is still beneficial and this possibility remains deserving of study.

3   BONE MARROW TRANSPLANTATION

Transplantation of bone marrow is now playing an increasingly well-defined role in the treatment of a variety of conditions. The procedure, however, presents a range of immunological problems that are not encountered during transplantation of other tissues. A fundamental difference is that the recipient's immune system as well as the haemopoietic marrow must be destroyed in order to allow successful colonization by the transplanted marrow, which will then provide both functions. Not surprisingly, successful engraftment of mismatched donor immunological function will result in attempted destruction of recipient tissues—a phenomenon known as *graft-versus-host disease* (GVHD). This can cause serious illness or fatality and must be curtailed by immunosuppressive therapy. Complicating the picture, however, is the possibility that a certain degree of GVHD also correlates with a reduction in relapse when transplantation is used for treatment of leukaemia. This phenomenon has come to be considered as the *graft-versus-leukaemia effect*.

Bone marrow transplantation is most successful between identical twins but is also effective between HLA-identical siblings and to a lesser degree between other family members sharing HLA haplotypes with the recipient. The use of matched unrelated donors is now increasing, but there are still a number of poorly understood problems to be faced, even when a high degree of HLA similarity is present.

Tissue typing and transfusion laboratories have an important and cooperative role to play in bone marrow transplantation programmes.[27,28] Their interests comprise:

(1) Determination of the optimum transfusion policies prior to transplantation.
(2) Tissue matching for HLA class I and class II antigens, and donor selection.
(3) Red cell serological studies, particularly when ABO-incompatible marrow is transplanted.

(4) Assessment of the progress of engraftment.
(5) Assessment of the recovery of immunological function.
(6) Selection and procurement of blood products for support during the recovery phase.
(7) Manipulation of bone marrow prior to transplantation in order to minimize the effects of ABO incompatibility and GVHD.

3.1 Applications of Bone Marrow Transplantation[29–32]

The conditions for which bone marrow transplantation is used include the following:

(1) *Severe aplastic anaemia and advanced myelodysplastic conditions:*[31–35] transplantation has now become the treatment of choice for those patients with a genotypically HLA-matched sibling. Long-term survivals of 60–80% are now possible. Graft rejection, although amenable to cyclosporin, is a significant problem.

Because of the likelihood of graft failure, GVHD and the need for high-intensity immunosuppression, the value of less-well matched grafts has not yet been established. In the absence of normal haemopoiesis, autologous grafts are not applicable. Because of the likelihood of alloimmunization and the consequences of accelerated graft rejection, pre-transplant blood transfusion should be avoided where possible.

(2) *Acute myeloid leukaemia:*[36,37] the continued improvements both in chemotherapy and in the success of bone marrow transplantation make the precise role of each somewhat less clearly established. Provided that well-matched sibling donor marrow is available, transplantation may now offer the best prospects for patients brought into their first remission. Projected 3-year survivals for this group are of the order of 60%, which may be better than obtainable by continued chemotherapy. The success rate appears to decline if transplantation is performed during second remission and is very poor if attempted for those in relapse.

(3) *Acute lymphoblastic leukaemias (ALL):*[38] a small subgroup of patients, particularly those with poor prognostic features at diagnosis who fare badly during conventional chemotherapy, may be better managed by transplantation. For patients without suitably matched donors autologous grafts or autologous peripheral blood stem cell grafts are now being utilized.

(4) *Chronic myeloid leukaemia (CML):*[29] Allogeneic bone marrow transplants, both related and unrelated, have been used successfully in CML. Transplants are more successful (e.g. greater than 50% 3-year disease-free survival rates) when carried out during the chronic phase, rather than during the period of acceleration towards blastic transformation. For patients without well-matched donors autologous or peripheral stem cell grafts are being utilized.

(5) *Patients with other haematological and non-haematological malignancies:*[47] transplantation and, in particular, autologous or peripheral blood stem cell transplants, are being increasingly used for a variety of malignant conditions. These

include non-Hodgkin's lymphoma, Hodgkin's disease, neuroblastoma, Ewing's sarcoma, ovarian carcinoma, carcinoma of the breast and melanoma.

(6) Patients with severe congenital *combined immunodeficiency syndrome*[39] have been successfully provided with both cellular and humoral immune competence by bone marrow grafting.

(7) Smaller groups of patients with *Fanconi anaemia, Wiskott–Aldrich syndrome, osteopetrosis* and other *inborn errors of metabolism* have benefited from marrow grafting.[40-43] Patients in the latter category who are particularly suitable are those with diseases such as mucopolysaccharidoses and sphingolipidoses, in which the deficient enzyme is produced by cells of bone marrow stem cell origin. Bone marrow transplantation also seems to improve the development of children with *osteopetrosis* by supplying normal osteoclasts so that bone growth and remodelling can continue.

(8) *Severe haemoglobinopathy*: bone marrow transplants using HLA-identical relatives have been utilized successfully for children with severe homozygous β-thalassaemia in order to avoid the long-term complications of blood transfusion and iron overload.[44] A similar approach has been utilized for severe sickle cell disease (HBSS). Despite encouraging early results the place of transplantation in the routine management of these conditions has by no means been fully resolved. Transplants should probably be reserved for children who are likely to be severely handicapped by their disease; however, it should also be performed early, before serious complications have arisen. Severe myeloablative treatment (e.g. high-dose busulphan and cyclosphamide) is required which may affect future growth and fertility,[45,46] although this has to be balanced against the morbidity of alternative forms of therapy.

3.2 Genetic Categories of Donor–Recipient Pairs

There are three major genetic categories of organ transplantation: syngeneic, allogeneic and autologous.

Syngeneic transplants are those in which an identical twin provides the grafts. The absolute genetic identity virtually assures that the graft will take and that there will be no immunological activity of the grafted marrow against host tissues (GVHD). Syngeneic transplants will obviously not be possible for inherited disorders, but will be highly suitable for patients with aplastic anaemia. Syngeneic marrow grafts 'take' well for patients with leukaemia but these may have a higher relapse rate than grafts from other close relatives.[48]

It seems likely that the lack of GVHD more readily permits re-emergence of leukaemic clones.

Allogeneic transplants are grafts provided from related or non-related,[14] but usually genetically similar, individuals. These can vary widely in the degree of disparity between HLA-A, -B, and -D loci as well as the as yet unidentified minor histocompatibility antigens. The most satisfactory matches are those between siblings who are genetically identical at least for the major HLA antigens, and will also share a high proportion of minor histocompatibility loci.

The following is an approximate preference order for graft selection:

(1) Siblings showing haplotype identity (these are usually genotypically matched): between 25% and 30% of patients are likely to have compatible sibling donors available.
(2) Relatives showing haplotype identity; i.e. HLA-A, -B, and -DR antigens matched with the recipient (these will be partly genotypically and partly phenotypically matched—e.g. antigens matched with the recipient, but which are not on the shared haplotype are likely to show differences at the biochemical level (see section 1.2, 'class II typing using DNA analysis')). Between 5% and 10% of patients may have such a family donor available.
(3) Unrelated donors fully antigen matched (e.g. HLA-A, -B and -DR phenotypic matches). The quality of matching can be maximized if splits and cross-reactive groups are considered. Phenotypic matched antigens may still differ at the biochemical level; the availability of such donors will depend on the frequency of phenotype occurrence within the population and may vary from around 1/2000 to being infinitely remote. A panel comprising 100 000 HLA-matched volunteers is likely to provide a reasonable match for about 45% of patients drawn from the same Caucasian population.[49]
(4) Unrelated matches in which one or more antigens are mismatched: the quality of HLA matching clearly determines transplantation success (see Table 7) although other variables (T cell depletion, immunosuppressive treatment, the nature of the original disease) are also important.

Although in some conditions, e.g. CML,[29] six antigen-matched (HLA-A, -B and -DR) unrelated donors have shown success rates close to that for matched family donors, the value of less well-matched transplants remains to be established.

Autologous transplants[37,50]

These entail collection, storage (often by freezing) and later reinfusion of the patient's own bone marrow. This is performed to allow myeloablative chemoradiotherapy to be given for the treatment of malignancy. This technique has proved beneficial for treatment of various haematological malignancies. In the case of acute leukaemias various combinations of cytotoxic agents and/or monoclonal tumour cell antibodies can be employed to remove residual neoplastic cells before reinfusion of the marrow. Tumour relapse may be more likely following autologous transplantation, possibly through lack of the graft versus leukaemia effect, difficulties in eradication of residual leukaemia and also as a result of rein-

Table 7 Post-transplantation problems influenced by HLA match quality

Graft rejection
Acute GVHD (> grade II)
Predisposition to infection
Relapse rate

fusion of leukaemia cells not eradicated from the processed marrow. Peripheral blood stem cells collected by leukapheresis after cytotoxic agent and recombinant growth factor stimulation are being used as a relatively novel form of autologous graft source and appear to have distinctive advantages (see section 3.11).

Umbilical cord blood as a source of haemopoietic precursor cells

A novel source of allogeneic (or occasionally syngeneic) haemopoietic precursor cells may be provided by umbilical cord blood salvaged at the time of delivery. Umbilical cord blood appears to contain higher proportions of primitive pluripotential stem cells than bone marrow. It has been shown to provide haemopoietic reconstitution without severe GVHD. If collected in sufficient amounts (which may prove difficult), HLA typed and cryopreserved, it may be possible to bank precursor cells against the needs of patients for whom a family donor is not available.[43,51]

3.3 Outcome Following Bone Marrow Transplantation[29]

The outcome of transplantation depends greatly on factors such as the nature of the primary diagnosis and the success in obtaining a suitably matched donor. The main causes of failure include:

(1) Recurrence of the original condition.
(2) Inadequate marrow dose: at least 2×10^8 nucleated cells per kilogram are required.
(3) Age of the bone marrow donor: patient survival is believed to be better where younger donors are used.
(4) Graft rejection: the likelihood of this can be related to quality of HLA match, lymphocytotoxic antibodies in pre-transplant sera and the presence of a refractory state to platelet transfusion. (Platelet refractoriness usually reflects HLA sensitization following previous transfusions.)
    The immunological factors affecting graft rejection will, in general, affect the prognosis most for patients with aplastic anaemia. These patients probably have normally reactive immune function or the disease in some cases may possibly be due to an underlying autoimmune process.
(5) GVHD (see section 3.8).
(6) Complications arising from immunosuppression and infection:[52] despite the use of prophylactic chemotherapy and barrier nursing/patient isolation procedures, a wide variety of serious opportunistic infections present a constant threat. Invasive candidiasis and aspergillosis are the principal fungal infections. *Pneumocystis* is a common cause of pneumonia. Cytomegalovirus (CMV) interstitial pneumonitis figures prominently as a cause of death. Other important infections include gastroenteritis of viral origin, e.g. CMV, adenovirus, Coxsackie and rotavirus infections. Herpes zoster and herpes simplex infections are also common problems. Bacterial infections include those due to *Staphylococcus aureus* (occasional severe infections), *Staphylococcus epidermidis* (a

frequent cause of bacteraemia arising from infection around intravenous lines), pneumococcal infections as well as a variety of Gram-negative septicaemias.

(7) Various long-term problems also face bone marrow transplant survivors.[53] These include reduced fertility, chronic GVHD with prolonged immuno-suppression, recurrent infections including interstitial pneumonitis, relapsed leukaemia in patients with this initial diagnosis and also secondary malig-nancies.

3.4 Sequence of Events During Transplantation

There are several phases that can usefully be identified during bone marrow graft procedures:

(1) *Before marrow grafting* blood components may be considered necessary for correction of anaemia and for treatment of bleeding or infective symptoms. Despite these clinical indications transfusions can have harmful consequences. At this time it seems most important to:

  (a) Avoid transfusions in aplastic patients if at all possible as these appear to cause HLA sensitization and jeopardize engraftment. If transfusions are unavoidable, random donors are preferred to family members but these still carry a risk of inducing broadly reactive HLA antibodies which may be cross-reactive with donor antigens. If red cells or platelets must be given they must be rendered leucocyte free (see chapter 3, section 1.5). Fortunately the adverse effect of previous transfusion does not seem to hold true for patients with leukaemia. These patients are relatively immu-nosuppressed compared with those with aplasia, in whom this aspect of immune responsiveness is normal.

  (b) Relatives of a family member who may be a potential graft donor should not be used as a source of blood products prior to transplantation. Rela-tives may possess minor histocompatibility antigens similar to those of the donor but which may be lacking in the patient and could therefore cause pre-sensitization.

(2) Immediately *prior to transplantation* various schedules of chemotherapy and radiotherapy, e.g. cyclophosphamide and total body irradiation, are applied to:

  (a) Ablate recipient bone marrow tissue.
  (b) Induce complete immunosuppression.
  (c) Destroy residual neoplastic tissues.

(3) For up to 4 weeks or more *following transplantation* there may be little effective output from the marrow. The patient will be severely pancytopenic and corre-spondingly vulnerable. There will be a degree of GVHD that will require con-tinued immunosuppressive therapy. A balance has to be struck between the suppression of GVHD and the risk of morbidity associated with the treatment by immunosuppressive agents. GVHD causes hepatic, renal, cutaneous and gastrointestinal damage. Immunosuppressive chemotherapy leads to mucositis and ulcerative lesions of the gastrointestinal tract. During this period there will be a need for blood product support.[54,55] Cellular components must be irradiated (see section 3.8) and should, at least for seronegative recipients, be

obtained from donors shown to be CMV antibody negative (chapter 24, section 7).

(a) The greatest need will be for *platelets*. Almost all patients need platelet transfusion. Prophylactic therapy is recommended to maintain counts above $10 \times 10^9/l$. Platelets from family donors are not prohibited during this period. If the patient shows evidence of refractoriness to random donor platelets then collections particularly from the bone marrow donor or from other family members or from HLA-matched cross-match compatible donors are more likely to be successful (see chapter 5, section 6).

(b) Virtually all patients will require *red cell transfusions*. Transfusions are usually given to maintain haemoglobin values of at least 8.5 g/dl. ABO-incompatible grafts appear to require greater transfusion support.

(c) There seems to be little need for *granulocyte transfusions*. Far from being beneficial their use has been associated with an increased risk of CMV transmission (see chapter 24, section 7) and, particularly in the pre-graft period, with sensitization to HLA antigens. Granulocyte preparations contain large numbers of viable lymphocytes which could cause GVHD; they must, therefore, always be irradiated.

Infections do, however, present a grave threat during this period, but many of the organisms would not be controlled by granulocyte transfusions. Interstitial pneumonitis, in many cases due to CMV infection, probably accounts for around 30–40% of post-transplant deaths.

(d) During this period, when infections are so frequent, complications such as disseminated intravascular coagulation, protein and fluid loss from gastroenteritis may necessitate the use of specific blood products (e.g. fresh plasma, cryoprecipitate or albumin solutions). Intravenous immunoglobulin has been claimed to have some protective effect against infections during the first 2 months following marrow ablative therapy, although the evidence is not very substantial.

(e) Attention to rigorous fluid balance is important because of the likelihood of renal, hepatic, cardiovascular or various other physiological or metabolic problems that render the patient less able to tolerate fluid overload.

(4) *Convalescent period*: for up to 1 year following successful engraftment both humoral and cellular immunity will still show some impairment.[56] Irradiated transfusions should be used for at least 6 months even where successful engraftment has taken place.

3.5 Selection of Bone Marrow Donors

Apart from transplants between identical twins, greatest success so far has been shown with grafts from siblings shown to be:

- HLA-A, -B, identical (class I antigens).
- HLA-D, -DR identical (class II antigens).

The majority of recipients (approximately 70%) will not have suitable sibling donors. A search may then be made first among willing family members and, if this is unproductive, from national panels of bone marrow volunteers.* The selection possibilities are outlined in section 3.2.

The sequence of events for identifying a potential donor includes the following:

(1) HLA typing of the recipient and testing the recipient serum for lymphocytotoxic antibodies.
(2) The study of HLA antigens amongst the immediate family members in the search for a satisfactory match.
(3) If this is not found then a search may be made amongst panels for unrelated volunteer bone marrow donors.
(4) Finally, choice of the most HLA-compatible volunteer donor.

Bone marrow panel donors will usually have been typed for class I antigens alone. Prospective donors must therefore be recalled for class II typing (see section 1.2, 'class II typing using DNA analysis'). The aim is to secure HLA-A, -B, -Cw, -DR and -DQ compatibility. Although the mixed lymphocyte reaction (MLR) has traditionally been used to enable final selection of donors, its usefulness has diminished as accuracy of DR typing particularly by DNA analysis, has increased. Amongst donors well matched for HLA-A, -B and -DR MLR tests may well recognize further differences, e.g. between DP locus products.

However, the clinical significance of such differences, for example as a predictor of GVHD, has not been adequately established. Other test systems, e.g. assay of cytotoxic or helper T lymphocyte precursor cell assays, are being studied for this purpose. DNA fingerprint-matching techniques are now also being used to establish final class II compatibility of prospective donor and recipient pairs. In addition to these laboratory procedures, the donor should also be assessed for physical fitness to donate and should receive counselling as a prerequisite for seeking fully informed consent. These procedures usually take some weeks, which acts as a major constraint to the use of unrelated donors. Patients must generally be in a sufficiently stable condition for this approach to be feasible. Attempts are being made to utilize faster alternative methods for establishing class II antigen compatibility (see section 1.2), and if applied successfully could open up the way to better utilization of unrelated donor panels.

In some patients with haematological malignancies, paucity of normal lymphocytes may make all serological HLA determinations, and in particular MLR testing, unreliable. DNA analysis should help to overcome this problem.

3.6 Red Cell Serological Studies

These are needed if an *ABO-incompatible donor* is to be used and may also be helpful in the detection of early evidence of engraftment.

ABO compatibility is surprisingly not necessary for successful engraftment. Early marrow precursor cells do not strongly express ABO antigens and are not

---

* Several countries have national panels of bone marrow volunteer donors. These include the Anthony Nolan Panel and British Bone Marrow Donor Appeal panels in the UK, and a National Marrow Donor Program in the USA (see Appendix A).

therefore seriously damaged by alloantibodies of the ABO system. As expected, however, there are risks of haemolytic transfusion reactions *at the time of grafting* when, for example, the red cells with group A marrow are given to group O recipients.[57,58]

In contrast, *delayed* haemolytic problems should be anticipated when group O bone marrow, with the capacity to form anti-A, anti-B, is transplanted into non-O recipients.

The following investigations are suggested:

- *ABO typing* including A subtyping of group A donors (in order to identify A_2 subtypes who may form anti-A_1).
- *Titration of anti-A, anti-B* in both donor and recipient serum at room temperature (for IgM agglutinins and haemolysins) and by antiglobulin methods at 37 °C (for IgG antibodies).

Prevention of haemolytic transfusion reactions (major ABO incompatibilities)

It may be necessary to aspirate up to 2 l of blood and marrow mixture from the donor and this clearly cannot be infused into the recipient without a risk of severe intravascular haemolysis. Two approaches are possible:

(1) *Removal of red cells from the donor marrow:*[59,60] this procedure is the favoured approach. Combined use of centrifugal cell washers, sedimenting agents such as hydroxyethyl starch or Ficoll gradients allows removal of almost all red cells while still retaining 60–70% of nucleated cells. The final volume of the marrow suspension can be reduced to below 200 ml for infusion. Marrow suspensions in this form are suitable for T cell removal procedures (see section 3.8). Potentially haemolytic donor antibodies are also removed by this process.
(2) *Plasmapheresis* of recipients with high antibody levels (e.g. agglutinating titres greater than 16): in practice it has proved difficult to reduce titres sufficiently to ensure that there will be no post-transfusion haemolysis.[61]

Following transplantation of ABO-incompatible marrow

Where donor marrow carries antigens not shared by recipient, e.g. A, B or AB donor, group O recipient, the following should be monitored:

(1) *Anti-A and anti-B titres:*[57] these antibodies are no longer produced by the ablated recipient marrow and the residues are absorbed by donor tissues. The titres fall progressively and are usually undetectable after 4 weeks.
(2) *The direct antiglobulin test on circulating red cells:* successful engraftment may be associated with a transient mild haemolytic state as residual anti-A or anti-B alloantibodies of the recipient are bound to newly formed red cells of donor marrow origin.
(3) *Reticulocyte counts* should be performed in addition to routine blood counts.

(4) *Red cell ABO status* to indicate the extent of replacement by donor marrow red cells: mixed field reactions are likely especially if transfusions have been given.

Transplantation into ABO- and/or Rh-incompatible recipients (minor incompatibilities)

Where the donor lacks recipient antigens, e.g. group O donor, A, B or AB recipient or Rh D-negative marrow to Rh-positive recipients, immunocompetent cells, transfused with the marrow graft, may form anti-A, B or anti-D respectively to produce a transient but sometimes severe 'autoimmune' haemolytic state affecting the original recipient red cells.[57,58] Donor marrow may also form antibodies to other potentially incompatible host blood group systems[62] for up to 1 year post transplantation.

Selection of blood for transfusion[63]

Red cell transfusions *must be compatible with the recipient's serum.* Group O red cell concentrates (which do not provide a further source of isoagglutinins) may have to be used during the first week or so. *Thereafter transfusions should be of the donor ABO group and all records should be amended to indicate acquisition of the new blood group. Platelet or plasma transfusions should where possible be compatible with the donor ABO group.*

Rh groups   Rh D-negative red cells should be given following an Rh D-negative marrow donation.

3.7   Monitoring Engraftment

After successful allogeneic transplantation, donor-derived haemopoietic cells should progressively replace those of recipient origin. Alternatively, there may be re-emergence of recipient cell lineages. If these show continuous progression relapse is likely; however, in some instances a stable state of chimerism appears to develop which may not necessarily be indicative of poor prognosis.

Routine blood counts and reticulocyte counts

Successful grafts show:

- Leucocyte counts greater than $1 \times 10^9/l$.
- Neutrophil counts greater than $0.5 \times 10^9/l$.
- Platelet counts greater than $30 \times 10^9/l$.
- Reticulocyte counts greater than 1%, usually between 2 and 3 weeks following transplantation.

The progress of engraftment is somewhat slower with T cell-depleted grafts.

Serological evidence

If extensive red cell phenotyping of both the donor and the recipient is performed before transplantation, the emergence of new cells of donor marrow origin may be detected. Red cell transfusions of course make this assessment more difficult. Study of the polymorphisms for other blood cells, for immunoglobulins or marrow donor origin, for red cell enzymes and for serum protein groups can provide evidence of establishment of the graft. Cytogenetic analysis can also be informative but more recently DNA analysis involving RFLP, PCR or Y chromosome-specific probes (for sex-mismatched grafts) and locus-specific mini-satellite probes[64] have been employed to permit sensitive detection of emergent minor cell populations.

Immunological recovery[56]

The severe post-transplant immunosuppression takes some months to recover fully. Lymphocytes usually reach $1 \times 10^9/l$ by 3 months. Cell-mediated immune function (e.g. PHA and MLR responses) and serum immunoglobulin concentrations usually normalize by 12–24 months. Recovery of immune competence remains severely impaired in the presence of chronic GVHD.

3.8   Graft-versus-host Disease and T Cell Removal[60,65-68]

GVHD from the transplant

GVHD is due to donor marrow T cells recognizing minor histocompatibility antigens of the recipient and responding by producing cytotoxic lymphocytes. These cause widespread tissue injury, and damaging effects are particularly evident in the skin, gastrointestinal tract, bone marrow, lymph nodes, liver and kidneys. Both *acute* and *chronic* forms occur.

Mild GVHD may have some value in suppressing residual leukaemic tissue and, for unexplained reasons, facilitating more prompt engraftment; but generally, acute GVHD presents a serious threat to survival, and various chemotherapeutic approaches (e.g. methotrexate, cyclosporin A) or immunological methods (e.g. antilymphocyte globulin, intravenous immunoglobulin) have been used to control it.

It has been shown that GVHD can be considerably ameliorated by removal of T cells from the donor marrow.[67] This has been accomplished by using:

(1) Heterologous (prepared from other species) complement-fixing and lytic anti-T-cell sera.
(2) Monoclonal complement-fixing and lytic anti-T-cell antibodies alone.
(3) A variety of other methods including 'cocktails' of monoclonal antibodies complexed with cell toxins, e.g. ricin, and plant lectins such as soya bean agglutinin.

Some delay in the speed of graft recovery has been noted with T cell-depleted marrow and there is a greater likelihood of rejection; these problems have tempered enthusiasm for routine T cell depletion. Since GVHD represents a major barrier to use of less 'compatible' tissue-matched donors, the procedure of T cell removal could, if these problems were to be overcome, offer great potential in widening the selection of possible donors. New donor T cells eventually differentiate from the transplanted marrow to restore normal immune function.

Intravenous immunoglobulin has also been shown to reduce morbidity due to acute GVHD in addition to its use for prophylaxis of septicaemia and interstitial pneumonia (see chapter 9).

GVHD from blood transfusions[69]

GVHD can also follow the transfusion of immunocompetent cells in blood components. For this reason all transfusions must be irradiated. Doses of 25 Gy are generally given. Secure arrangements must be established for ensuring that all potentially 'risky' blood components are labelled to show that they have been irradiated.

GVHD is not normally a risk of autologous marrow transplants, but it may happen following administration of unirradiated blood components to patients who have been immunosuppressed and transplanted, especially if total nodal irradiation has been given.

3.9   Collection of the Bone Marrow Graft[70]

This is obtained by means of multiple needle aspirations principally from the posterior iliac crest and also, if necessary, from the anterior iliac spine and the sternum. A dose of at least 3×10^8 nucleated cells per kilogram is desirable. Cell counts can be determined during the graft collection, but it is necessary to make allowance for the nucleated cell count of the peripheral blood which inevitably contaminates the marrow sample. Volumes of between 200 ml and 2 l may be required to obtain sufficient nucleated cells. The heparinized marrow cell suspension is filtered and transferred to specially designed plastic blood pack assemblies to allow subsequent manipulations.

Table 8   Assessment of the collected marrow sample

Total volume
Red cell count/Hct
Mononuclear cell count
Haemopoietic progenitor cell assays
(e.g. CFU-GM/BFU-E)
Immuno-phenotyping assay of CD34-positive cells
Bacterial culture

CFU-GM, granulocyte–macrophage colony-forming unit; BFU-E, erythroid burst-forming unit.

In view of the fact that recipients are immunosuppressed and neutropenic, and that febrile episodes are common in the post-graft period, it is important to take all feasible measures to avoid microbial contamination.

3.10 Potential Donor Problems[71]

The risks and possible complications of the procedure should be clearly explained to the prospective donor in order to allow them to give fully informed consent. Marrow collection is usually performed under general anaesthesia but spinal block epidural anaesthesia can be used.

In a large analysis of over 1000 marrow donations:[71]

- 0.5% had life-threatening complications (cerebrovascular accidents, cardio-pulmonary problems, septicaemia).
- 10% had considerable local pain, sometimes transient neuropathia due to haematoma.
- 10% had post-operative febrile episodes.

Autologous blood (one or two units) is sometimes collected from the donor during the preceding 2 weeks and reinfused postoperatively to compensate for the volume lost at the time of marrow collection. In this series random donor blood was also required for some donors.

3.11 Peripheral Blood Haemopoietic Stem Cell Transplantation[72]

Normally, peripheral blood contains very small numbers of the pluripotential stem cells capable of long-term haemopoietic reconstitution. Their numbers can be greatly increased in patients following cytotoxic therapy or by the use of recombinant myeloid growth factors and even more so by a combination of both. In principle the approach involves:

(1) *Stem cell mobilization*: rebound of marrow proliferative activity after cytotoxic therapy (e.g. cyclophosphamide 1.5–$7 \, \text{g/m}^2$) is followed by release of large numbers of pluripotential cells (granulocyte–macrophage colony-forming units CFU-GM) into the circulation. Recombinant growth factors, most typically rHu G-CSF or rHu GM-CSF (recombinant granulocyte or granulocyte–macrophage stimulating factor) factor can be used to flush out even larger increases of precursor cells so that leukapheresis yields can reach those of conventional bone marrow harvests.

(2) *Stem cell collection*: the lymphocyte fraction of peripheral blood is harvested by suitably modified leukapheresis procedures and stored frozen until required. Several consecutive collections are usually undertaken to ensure an adequate CFU-GM/CD34-positive cell yield. Timing of the collection following bone marrow stimulation is problematic. Stem cell assays cannot be employed on a day-to-day basis as a guide to the most fruitful collection time. A rising mononuclear cell count can be a surrogate marker for the arrival of adequate

numbers of peripheral blood stem cells. CD34 cells, which are identified by immunophenotyping, appear to equate closely with CFU-GM precursors. Assay of CD34 cells might therefore give a good indication of the time to harvest peripheral blood stem cells.

Peripheral blood stem cell grafts appear to offer several advantages:

(1) Easier, safer and less traumatic collections.
(2) Haemopoietic reconstitution occurs more quickly (e.g. neutrophils $>0.5 \times 10^9$ by day 11, and platelet counts $>50 \times 10^9$ by day 13, i.e. about 10 days earlier than seen with autologous bone marrow transplants).
(3) The earlier bone marrow recovery reduces clinical morbidity and consequently the need for blood product support and the duration of hospital stay.
(4) There may be less risk of tumour cell contamination than with autologous bone marrow transplants.

Peripheral blood stem cell collections are now extensively used for autologous transplantation. Their role in volunteer allogeneic transplantation has not yet been established. Occasionally peripheral blood stem cells (PBSC), collected after growth factor stimulation, have been used to provide a second dose of stem cells when bone marrow engraftment is delayed. Although the collection technique, e.g. by leukapheresis, would be undoubtedly preferred by volunteer donors, safety of the routine use of growth factors needs to be agreed.

4 TRANSPLANTATION OF OTHER ORGANS

Experience is now steadily growing of successful cardiac transplants, combined heart–lung transplants as well as those involving pancreatic tissues[73] and the liver.[74,75] While there may well be differences in tissue-matching requirements for different organs there is as yet too little clinical information to draw firm conclusions. It must be assumed, therefore, that donor selection procedures should, under ideal circumstances, follow those established for renal transplantation. Many organ transplants are performed as an emergency life-saving procedure when clinically satisfactory grafts become available. Under such circumstances the quality of HLA matching is usually regarded as being of secondary importance.

4.1 Cardiac Transplantation

ABO compatibility is essential for cardiac transplants[76] and the lymphocytotoxic cross-match should be negative; retrospective analyses have shown prognosis of cardiac transplants to correlate with HLA -A, -B and particularly with -DR match quality.[77,94] As with renal transplants, positive cross-matches are liable to result in hyperacute rejection. Patients have, however, been grafted in the presence of positive cross-matches, but measures such as plasma exchange and more intensive immunosuppression are necessary.[78] Blood component usage for heart transplants and heart–lung transplants are substantial, particularly where patients have coagulopathy secondary to hepatic congestion and patients in whom previous cardiothoracic surgery or transplantation has been performed. Improvements in technical proficiency have reduced mean blood component usage. Recently published experience from the USA[75] provided mean figures of eight red cell units, four FFP units and five platelet concentrates with a simultaneous reduction in the demands for *fresh* blood!

4.2 Liver Transplantation

Liver transplantation is applied increasingly to the treatment of those chronic liver disorders that culminate in irreversible liver failure. A smaller proportion of cases of subacute or fulminant hepatic failure have also been successfully transplanted. In all instances transplantation is used only as a last resort, after failure of all other possible lines of treatment. Overall success rates seem to be higher in younger patients. One-year survivals have been reported to be of the order of 44%[80] to 72%[81] which is substantially better than those expected without transplantation. However, peri-operative mortality, in many cases due to blood loss, has been as high as 40% in combined data from European and American transplant centres.

Blood transfusion support

Liver transplantation programmes have a major effect on transfusion services, mainly because of the massive blood transfusion support that is required. Blood consumption figures of 20–40 units per case were not unusual in the early years of liver transplantation programmes and were supplemented by 10–20 donor units of both fresh frozen plasma and platelet concentrates. Mean red cell usage has now improved to around 10–20 units per case.[82] Substantial improvements in blood conservation had been achieved using high-capacity red cell salvage procedures; the techniques may be life-saving if massive exsanguination occurs.

Blood loss figures have been shown to correlate inversely with survival; in one centre median figures of 7.5 l and 25 l occurred in survivors and non-survivors respectively,[83] and similar findings have been reported by others.[84] In some instances severe haemorrhagic diathesis, due to excessive fibrinolysis, occurs during the anhepatic phase of surgery.[85] Poor pre-surgical coagulation status appears to indicate an adverse prognosis and in some patients restoration of blood perfusion of the transplanted liver appears to have precipitated coagulation failure and massive bleeding.

Recipients are frequently transplanted only when they reach a critical state (all other treatments having failed); this, coupled with the difficulties of organ procurement, has meant that the timing of transplants has often been unpredictable. Adding this problem to the tremendous variability in need for blood and fresh components restricts the procedure of liver transplantation to the relatively few hospitals that can obtain large quantities of transfusion materials at short notice. It is absolutely essential that careful planning to ensure the availability of blood precedes the inception of liver transplantation programmes. Failure to do this is irresponsible and places blood supplies to all other hospital patients severely at risk. In order to avoid the massive drain on transfusion materials, and misuse of voluntary donations, it is necessary to try to determine the factors which identify high-risk operative cases. These might include those with severe chronically impaired coagulation tests, and certainly those involving a significant degree of disseminated intravascular coagulation. Patients with primary biliary cirrhosis or carcinoma have been found to need only half the amount of blood transfusion support that was required for those with hepatitis, cirrhosis or sclerosing cholangitis complicated by portal hypertension.[84]

Bleeding from oesophageal varices or intestinal bleeding from other causes are common problems faced by potential graft recipients.

The *coagulation disturbances* of liver disease have been discussed in chapter 18, section 4. Clearly attempts to maintain adequate haemostatic performance should follow the principles discussed for management of acute blood loss (chapter 11) and massive transfusion (chapter 12), subject to the availability of fresh blood components.

Serological management should also follow that suggested for massive acute blood loss (chapter 12, section 5.3). Where alloantibodies are present their existence may be safely disregarded after exchange of one blood volume if massive loss continues.[84] However, when the rate of blood replacement slows and the end of transfusion seems in sight, substitution of 'antigen-negative' blood may again be appropriate.

ABO compatibility is normally sought for liver transplants. ABO mismatched grafts have been performed, but survival is substantially worse.[86]

Transient haemolytic episodes have been seen in non-group O recipients given group O transplants.[87] These have been ascribed to ABO alloantibodies produced by group O donor lymphocytes and are similar to those reported following renal transplantation[13] and splenic transplantation.[88] Because of the high incidence (25–50%) of this phenomenon, prophylactic use of donor type red cells during surgery has been suggested.[89] Immune haemolysis due to antibodies in Rh as well as non-Rh blood group systems[90,91] has been reported in ABO-compatible matches. Haemolysis has generally occurred within 1–2 weeks following transplantation and subsided after a further 2–3 weeks.

Fortunately, HLA match quality does not appear to influence graft survival. The finding of a positive cross-match is important[92] and although for practical reasons it cannot determine whether grafts are used or not, it may have a bearing on how much immunosuppressive treatment is needed.

4.3 Corneal Transplantation

Corneal transplantation has been an established procedure for many years, and even in this situation there is some evidence that better outcome is achieved for high-risk patients (i.e. previous graft failures) when good HLA matching is achieved).[79]

REFERENCES

1 Terasaki, P.I. (1991) Histocompatibility testing in transplantation. *Arch. Pathol. Lab. Med.*, **115**: 250–254.

2 Ratner, L.E., Gregg, A.H. and Hanto, D.W. (1991) Immunology of renal allograft rejection. *Arch. Pathol. Lab. Med.*, **115**: 283–287.

3 Bodmer, J.G., Marsh, S.G.E., Albert, E.D. *et al.* (1994) Nomenclature for factors of the HLA system. *Tissue Antigens*, **44**: 1–18.

4 Bidwell, J. (1994) Advances in DNA-based HLA-typing methods. *Immunology Today*, **15**: 303–307.

5 Tiercy, J.M., Jeannet, M. and Mach, B. (1990) A new approach for the analysis of HLA class II polymorphism: 'HLA oligotyping'. *Blood Rev.*, **4**: 9–15.

6 Olerup, O. and Zetterquist, H. (1992) HLA-DR typing by PCR amplification with sequence-specific primers (PCR-SSP) in 2 hours: an alternative to serological DR typing in clinical practice including donor–recipient matching in cadaveric transplants. *Tissue Antigens*, **39**: 225–235.

7 Tiwari, L. and Terasaki, P.I. (1985) *HLA and Disease Associations*. New York: Springer-Verlag.

8 Lundgren, G., Albrechtsen, D., Flatmark, A. *et al.* (1986) HLA-matching and pre-transplant blood transfusions in cadaveric renal transplantation: a changing picture with cyclosporin. *Lancet*, **ii**: 66–69.

9 Persijn, G.G., Schreuder, G.M. Th., Hendriks, G.F.H., Cohen, B., D'Amaro, J. and van Rood, J.J. (1986) Cyclosporin, HLA matching, and transfusions in kidney transplants. *Lancet*, **ii**: 915.

10 Opelz, G. (1988) Importance of HLA antigen splits for kidney transplant matching. *Lancet*, **ii**: 106–107.

11 Takemoto, S., Terasaki, P.I., Cecka, J.M., Cho, Y.W. and Gjertson, D.W. (1992) Survival of nationally shared, HLA-matched kidney transplants from cadaveric donors. *N. Engl. J. Med.*, **327**: 834–839.

12 Gjertson, D.W., Terasaki, P.I., Takemoto, S. and Mickey, M.R. (1991) National allocation of cadaveric kidneys by HLA matching: projected effect on outcome and costs. *N. Engl. J. Med.*, **324**: 1032–1036.

13 Bevan, P.C., Seaman, M., Tolliday, B. and Chalmers, D.G. (1985) ABO haemolytic anaemia in transplanted patients. *Vox Sang.*, **49**: 42–48.

14 Kerman, R.H. (1991) The role of crossmatching in organ transplantation. *Arch. Pathol. Lab. Med.*, **115**: 255–259.

15 Wick, M.R., Delong, E.N. and Moore, S.B. (1985) Passively acquired antibody directed human erythrocytes seen during therapy with Minnesota antilymphoblast globulin. *Vox Sang.*, **48**: 229–234.

16 Ballas, S.K., Draper, E.K. and Dignam, C.M. (1985) Pre-transfusion testing problems caused by anti-lymphocyte globulin and their solution. *Transfusion*, **25**: 254–256.

17 Editorial (1989) Antibodies as a barrier to kidney transplantation. *Lancet*, **ii**: 357.

18 *UKTSSA Users' Bulletin* (1993) Organ donation 1989–1992: where is the decline? Issue no. 8.

19 Palmer, A., Welsh, K., Gjorstrup, P., Taube, D., Bewick, M. and Thick, M. (1989) Removal of Anti-HLA antibodies by extracorporeal immunoadsorption to enable renal transplantation. *Lancet*, **ii**: 10–12.

20 Opelz, G. (1985) Current relevance of the transfusion effect in renal transplantation. *Transplant. Proc.*, **17**: 1015–1021.

21 Ross, W.B. and Yap, P.L. (1990) Blood transfusion and organ transplantation. *Blood Rev.*, **4**: 252–258.

22 Moore, S.B., Sterioff, S., Pierides, A.M., Watts, S. and Ruud, C. (1984) Transfusion-induced alloimmunization in patients awaiting renal allografts. *Vox Sang.*, **47**: 354–361.

23 van Twuyer, E., Mooijaart, R.J.D., ten Berge, I.J.M. *et al.* (1991) Pretransplantation blood transfusion revisited. *N. Engl. J. Med.*, **325**: 1210–1213.

24 Lazda, V.A., Pollak, R., Mozes, M.F., Barber, P.L. and Jonasson, O. (1990) Evidence that

HLA class II disparity is required for the induction of renal allograft enhancement by donor-specific blood transfusions in man. *Transplantation,* **49:** 1084–1087.

25 Nagarkatti, P.S., Joseph, S. and Singal, D.P. (1984) Blood transfusion and antiidiotypic immunity. *Transplant. Proc.,* **16:** 1407–1409.

26 Opelz, G. (1989) The role of HLA matching and blood transfusions in the cyclosporine era. *Transplant. Proc.,* **21:** 609–612.

27 McCullough, J. (1991) The role of the blood bank in transplantation. *Arch. Pathol. Lab. Med.,* **115:** 1195–1200.

28 Anasetti, C. (1991) The role of the immunogenetics laboratory in marrow transplantation. *Arch. Pathol. Lab. Med.,* **115:** 288–292.

29 Stroncek, D.F. (1991) Review: results of bone marrow transplants from unrelated donors. *Transfusion,* **32:** 180–189.

30 Kernan, N.A., Bartsch, G., Ash, R.C. *et al.* (1993) Analysis of 462 transplantations from unrelated donors facilitated by the National Marrow Donor Program. *N. Engl. J. Med.,* **328:** 593–602.

31 Hows, J.M. (1991) Paediatric bone marrow transplantation using donors other than HLA genotypically identical siblings. *Arch. Dis. Child.,* **66:** 546–550.

32 Gajewski, J., Cecka, M. and Champlin, R. (1990) Bone marrow transplantation utilizing HLA-matched unrelated marrow donors. *Blood Rev.,* **4:** 132–138.

33 Locatelli, F., Porta, F., Zecca, M. *et al.* (1993) Successful bone marrow transplantation in children with severe aplastic anaemia using HLA partially matched family donors. *Am. J. Hematol.,* **42:** 328–333.

34 de Witte, T. (1993) Bone marrow transplantation for myelodysplastic syndrome and secondary leukaemias. *Br. J. Haematol.,* **84:** 361–364.

35 Greinix, H.T., Storb, R., Sanders, J.E. *et al.* (1993) Long-term survival and cure after marrow transplantation for congenital hypoplastic anaemia (Diamond–Blackfan syndrome). *Br. J. Haematol.,* **84:** 515–520.

36 Ljungman, P., de Witte, T., Verdonck, L. *et al.* (1992) Bone marrow transplantation for acute myeloblastic leukaemia: an EBMT Leukaemia Working Party prospective analysis from HLA typing. *Br. J. Haematol.,* **84:** 61–66.

37 Pendry, K., Alcorn, M.J. and Burnett, A.K. (1993) Factors influencing haematological recovery in 53 patients with acute myeloid leukaemia in first remission after autologous bone marrow transplantation. *Br. J. Haematol.,* **83:** 45–52.

38 Herzig, R.H., Bortin, M.M., Barrett, A.J. *et al.* (1987) Bone marrow transplantation in high-risk acute lymphoblastic leukaemia in first and second remission. *Lancet,* **i:** 786–789.

39 Friedrich, W., Vetter, U., Heymer, B. *et al.* (1984) Immunoreconstitution in severe combined immunodeficiency after transplantation of HLA-haploidentical, T-cell-depleted bone marrow. *Lancet,* **i:** 761–764.

40 Baranger, J.A. (1984) Marrow transplantation in genetic disease. *N. Engl. J. Med.,* **311:** 1629–1630.

41 Pyeritz, R.E. (1984) Treatment of inborn errors of metabolism by transplantation. *Nature,* **312:** 405–406.

42 Fischer, A., Friedrich, W., Levinsky, R. *et al.* (1986) Bone marrow transplantation for immunodeficiencies and osteopetrosis: European survey, 1968–1985. *Lancet,* **ii:** 1080–1083.

43 Kohli-Kumar, M., Shahidi, N.T., Broxmeyer, H.E. *et al.* (1993) Haemopoietic stem/progenitor cell transplant in Fanconi anaemia using HLA matched sibling umbilical cord blood cells. *Br. J. Haematol.,* **85:** 419–422.

44 Lucarelli, G., Galimberti, M., Polchi, P. *et al.* (1993) Marrow transplantation in patients with thalassemia responsive to iron chelation therapy. *N. Engl. J. Med.,* **329:** 840–844.

45 Davies, S.C. (1993) Bone marrow transplant for sickle cell disease: the dilemma. *Blood Rev.,* **7:** 4–9.

46 Vermylen, C. and Cornu, G. (1993) Bone marrow transplantation in sickle cell anaemia. *Blood Rev.,* **7:** 1–3.

47 Gorin, N.C., Gale, R.P. and Armitage, J.O. (1989) Autologous bone marrow transplants: different indications in Europe and North America. *Lancet,* 317–318.

48 Gale, R.P. and Champlin, R.E. (1984) How does bone marrow transplantation cure leukaemia? *Lancet*, **ii**: 28–30.
49 Beatty, P.G., Dahlberg, S., Mickelson, E.M. *et al.* (1988) Probability of finding HLA-matched unrelated marrow donors. *Transplantation*, **45**: 714–718.
50 Gale, R.P. and Butturini, A. (1989) Autotransplants in leukaemia. *Lancet*, **ii**: 315–317.
51 Hows, J.M., Bradley, B.A., Marsh, J.C.W. *et al.* (1992) Growth of human umbilical-cord blood in longterm haemopoietic cultures. *Lancet*, **340**: 73–76.
52 Watson, J.G. (1983) Problems of infection after bone marrow transplantation. *J. Clin. Pathol.*, **36**: 683–692.
53 Deeg, H.J., Storb, R. and Thomas, E.D. (1984) Bone marrow transplantation: a review of delayed complications. *Br. J. Haematol.*, **57**: 185–208.
54 Smith, O.P., Prentice, H.G., Hazlehurst, G., Brozovic, B., Hoffbrand, A.V. and Mehta, A.B. (1991) Blood product support in patients undergoing chemotherapy and autologous or allogeneic bone marrow transplantation for haematological malignancies. *Clin. Lab. Haematol.*, **13**: 107–114.
55 Anderson, K.C. (1992) The role of the blood bank in hematopoietic stem cell transplantation. *Transfusion*, **32**: 272–280.
56 Lum, L.G. (1987) The kinetics of immune reconstitution after human marrow transplantation. *Blood*, **69**: 369–380.
57 Wernet, D. and Mayer, G. (1992) Isoagglutinins following ABO-incompatible bone marrow transplantation. *Vox Sang.*, **62**: 176–179.
58 Hows, J., Beddow, K., Gordon-Smith, E. *et al.* (1986) Donor-derived red blood cell antibodies and immune hemolysis after allogeneic bone marrow transplantation. *Blood*, **67**: 177–181.
59 Winston, G.H., Champlin, R.E., Feig, S.A. and Gale, R.P. (1984) Transplantation of ABH incompatible bone marrow: gravity sedimentation of donor marrow. *Br. J. Haematol.*, **57**: 155–162.
60 Jones, H.M., Linch, D.C., Marcus, R.E., Singer, C.R. and Goldstone, A.H. (1984) Red cell removal from donor bone marrow. *Br. J. Haematol.*, **58**: 553–555.
61 Ockelford, P.A., Hill, R.S., Nelson, L., Blacklock, H.A., Woodfield, D.G. and Matthews, J.R.D. (1982) Serological complications of a major ABO incompatible bone marrow transplantation in a Polynesian with aplastic anaemia. *Transfusion*, **22**: 62–65.
62 Ting, A., Pun, A., Dodds, A.J., Atkinson, K. and Biggs, J.C. (1987) Red cell alloantibodies produced after bone marrow transplantation. *Transfusion*, **27**: 145–147.
63 Lasky, L.C., Warkentin, P.I., Kersey, J.H., Ramsay, N.K.C., McGlave, P.B. and McCullough, J. (1983) Haemotherapy in patients undergoing blood group incompatible bone marrow transplantation. *Transfusion*, **23**: 277.
64 Katz, F., Hann, I., Kinsey, S., Ball, S., Morgan, G. and Chessells, J. (1993) Assessment of graft status following allogeneic bone marrow transplantation for haematological disorders in children using locus-specific minisatellite probes. *Br. J. Haematol.*, **83**: 473–479.
65 Ekblom, M., Ruutu, T., Volin, L., Leskinen, R., Renkonen, R. and Hayry, P. (1984) Immunological monitoring of bone marrow transplant recipients. *Scand. J. Haematol.*, **33**: 113–122.
66 Bross, D.S., Tutschka, P.J., Farmer, E.R. *et al.* (1984) Predictive factors for acute graft-versus-host disease in patients transplanted with HLA identical bone marrow. *Blood*, **63**: 1265–1270.
67 Janossy, G. (1984) 'Purging' of bone marrow and immunosuppression. *Br. Med. J.*, **290**: 658–660.
68 Denman, A.M. (1985) Graft versus host diseases: new versions of old problems? *Br. Med. J.*, **290**: 658–660.
69 Linden, J.V. and Pisciotto, P.T. (1982) Transfusion-associated graft-versus-host-disease and blood irradiation. *Transfusion Med. Rev.*, **6**: 116–123.
70 BCSH (1994) Guidelines for the collection, processing and storage of human bone marrow and peripheral stem cells for transplantation. In: Wood, J.K. (ed.), *Standard Haematology Practice*, Vol. 2. Oxford: Blackwells.

71 Buckner, C.D., Clift, R.A., Sanders, J.E. *et al.* (1984) Marrow harvesting from normal donors. *Blood*, **64**: 630–634.
72 Craig, J.I.O., Turner, M.L. and Parker, A.C. (1992) Peripheral blood stem cell transplantation. *Blood Rev.*, **6**: 59–67.
73 Sells, R.A. and Brynger, H. (1987) Progress in pancreatic transplantations. *Lancet*, i: 1024–1025.
74 Neuberger, J. (1987) When should patients be referred for liver transplantation? *Br. Med. J.*, **295**: 565.
75 Hunt, B.J., Sack, D., Amin, S. and Yacoub, M.H. (1992) The perioperative use of blood components during heart and heart–lung transplantation. *Transfusion*, **32**: 57–62.
76 Terasaki, P.I. (1991) Red cell crossmatching for heart transplants. *N. Engl. J. Med.*, **325**: 1748–1749.
77 Hendriks, G.F.J., v. Steenberge, E.P.M., Schreuder, G.M.Th. *et al.* (1988) Treatment with cyclosporin and risks of graft rejection in male kidney and heart transplant recipients with non-O blood. *Br. Med. J.*, **297**: 888–890.
78 Ippoliti, G., Lazzaro, A., Martinelli, L. and Vigano, M. (1988) Heart transplantation and performed cytotoxic antibodies. *Lancet*, i: 51–52.
79 Sanfilippo, F., MacQueen, J.M., Vaughn, W.K. and Foulks, G.N. (1986) Reduced graft rejection with good HLA-A, and B matching in high-risk corneal transplantation. *N. Engl. J. Med.*, **315**: 29–35.
80 Bismuth, H., Ericzon, B.G., Rolles, K. *et al.* (1987) Hepatic transplantation in Europe. First report of the European Liver Transplant Registry. *Lancet*, ii: 674–676.
81 Busuttil, R.W., Memsic, L.D.F., Quinones-Baldrich, W., Hiatt, J.R. and Ramming, K.P. (1986) Liver transplantation at UCLA: program development, organization, initiation, and early results. *Am. J. Surg.*, **152**: 75–80.
82 Lewis, J.H., Bontempo, F.A., Cornell, F. *et al.* (1987) Blood use in liver transplantation. *Transfusion*, **27**: 222–225.
83 Krom, R.A.F., Gips, C.W., Houthoff, H.J. *et al.* (1984) Orthotopic liver transplantation in Groningen, The Netherlands (1979–1983). *Hepatology*, **4**: 61–65.
84 Butler, P., Israel, L., Nusbacher, J., Jenkins, D.E. and Starzl, T.E. (1985) Blood transfusion in liver transplantation. *Transfusion*, **25**: 120–123.
85 Dzik, W.H., Arkin, C.F., Jenkins, R.L. and Stump, D.C. (1988) Fibrinolysis during liver transplantation in humans: role of tissue type plasminogen activator. *Blood*, **71**: 1090–1095.
86 Gugenheim, J., Samuel, D., Reynes, M. and Bismuth, H. (1990) Liver transplantation across ABO blood group barriers. *Lancet*, **336**: 519–523.
87 Ramsey, G., Nusbacher, J.M., Starzle, T.E. and Lindsay, G. (1984) Isohemagglutinins of graft origin after ABO-unmatched liver transplantation. *N. Engl. J. Med.*, **311**: 1167–1170.
88 Salamon, D.J., Ramsey, G., Nusbacher, J., Yang, S., Starzle, T.E. and Israel, L. (1985) Anti-A production by a group O spleen transplanted to a group A recipient. *Vox Sang.*, **48**: 309–312.
89 Triulzi, D.J., Shirey, R.S., Ness, P.M. and Klein, A.S. (1992) Immunohematologic complications of ABO-unmatched liver transplants. *Transfusion*, **32**: 829–833.
90 Hyma, B.A., Moore, S.B., Grande, J.P. *et al.*' (1988) Delayed immune hemolysis in a patient receiving cyclosporine after orthotopic liver transplantation. *Transfusion*, **28**: 276–279.
91 Kim, B.K., Whitsett, C.F. and Hillyer, C.D. (1992) Donor origin Rh antibodies as a cause of significant hemolysis following ABO-identical orthotopic liver transplantation. *Immunohematology*, **8**: 100–101.
92 Katz, S.M., Kimball, P.M., Ozaki, C. *et al.* (1994) Positive pretransplant crossmatches predict early graft loss in liver allograft recipients. *Transplantation*, **57**: 616–620.
93 Scornik, J.C., Brunson, M.E., Schaub, B., Howard, R.J. and Pfaff, W.W. (1994) The crossmatch in renal transplantation. *Transplantation*, **57**: 621–625.
94 De Mattos, A.M., Head, M.A., Everett, J. *et al.* (1994) HLA-DR mismatching correlates with early cardiac allograft rejection, incidence, and graft survival when high-confidence-level serological DR typing is used. *Transplantation*, **57**: 626–630.

Part G
TRANSFUSION
COMPLICATIONS

23
Harmful Effects of Transfusion

Until the advent of acquired immunodeficiency syndrome (AIDS) as a transfusion problem, the safety of blood transfusion was all too often taken for granted. Indeed, even taking this new development into account, transfusion still appears to be relatively safe compared with the risks of many other concurrent medical or surgical treatments that a patient may be receiving. It is, however, not entirely risk free even when all reasonable precautions are taken to reduce mishaps. Transfusions should, therefore, only be given when a clear benefit to the patient can be anticipated. It is most important that all adverse reactions are fully documented, and signed records should be made of all clinical observations and of the results of investigations that are carried out to determine their causes. Since a degree of risk is inescapable with any transfusion procedure, it is best to ensure that patients are fully informed about the need for transfusion whenever possible.

The major categories of transfusion complications include the following:

(1) *Transmitted infection*: blood is potentially an effective vehicle for transmission of a considerable variety of infective organisms. This topic is covered in chapter 24.
(2) *Haemolytic transfusion reactions*: these are mainly due to the destruction of incompatible donor red cells by antibodies in the recipient's circulation.
(3) *Non-haemolytic transfusion reactions*: these usually result from reactions between various other antigenic constituents in donor blood (e.g. leucocytes or plasma proteins) and pre-formed antibodies in the recipient's circulation.
(4) *Iron overload*: this is an almost inescapable consequence of long-term transfusion regimens. Its progression can, however, be considerably slowed if not arrested by iron chelation therapy (see chapter 4, section 2.1).
(5) *Volume overload*: the very old and the very young, the severely anaemic, and those already in cardiac failure must be transfused with particular care. This is discussed in chapter 18, section 2.
(6) *Adult respiratory distress syndrome*: Pulmonary damage from microaggregates of fibrin, leucocytes and platelets has been blamed for pulmonary failure and death during massive transfusions. The various mechanisms causing pulmonary damage are considered in chapter 13.
(7) *Massive transfusion risks*: these include a variety of haemostatic or metabolic complications and are discussed in chapter 13.

1 RISKS OF DEATH FROM TRANSFUSION

The 328 fatalities that could be ascribed to transfusion over a 10-year period (1976–1985) in the USA have recently been analysed.[1] The overall fatality rate was 3.5 per million units. One hundred and sixty-four were clearly acute haemolytic reactions and of these 131 (48% of the total) were ABO or presumed ABO reactions; around 8% were due to other antibodies and the residue to mishandled and

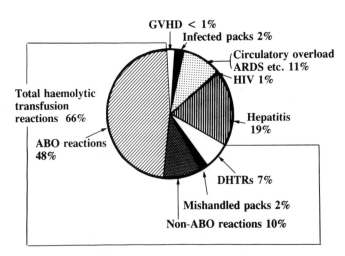

Figure 1   Pie diagram showing principal causes of death

damaged blood or to uncertain causes. Delayed haemolytic reactions accounted for 26 deaths (7%), these usually occurring up to 16 days following transfusion. Deaths from hepatitis in this survey accounted for 19% (68 cases; hepatitis B 26 cases, non-A non-B hepatitis 42 cases) and AIDS 1% (three cases) but these were regarded by the author as almost certainly an underestimate of the true frequency. Respiratory failure, presumably due either to circulatory overload or anaphylactoid reactions, accounted for 39 deaths (11%), while infected packs (seven cases) and graft-versus-host disease (one case) accounted for the remainder.

This analysis probably slightly underestimates the risks of fatalities since those deaths in which the causes were multiple, and in which transfusion may have only played a part, are probably not reported.

Breakdown of the organizational errors leading to acute haemolytic fatalities[1] showed nearly 54% to be due to administration of blood to the wrong patient, either in the theatre or at the bedside; 96% were due to erroneous identification of samples or request forms during blood collection or ordering. On 29% of occasions confusion occurred within the laboratory; in 13% of these serological mistakes were to blame. In 8% of all cases the source of the error was not clearly ascertained.

A more recent analysis of 104 transfusion errors in New York State[2] confirms that organizational errors remain a serious concern. The likely true incidence of ABO errors (taking account of the presumed non-reporting of 'compatible' ABO mismatches) was estimated to be as high as one in 12 000 red cell transfusions. In fact 54 (one in 33 000) ABO mismatches were reported and the fatality rate was one in 33 000. A recent analysis in the UK[3] showed compliance with management procedures to be the weakest link. All five reported incidents were due entirely to failure to adhere to established safety procedures and again it was concluded that the true frequency of critical incidents is almost certainly higher than that reported.

2 HAEMOLYTIC TRANSFUSION REACTIONS

2.1 Causes

These vary in severity from those that have dramatic, sometimes fatal, consequences to others which become evident only as incidental findings. The potential is, nevertheless, always serious and transfusion procedures must be designed to reduce the risks as far as is practically possible.[69] Haemolytic transfusion reactions detected at the Mayo Clinic occurred at an incidence of around one in 6000 transfusions, with a fatality rate of one in 33 500 transfusions.[4] A noteworthy feature, however, was the low incidence of ABO incompatibilities compared with the more general experience.[1] Serious reactions were largely confined to antibodies of the Kell, Duffy, Kidd and Rh systems. Obviously, the reported incidences depend to a very considerable extent on factors such as the efficiency of notification and the success in determining the causes in each case. While haemolytic transfusion reactions are usually due to antibody-mediated haemolysis of donor blood, this is not always so and other causes must also be considered.

(1) *Mishandled blood packs*: these may be overcooled or overheated through improper storage. Blood should only be stored in refrigerators which have been designed and approved for the purpose. These must include temperature control between $2\,^{\circ}C$ and $6\,^{\circ}C$, together with a continuously monitored warning alarm system. In the UK BS4376 (1991) applies. Poorly designed blood warmers can also damage blood during administration. The supernatant plasma may show haemolysis if blood has been damaged during storage.

(2) The red cells may have been mixed with *hypotonic intravenous fluids*. Dextrose in water or hypotonic saline must not be added to blood,[5] neither should *calcium*-containing solutions such as Ringer's lactate; 0.9% (isotonic) saline is the only acceptable fluid for mixing with blood.

(3) *Infected blood packs* may show visible haemolysis. Transfusion of these is likely to have fatal consequences (see chapter 24, section 13).

(4) Haemolysis of the donor red cells more frequently follows *serological* causes. Of these ABO-mismatched transfusions far outweigh any other as causes of death; these errors should be preventable by strict adherence to correctly laid down identification procedures for blood sample collection and for administration of blood units.

 Almost without exception it is the presence of antibodies in the recipient's circulation that is responsible for causing destruction of incompatible donor red cells. Antibodies in donor blood may be disregarded during routine cross-matching procedures and are of virtually no significance during transfusion. Screening of donor plasma for antibodies may be worthwhile (but only rarely) in otherwise inexplicable cases of haemolytic transfusion reaction.

(5) Haemolysis of the recipient's cells may appear to be precipitated by transfusion in patients with *paroxysmal nocturnal haemoglobinuria* or *glucose 6-phosphate dehydrogenase deficiency*.

2.2 Sites of Red Cell Destruction

The modes of a red cell destruction by antibodies are described in chapter 2, section 5.

(1) Complement-fixing antibodies causing *intravascular haemolysis* produce the most severe symptoms. As much as 1000 ml of ABO-incompatible blood may, for example, be destroyed almost as rapidly as it is transfused. Antibodies that do not fix complement, or where complement activation does not proceed beyond the C3b stage, lead to clearance of the incompatible cells from the circulation by reticuloendothelial macrophages. Paradoxically, some Rh antibodies which do not fix complement *in vitro* do appear to be capable of intravascular haemolysis.[6–8]

(2) *Extravascular haemolysis*: this is usually a slower process occurring over some hours. The reticuloendothelial system may sometimes be overwhelmed by large volumes of incompatible cells, and in these circumstances some fragile damaged cells may continue to circulate for a while and some intravascular lysis may occur.

Unfortunately, apart from the realization that 'room temperature only' antibodies are not clinically destructive, the *in vitro* behaviour of antibodies correlates only loosely with their clinical effects. This sometimes acts for the good as on occasions potentially fatal transfusions of group A blood to group O recipients have simply disappeared and been clinically entirely uneventful!

(3) *Delayed haemolytic transfusion reaction* is the term given to the slower haemolysis of donor blood which usually begins within 2–10 days following transfusion. It is described more fully in section 2.6.

2.3 Consequences of Haemolytic Transfusion Reactions[9]

The symptoms described below will usually be most pronounced during severe intravascular haemolysis, less so for extravascular haemolysis and even less evident during delayed reactions.

Patients under *anaesthesia* obviously cannot display symptoms, and recognition of haemolytic reactions may therefore be delayed. Unexplained *hypotension* is an important warning sign. However, hypotension caused by a haemolytic transfusion reaction may be difficult to distinguish from that due to inadequate blood volume replacement.

The effect of the volume transfused

Serious symptoms usually require transfusion of over 25 ml; there may, however, be warnings before this. Minor pyrexial or 'flu-like' symptoms can be noticed with transfusion of as little as 1 ml of blood. For this reason it is most important to begin all non-emergency transfusions slowly, e.g. not more than 1 ml/kg per hour in the first 15 minutes.

Small volumes of incompatible blood are sometimes destroyed more rapidly than larger volumes, presumably because the latter absorb the antibody, dilute the number of antibody molecules available per red cell, or overwhelm the limited phagocytic capacity of the reticuloendothelial tissue.

Symptoms and signs

(1) Pyrexia and rigors.
(2) Faintness and dizziness.
(3) Increased pulse and respiration rate, hypotension.
(4) Pallor and sweating.
(5) Headaches, chest or lumbar pain.
(6) Local pain at the infusion site.
(7) Cyanosis.

In addition to these, disseminated intravascular coagulation and renal failure due to acute tubular necrosis are dangerous sequelae of massive haemolysis.

Pathogenesis

The various symptoms and signs listed above stem from a rather complex set of events. Two aspects predominate:

(1) Disrupted red cells liberate *thromboplastic constituents*, principally stromal lipoproteins, which initiate intravascular coagulation.
(2) Massive *antigen–antibody* reactions and *complement activation* result in formation of anaphylotoxic fragments, e.g. C3a and C5a.

Disseminated intravascular coagulation and complement activation function in various ways to produce pharmacological and pathological havoc. Microthrombi form in the renal afferent arterioles and glomerular capillaries, leading to renal damage. Renal perfusion is further impaired following the release of the vasoconstrictor agent serotonin from damaged platelets. Activated complement products cause histamine release from mast cells, activation of the kinin system to produce bradykinin and of Hageman factor (Factor XIII) to initiate the coagulation mechanism. Increased capillary permeability causes loss of intravascular fluid and this aggravates the hypotension due to the vasodilator effects of bradykinin formation. Hypotension provokes a sympathetic nervous system response (catecholamine release) in the form of vasoconstriction of the visceral circulation along similar lines to the hypotension following acute blood loss. Renal perfusion is thereby further jeopardized, making serious renal failure more likely.

Disturbances to the autonomic nervous system and smooth muscle contraction account for nausea, vomiting, diarrhoea and incontinence of urine and faeces.

2.4 Biochemical Effects of Red Cell Destruction

Intravascular destruction of red cells leads to liberation of free *haemoglobin* in the plasma and of stromal and membrane fragments. Small amounts of haemoglobin are bound by plasma *haptoglobin* (which then becomes reduced in concentration). Haemoglobin is also degraded, the haem binding to albumin to form the pigment *methaemalbumin*, which is detectable spectroscopically and colours the plasma brown. Free plasma haemoglobin levels exceeding 1000 mg/l are followed by visibly obvious excretion in the urine. A late effect of haemoglobinuria is *haemosiderin* in renal tubular cells, produced as a result of reabsorption and later catabolism of haemoglobin molecules. This can be detected by staining for iron in renal tubular cells of the urinary sediment.

Red cells destroyed in extravascular (reticuloendothelial) tissues mainly result in increased plasma *bilirubin* levels. These occur around 6 hours following the onset of haemolysis. Hepatic metabolism of bilirubin leads to increased excretion of urobilinogen in the urine (where it is oxidized to the dark-brown pigment urobilin) and also in the bowel.

2.5   Action to be Taken in the Event of a Serious Haemolytic Transfusion Reaction

(1) *STOP the blood transfusion* but replace with crystalloids or 5% albumin to maintain blood pressure and urine output.

(2) Consult the haematology laboratory. *The senior physician in charge of the case should be notified if it appears that a serious haemolytic transfusion reaction has occurred.*

(3) Institute blood pressure, pulse and urine output chart; catheterize if apparently anuric after 1 hour.

(4) Further management will depend upon results of serology tests, coagulation studies and presence of any evidence that renal damage has occurred.

    (a) If there is evidence that *disseminated intravascular coagulation* has occurred it may be necessary to transfuse fresh blood components, e.g. fresh frozen plasma and platelets. If more than 200 ml of blood have been given and intravascular haemolysis seems to have occurred, heparin should be given as prophylaxis against disseminated intravascular coagulation. Loading doses of 5000 units are usual, followed by 1500 units hourly.

    (b) If a *serious haemolytic transfusion reaction* has taken place the following action may be necessary in anticipation of the development of renal failure:

        (i)   Give 200 ml 20% mannitol i.v.* together with saline or colloids to maintain blood pressure.

        (ii)   Balance intravenous fluids with hourly urine output, in an attempt to maintain an output of 0.5 ml/kg per hour.

        (iii)   If this cannot be achieved, frusemide e.g. 250 mg i.v., may be given.

    (c) *At the bedside the following samples/materials should be obtained*:

        (i)   The blood pack together with the administration set and any other intravenous fluids being given concurrently. Any previously administered blood packs should also be sent to the laboratory.

        (ii)   Blood samples:
- For full blood count including platelets.
- Clotted blood for serological investigation.
- Coagulation test samples.
- Blood cultures.

        (iii)   Aliquots of all urine samples.

    (d) *The laboratory plan is designed to*:

        (i)   Establish that a haemolytic, as opposed to a non-haemolytic, transfusion reaction has occurred.

        (ii)   Exclude *infection* of the blood pack.

        (iii)   Ensure that no *mishandling* of the blood or misuse of coincidental intravenous fluids has occurred.

---

* Note the use of mannitol is not espoused by all renal physicians. Frusemide or ethacrynic acid diuretics are regarded by many as the mainstay for preserving renal output. In any event the advice of a renal physician should be sought at the earliest opportunity if there seems any chance that renal failure might develop.

(iv) If the reaction is completely inexplicable, diagnosis of paroxysmal nocturnal haemoglobinuria or glucose 6-phosphate dehydrogenase deficiency must be considered.

(e) *Laboratory analysis*:

(i) A rapidly centrifuged blood sample (e.g. as for haematocrit determination) will show whether there is any *free plasma haemoglobin*. If there is no plasma discoloration a serious haemolytic transfusion reaction is unlikely to have occurred. Haemoglobin concentrations of 250 mg/l are just visibly recognizable; this amount would correspond to intravascular destruction of only a few millilitres of red cells.

(ii) A *clerical check* must be performed on all the identity details attached to:

- The pre-transfusion blood sample.
- Blood pack compatibility labels.
- Post-transfusion blood samples.

(iii) The *ABO and Rh D* group should be performed on all of the above samples. *If any possibility that a clerical mistake, or a sample handling or blood grouping error has occurred all issues from the blood bank should be halted until it is clear that no other patients are involved.*

(iv) A full *compatibility test* should be performed using both the pre-transfusion and post-transfusion serum samples and red cells from each of the blood packs administered. It may be necessary to include the most sensitive screening and compatibility techniques available, e.g. enzyme-pre-treated cells, low ionic strength antiglobulin tests. In cases of difficulty samples may need to be sent to the local serological reference centre.

(v) The *direct antiglobulin* test should be performed on the recipient's pre-transfusion red cells (if available) and the post-transfusion cells.

(vi) A 2% suspension of the patient's blood in saline should be examined for *visible agglutinates*; also examine the plasma spectroscopically for *haemoglobin* and *methaemalbumin*.

(vii) Inspect urine samples for *haemoglobinuria*. Evidence that a previous episode of haemoglobinuria has occurred can be obtained by staining for haemosiderin in renal tubular cells. This is performed on the centrifuged deposit from urine samples.

(viii) Examine later specimens for *serum bilirubin* and urine and urine urobilinogen. Bilirubin levels are increased by 6 hours following haemolysis.

(ix) If *antibodies* are found these should be identified using an identification panel. Both the patient's and the donor cells should be typed for the antigen concerned. Use the appropriate specific antisera, e.g. anti-K, to examine post-transfusion blood for surviving K^+ cells if a reaction due to anti-K is suspected. If surviving 'incompatible' cells are present there has probably been no clinically significant transfusion reaction!

(x) The *haemoglobin concentrations pre and post transfusion* should be compared. Failure to obtain the anticipated rise (e.g. approximately 1 g haemoglobin per unit transfused) in the absence of bleeding is supportive evidence for a haemolytic transfusion reaction.

(xi) If *bacterial contamination* is suspected samples should be collected aseptically from the blood bag residue; a sealed segment of tubing and blood should also be obtained from the patient. Culture these in blood agar and thioglycolate media at 4 °C, room temperature and 37 °C, using a quantitative technique, so that an estimate of the number of organisms per millilitre is obtained. Examine a Gram-stained film of the bag contents; this will, however, only show a positive result if rampant proliferation of bacteria has occurred in the blood pack.

(xii) Examine later serum samples for evidence of a *rising antibody titre*; a prompt rise indicates that antibodies that were previously present have been boosted by the recent transfusion.

2.6 Delayed Haemolytic Transfusion Reactions

This term defines the haemolysis which occurs only after a period of time, usually between 5 and 10 days, has elapsed since the transfusion. The frequency of such reactions has been estimated to be between $1/1000$[11] and $1/12\,000$ units transfused.[10]

Mild reactions are likely to be missed, especially if they occur in patients who have other reasons for jaundice or falling haemoglobin levels. It is likely that delayed haemolysis is an under-diagnosed event, most episodes occurring in patients who receive repeated transfusions.

The signs and symptoms are not always strikingly obvious but nevertheless it should not be concluded that all delayed reactions are insignificant. Prospective studies have demonstrated that most cases show only laboratory signs of haemolysis.[11] Three important consequences of delayed reactions deserve consideration:

(1) The patient will not derive full benefit from the transfusion.
(2) The metabolic effects of haemolysis may exacerbate underlying problems in patients who are already seriously ill. Renal failure may, for example, be precipitated.
(3) Abnormal haematological and biochemical findings resulting from the haemolysis may necessitate extra investigations until their cause is determined.

Delayed haemolytic reactions can present in several ways.

(1) Clinical signs of a haemolytic transfusion reaction similar to, although less acute than, those described for immediate reactions.
(2) An unexplained fall in haemoglobin values as the transfused blood is destroyed.
(3) Appearance of jaundice, renal failure or the biochemical features associated with immediate transfusion reactions.
(4) Detection of positive direct antiglobulin tests (IgG usually, C3d less

commonly) or unexpected alloantibodies in post-transfusion blood samples. Positive direct antiglobulin reactions are sometimes persistent—well beyond the expected time of cell clearance, for reasons which are not fully explained.[11,12]

Investigation of suspected delayed haemolytic reactions

Delayed reactions are usually due to boosting and emergence of antibodies that were undetectable at the time of the original transfusion. Investigations therefore follow the lines described earlier for transfusion reactions. The practice of keeping pretransfusion sera for a least 2 weeks provides a valuable chance to repeat earlier tests as well as the opportunity to compare pre-transfusion and post-transfusion serum samples. If antibodies are discovered, it may well be worthwhile obtaining further blood samples from the donors concerned in the transfusion to enable complementary studies of the corresponding antigens.

It is possible to overestimate the clinical significance of laboratory findings. If, for example, the 'incompatible' cells are still present in significant numbers in the recipient's circulation it will be unlikely that there has been sufficient haemolysis to affect the patient's clinical condition. There should be clear evidence of incompatible red cell destruction before it is concluded that the serological results are clinically important.

Antibodies associated with delayed haemolytic transfusion reactions

These reactions generally occur as a result of boosting (anamnestic responses) of antibodies.[7,8,10,13,14] Anti-Kidd (anti-Jk^a and -Jk^b) are classical culprits. These are notoriously difficult to detect, may disappear rapidly only to return and cause severe haemolysis a few days after what appear to be apparently compatible transfusions.

Antibodies of the Rh, Kell and Duffy systems have also been associated with these reactions.

3 NON-HAEMOLYTIC REACTIONS

These do not involve red cell destruction but arise from immunological reactions between antibodies in patient's plasma and various other antigenic constituents of donor blood. They are classified clinically (in increasing order of severity) as:

- Urticarial reactions.
- Febrile reactions.
- Serum sickness-type reactions.
- Pulmonary oedema of non-cardiac origin.
- Anaphylactoid reactions.

Although these distinct symptom categories can be recognized, the underlying aetiological factors share immunological features in common, and it is to be expected that a degree of overlap in the clinical symptomatology will occur. Reactions are far the most common with granulocyte preparations[15] and tend to diminish in frequency and severity as the leucocyte and plasma protein content of the transfusion is reduced. Not surprisingly, therefore, it has been shown that most of these reactions are due to antigen–antibody reactions involving leucocytes or plasma proteins. The reported frequency of such reactions is probably of the order of 1% of all transfusion episodes, but it is highly likely that many of the milder reactions are treated symptomatically and never notified. Non-haemolytic transfusion reactions occur most frequently in multi-transfused patients or more generally in those who have been previously transfused or pregnant, either event presumably providing an antigenic stimulus to the initial antibody formation.

Urticarial reactions

Erythema, urticaria and pruritus, occurring within a few minutes of the start of transfusion, are symptoms of histamine and serotonin release as a result of antigen–antibody reaction. The transfusion rate should be slowed and intravenous antihistamines (e.g. chlorpheniramine 10–20 mg) given. If after 30 minutes there is no progression of symptoms, the transfusion may be continued normally. No further investigation is required. Repeated episodes merit prophylactic antihistamines.

Febrile transfusion reactions

Febrile transfusion reactions are observed in as many as 2% or so of routine red cell transfusions and are even more common (up to 21%)[16] as complications of platelet transfusion.

A rapid temperature rise of up to 1–2 °C accompanied by chills and rigors may be the early warning of haemolytic transfusion reaction or, if as is more usual, it is due to a non-haemolytic reaction, symptoms may progress no further. Although these symptoms have been ascribed to leucocyte–leucocyte antibody reactions, there is increasing evidence that storage-related release of leucocyte cytokines and/or vasoactive substances maybe to blame (see section 3.1).

In unexpected or severe reactions the transfusion should be discontinued, and blood units and samples should be collected for serological investigation.

Common practice is to give aspirin 600 mg orally and substitute the transfusion with isotonic saline. If after a few hours the fever subsides, the red cell serological findings are negative and there is no clinical cause for concern, the next blood unit can be given.

Repeated mild reactions necessitate prophylactic aspirin. More severe reactions necessitate leucocyte depletion of blood components as described in chapter 3, section 1.5.

Serum sickness reactions

These take place within a few days of transfusion and comprise fever, myalgia, arthritis, pleural and pericardial effusions. Sometimes vomiting as well as abdominal and lumbar pain occur. The symptoms are self-limiting and usually reflect immune complex formation between recipient antibodies and donor immunoglobulins which act as alloantigens.[17] Steroids have been used for treatment and only plasma-free products should be transfused thereafter.

Acute pulmonary oedema

Pulmonary oedema is most often due to cardiac failure as a result of a too rapid rate of transfusion or circulatory overload. When this is not the case, the pulmonary oedema appears to be due to a form of severe anaphylactic reaction biased towards pulmonary damage. The precipitating event may be the occurrence of complement-mediated disruption of leucocyte/antileucocyte agglutinates trapped in the pulmonary circulation. Usually the reactions can be ascribed to potent leucocyte antibodies of donor blood damaging the circulating and marginating leucocytes of the recipient.[18]

The phenomenon may be seen following transfusion of any blood components containing plasma. Investigations have shown that implicated donors are almost invariably multiparous (more than three 3 pregnancies) women, and specific incompatibilities between donor HLA or neutrophil antibodies and recipient leucocyte antigens can be demonstrated.

Degranulation of leucocytes and release of their proteolytic enzymes, and liberation of allergic reaction by-products, e.g. activated C3a and C5a, are the events presumed to cause damage to pulmonary capillaries; capillary permeability is increased and leads to the acute onset of oedema.

This unusual but dramatic event has become known as *transfusion-related acute lung injury* (TRALI). The symptoms comprise:

- Dyspnoea.
- Cyanosis.
- Fever.
- Circulatory collapse.

Sometimes there is a copious outpouring of plasma-like oedema fluid into the bronchial tree.

Patchy bilateral pulmonary infiltrates are typically seen on chest X-ray.

Treatment of acute pulmonary distress   There is really no certainty about treatment measures, especially for those dramatic emergencies that usually come as a complete surprise. Obviously therapy is tailored to the predominant symptom and also depends on whatever other medical or surgical treatment is already in progress. Transfusion-related acute lung injury may, for example, be so severe as to require oxygen and mechanical ventilation. Circulatory collapse has been attributed to low-output cardiac failure, in which case administration of intra-venous fluids and avoidance of diuretics (in spite of the pulmonary oedema) restores left atrial filling pressures and cardiac output.[19] The treatment measures used for the more typical anaphylactic reactions (see below) may also be required.

If the acute emergency can be controlled the symptoms usually subside completely although full resolution may take several days.

Anaphylactoid reactions

Dramatic and severe symptoms may occur within minutes of the start of transfusion of blood or plasma products. These must be recognized promptly as fatalities can occur.

The typical symptoms are more widespread in their distribution than those described above and lack the copious pulmonary oedema. They include:

- Respiratory distress, bronchospasm.
- Hypertension initially, which may be followed by hypotension.
- Subcutaneous oedema.
- Nausea, vomiting and diarrhoea.

Treatment measures that *may* be required:

(1) Stop the transfusion and give isotonic saline or Ringer's lactate.
(2) Antihistamine (e.g. chlorpheniramine (10–20 mg i.v.))
(3) Give corticosteroids, e.g. 100 mg hydrocortisone, or, for drastic reactions, 0.5–1.0 g methylprednisone i.v.
(4) Oxygen.
(5) Give diuretics, e.g. frusemide 250 mg i.v.

These signs and symptoms are caused by the by-products of antigen–antibody reaction and complement activation similar to those occurring during haemolytic transfusion episodes.

Allergic reactions to donor plasma proteins, or less frequently to leucocyte antigens, are usually implicated. If, after recovery, further transfusions must be given they should consist of washed leucocyte-poor red cells (see chapter 3, section 1.5) and be given slowly with extreme caution; 5% albumin should be safe, but should be given with similar care.

An attempt should be made to determine the cause, as described below.

3.1 Causes of Non-haemolytic Transfusion Reactions

Leucocyte antibodies[20]

The aetiological role of these antibodies is most conclusively proven when clinical reactions are shown in a controlled manner to be prevented by transfusion of leucocyte-free blood. The serological confirmation that clinically important antibody-mediated leucocyte destruction has occurred is less straightforward.

Lymphocytotoxic and leucoagglutinating antibodies, as well as positive immuno-fluorescence tests for lymphocyte, granulocyte and platelet alloantibodies, can, in varying proportions, be found in most multi-transfused patients. They are most frequently found in those suffering febrile reactions but are also fairly common in patients without reactions. Laboratory findings do not therefore correlate well with clinical symptoms. Broadly reactive lymphocytotoxic or leucoagglutinating antibodies can be demonstrated in around 60% of patients with these transfusion reactions—an incidence which is, however, only twice that seen in control patients with a similar transfusion history but not showing clinical reactions.[15]

Around 50% of patients have been shown to have granulocyte specific antibodies. Several granulocyte-specific antigens have been identified and designated, e.g. NA1, NA2, NB. Most appear to be of relatively high frequency; patients with these antibodies would therefore be expected to have reactions with a majority of transfused donor units. Techniques for detection of these granulocyte-specific reactions are restricted to reference laboratories.

Antibodies to platelet-specific antigens

Antibodies to platelet-specific antigens are most frequently found in association with leucocyte antibodies but are very occasionally the only abnormality found in non-haemolytic transfusion reactions. Various antigen systems, e.g. HPA-1 (Pl^A), HPA-2, have been identified. HPA-1a antibodies are of the greatest interest as a cause of neonatal thrombocytopenia due to maternal alloimmunization (see chapter 20, section 3.1), or as a cause of post-transfusion purpura (section 4.3).

IgA antibodies

Around one in 500 people appear to be almost totally IgA deficient. In these people IgA antibodies can be stimulated by transfusion and as a result subsequent transfusions may be accompanied by severe anaphylactoid reactions[21,22] or even fatality.[22]

Profound circulatory collapse with cyanosis and precordial pain were observed in one case after as little as 15 ml.[23] Future transfusions for such patients should be with:

(1) *Washed red cells*: the residual IgA should be reduced to below 0.5 mg/l.[24] Or
(2) *Donations from IgA-deficient donors.*
(3) *IgA-depleted blood products*: most blood products contain traces of IgA; the IgA content of products prepared by the protein fractionation centre of the Scottish NBTS has been published.[25]

    At least one IgA-depleted intravenous immunoglobulin preparation is available.[26]

IgA deficiency can be diagnosed by immunodiffusion or haemagglutination techniques. In immunized subjects precipitin lines can be demonstrated between anti-IgA in the IgA-deficient serum and the IgA in serum from normal donors. The usual criterion for IgA deficiency is an IgA level below 50 mg/l; a high proportion of 'deficient' patients in fact have levels even below 1.0 mg/l. Between 10% and 40% of these people can be shown to have IgA antibodies.

Antibodies have also been found against the subclasses A1 and A2 of IgA found in individuals homozygous for the alternative allotype.[27] Clinical reactions due to subclass-specific IgA antibodies are usually less severe than those occurring in patients with class-specific antibodies and total IgA deficiency.

IgG allotypes

IgG also exists in various allotypes. Antibodies against the heavy chain Gm antigen may be uncommon causes of mild reactions.

Genetic polymorphisms

Genetic polymorphisms of other serum proteins, e.g. the complement component C4, have been shown to be associated with transfusion reactions.[28]

Cytokines and vasoactive substances in transfused products

Febrile reactions to platelet transfusions have been linked to concentrations of cytokines, e.g. tumour necrosis factor (TNF), interleukin 1 (IL-1) interleukin 6 (IL-6), as well as vasoactive substances such as histamine and bradykinin. These substances appear to be released from leucocytes during storage of platelet concentrates.[29–31]

3.2 Prophylactic Management: Patients with Non-haemolytic Transfusion Reactions

Because of the many causes of non-haemolytic febrile transfusion reactions (NHFTR) it is not surprising that prevention cannot necessarily be achieved by any single measure alone. Efficient leucocyte depletion, particularly if carried out before storage (see chapter 4), can reduce reaction rates. It clearly cannot be effective for reactions in platelet recipients where platelet-specific antibodies have a role, and if allergic reactions to plasma are occurring attempts must be made to minimize the plasma component of donations.

4 OTHER PROBLEMS ASSOCIATED WITH TRANSFUSION

4.1 Graft-versus-host disease[32]

Because it is almost invariably fatal it is fortunate that *graft-versus-host disease (GVHD)* is a rare complication of transfusion. This condition is caused by *donor*

T-lymphocytes performing their normal role of immunological attack against foreign tissues; in this instance, however, the target tissues are those of the transfusion recipient. The *skin, gastrointestinal tract, liver, kidneys, bone marrow* and *lymph nodes* are particularly severely affected. The problem is typically associated with recipients who are in themselves immunodeficient and hence unable to mount their own immunological defences against the viable transfused leucocytes. Recently GVHD has been recognized as a quite unexpected sporadic occurrence in transfused patients who are not immunodeficient. In such instances it has almost invariably been found that donors are homozygous for a haplotype or more particularly an extended haplotype spanning the entire major histocompatibility complex shared by the recipient.[33]

In such instances, donor lymphocytes are not recognized as foreign and hence engraft themselves and proceed to mount an immune reaction against the recipient's tissues.[34,35] GVHD is a potential but exceptionally uncommon risk of transfusion to *premature neonates*[36,37] and *immunocompromised patients*.[38,39]

GVHD constitutes a major problem in *bone marrow transplantation* and is considered in more detail in chapter 22, section 3.8. GVHD shows as *fever, erythematous* and eventually *desquamating skin rashes, profuse diarrhoea and hepatitis*, usually within 1 month following transfusion. There will characteristically be *pancytopenia* in post-transfusion cases, but not in those following marrow transplantation, since in these latter cases the bone marrow cells are of donor origin. Irradiation of blood components kills the lymphocytes responsible for GVHD and is the only effective prophylactic measure.[40]

The rarity and unpredictability of transfusion-associated GVHD makes recommendations for its prophylaxis difficult. The susceptibility of individual patients is almost certainly determined by the interplay of three variables: *the dose of lymphocytes, the degree of immunosuppression* and, finally, *antigenic disparity*, or lack of it between donor and recipient.

Patients that *must* receive only irradiated materials include:

- Bone marrow transplant recipients (until immunocompetence is restored).
- Patients with congenital cellular immunodeficiencies.

Irradiated components are *advisable* for:

- Intrauterine transfusions (IUT).
- Exchange transfusion (if previous IUT have been given). (There is too little evidence to commend use of irradiated components for all very low birth weight (< 1500 g) neonates.)
- Recipients of donations from close blood relatives.

They may be *considered* for severely immunosuppressed patients, e.g. those with *Hodgkin's disease* (possibly because of an intrinsic T cell deficiency) receiving intensive therapy. Although instances of GVHD have been reported for other intensively treated patients, including those with haematological[41] and non-haematological malignancies,[42] the risk level appears too small to justify dogmatic recommendations. Transfusion-associated GVHD in immunocompetent subjects appears to be a significant problem in more genetically homogeneous populations such as the Japanese, in which the risk of receiving blood from an

HLA homozygous but unrelated donor appears to be as high as around one in 1000.

The diagnosis of GVHD can be easily overlooked since its symptoms may often be confused with those from the patient's underlying disease. Skin biopsy shows characteristic changes of cell necrosis with vacuolation of cytoplasm and surrounding lymphocytic infiltration. More conclusive evidence of foreign cell engraftment is gained by DNA HLA typing which may also enable identification of the implicated donation.[43,44]

The *materials* that require irradiation certainly include all cellular components, particularly those such as platelet concentrates and granulocyte preparations in which lymphocyte contamination may be high. Although fresh frozen plasma may contain a few viable lymphocytes the need for its irradiation has not yet been clearly established.

The most frequently used *dose* is 25 Gy (2500 rad).[45] This is adequate to abolish mixed lymphocyte culture reactivity (probably the most relevant *in vitro* indicator) and is also sufficient to remove most lymphocyte proliferative capacity and responsiveness to mitogen stimulation. This dose does not appear to damage the function of red cells, platelets or granulocytes.

Blood components should be *labelled* as having been irradiated. Local policies should also make it clear that unused irradiated components can safely be transfused to other patients. An important caution applies, however. Irradiation of red cells impairs membrane function and causes K^+ leakage into supernatant plasma.[46,47]

This might be dangerous for large transfusions in neonates, and for these use of blood within 48 hours following irradiation is advised.

4.2 Alloimmunization to Red Cell Antigens

Alloimmunization as a result of transfusion is considered in chapter 4, section 2.3.

4.3 Post-transfusion Purpura[48,49]

Severe thrombocytopenia is occasionally observed 5–10 days after the transfusion of blood or platelet concentrates. In the majority of cases this appears to occur in people negative for the HPA-1a platelet antigen who become sensitized to this alloantigen through *pregnancy* or occasionally from *previous transfusions*. Less commonly, immunization to other platelet antigens has been described. The challenge of a repeat transfusion of incompatible platelets anamnestically boosts alloantibody and this appears to damage both transfused as well as *autologous platelets*. By the time antibodies can be detected most donor platelet material has, in fact, already left the circulation.

The destruction of autologous platelets is enigmatic; possibly these are damaged by immune complexes. There is evidence, including for example the apparently beneficial effect of intravenous immunoglobulin, suggesting that an autoantibody is produced simultaneously with the anti-HPA-1a. Spontaneous recovery of thrombocytopenia is the rule; this usually takes place within 3–5 weeks. On rare occasions the condition has been fatal and it should, therefore, be considered no less seriously than other forms of thrombocytopenia. A very few cases of post-transfusion purpura due to passive antibody transfer have been described.[50] In such instances thrombocytopenia is usually noticed within a few hours following transfusion. Donors have usually been *multiparous women*, presumably sensitized during pregnancy, carrying persistently high-titre platelet-specific antibodies. It would seem reasonable, therefore, to exclude all potential donors who have a known history of platelet alloimmunization unless their safety has been confirmed by antibody screening.

The condition is not easy to treat; administration of random donor platelets is clearly unhelpful; even HPA-1a-negative donations are not usually effective, which may be supportive evidence for the presence of a relatively non-specific coexisting autoantibody. Plasmapheresis may be effective; high-dose steroids have been useful but the most promising approach so far seems to be *intravenous immunoglobulin*. Treatment should be reserved for patients with symptomatic thrombocytopenia or where platelet counts seem likely to fall to hazardous levels.

4.4 Immunosuppressive Effects of Blood Transfusion: Relationship to Tumour Recurrence and Post-operative Infection

The beneficial effects of blood transfusion on renal allograft survival, particularly convincing prior to the introduction of cyclosporin, has provided compelling clinical evidence that allogeneic transfusions modify the behaviour of the recipient immune system. Although various hypotheses have been advanced in explanation, the mechanism for this effect remains largely conjectural (see chapter 22, section 2.3). Blood transfusion has, however, been shown to produce a number of well-recognized immunosuppressive effects.[51-53] These include:

• Reduced natural killer cell activity.
• Inhibition of cell-mediated immune functions.

Depressed cellular immune function is revealed by reduced lymphocyte responses to antigens and mitogens, these being possibly a consequence of enhanced suppressor cell functions or anti-idiotype antibody regulatory mechanisms.

Some of these changes appear to persist months or even years after transfusion. The relationship between blood transfusion and immunosuppression has been examined in a number of clinical settings, including cancer recurrence following surgery and post-operative infection.

Blood Transfusion and Post-operative Infection[54-58]

The relationship between peri-operative blood transfusion and post-operative infection has been examined in such diverse situations as *colorectal surgery, cardiac bypass surgery* and *abdominal trauma*. Transfused patients have, it is claimed, a greater frequency of wound infections, urinary tract infections, pneumonia, peritonitis etc. These claims are challenged for the same reasons as the putative link between blood transfusion and cancer, namely that the transfusions are, in essence, a marker for a variety of other factors, each being a credible risk factor for establishment of infection. Animal studies have been conducted in attempts to determine whether allogeneic transfusions increase mortality following microbial inoculation but the results of these studies do not universally support the hypothesis. In addition to the possible immunosuppressive effects, transfusion could affect the susceptibility to infection in other ways. Transfusions usually contain substantial amounts of senescent red cells, leucocytes and platelet debris, and these are likely to transiently saturate the capacity of the reticuloendothelial system, thereby diminishing its ability to clear circulating bacteria. It has also been postulated that transient abundance of iron as senescent red cell haemoglobin is catabolized may favour microbial proliferation. These and other postulated mechanisms lend some scientific support to the casual link between transfusion and infection. The true relationship between these two events awaits larger and well-controlled prospective studies.

Blood transfusions and cancer

The possibility that *transfused patients* were more likely to have recurrence of their original surgically resected tumour has been examined repeatedly since the first disquieting evidence was produced in the early 1980s. Originally investigated in colorectal surgery patients, subsequent studies have investigated cancers of a variety of other systems, including the lung, prostate, breast, vulva, stomach and kidney.[59-66] Studies have been mainly retrospective, measuring tumour recurrence or survival, and have attempted as far as possible to examine blood transfusion as an isolated variable, recognizing the likelihood of the need for blood transfusion being associated with tumour staging, difficulty of surgical resection and the general physical condition of patients, all of which might be expected to have a bearing on outcome. In general, studies appear to suggest either statistically significant adverse transfusion effects or, failing that, an overall trend supporting the hypothesis, and indeed a survey of studies from 1982 to 1990 claimed to show clear evidence that blood transfusion increased the probability of tumour recurrence or death from cancer. The evidence is, however, not entirely one-sided, and other reports[65,66] have failed to confirm the association between blood transfusion and poor prognosis. Furthermore, patients presenting with cancer are not more likely to have had a previous history of blood transfusion, as might be expected if transfusion significantly diminished the level of immunological surveillance against neoplasia. Uncertainty also surrounds the nature of the constituent of blood which might be deleterious. Attention has focused on both the leucocyte content of blood and also on plasma as responsible for immunomodulation,[67] evidence being available from animal experimental studies to support either contention. The apparent attenuation of endogenous immune recognition and hence tumour suppression as a result of allogeneic blood transfusion has been used to support the case for utilizing autologous blood transfusion whenever practicable. The value of this strategy has, however, been cast in doubt by studies in which no differences could be found between patients given autologous transfusion and allogeneic blood.[68]

From these studies, it has been concluded that the act of blood transfusion or the circumstances requiring it were in fact the important determinant.

Despite considerable effort, proof of the association between blood transfusion and neoplasia remains elusive. Nevertheless, until the uncertainty is resolved, this concern is yet another reason for giving transfusion only when clearly necessary.

REFERENCES

1 Sazama, K. (1990) Reports of 355 transfusion-associated deaths: 1976 through 1985. *Transfusion*, **30**: 583–590.
2 Linden, J.V., Paul, B. and Dressler, K.P. (1992) A report of 104 transfusion errors in New York State. *Transfusion*, **32**: 601–606.
3 Murphy, W.G. and McClelland, D.B.L. (1989) Deceptively low morbidity from failure to practice safe blood transfusion: an analysis of serious blood transfusion errors. *Vox Sang.*, **57**: 59–62.
4 Pineda, A.A., Brzica, S.M. and Taswell, H.F. (1978) Haemolytic transfusion reaction: recent experience in a large blood bank. *Mayo Clin. Proc.*, **53**: 378.
5 Easton, D.J. and Ternoey, C.M. (1985) Haemolysis of donor cells in 'two-thirds–one-third' solution. *Transfusion*, **25**: 85.
6 Chaplin, H. (1984) The implication of red cell-bound complement in delayed haemolytic transfusion reactions. *Transfusion*, **24**: 185–187.
7 Pickles, M.M., Jones, M.N., Egan, J., Dodsworth, H. and Mollison, P.L. (1978) Delayed haemolytic transfusion reactions due to anti-C. *Vox Sang.*, **35**: 32–35.
8 Molthan, L., Matulewicz, T.J., Bansal-Carver, B. and Benz, E.J. (1984) An immediate haemolytic transfusion reaction due to anti-C: and a delayed haemolytic transfusion reaction due to anti-Ce+e: haemoglobinemia, haemoglobinuria and transient impaired renal function. *Vox Sang.*, **47**: 348–353.
9 Webster, B.H. (1980) Clinical presentation of haemolytic transfusion reactions. *Anaesth. Intens. Care*, **8**: 115–119.
10 Pineda, A.A., Taswell, H.F. and Brzica, S.M. (1978) Delayed haemolytic transfusion reaction: an immunologic hazard of blood transfusion. *Transfusion*, **18**: 1–7.
11 Ness, P.M., Shirey, R.S., Thoman, S.K. and Buck, S.A. (1990) The differentiation of delayed serologic and delayed haemolytic transfusion reactions: incidence, long-term serologic findings, and clinical significance. *Transfusion*, **30**: 688–693.
12 Salama, A. and Mueller-Eckhardt, C. (1984) Evidence for complement activation involving allogeneic and autologous red cells. *Transfusion*, **24**: 188–193.
13 Moore, S.B., Taswell, H.F., Pineda, A.A. and Sonnenberg, C.L. (1980) Delayed haemolytic transfusion reactions. *Am. J. Clin. Pathol.*, **74**: 94–97.
14 Solanki, D. and McCurdy, P.R. (1978) Delayed haemolytic transfusion reactions. *JAMA*, **239**: 729–731.
15 Decary, F., Ferner, P., Giavedoni, L. *et al.* (1984) An investigation of non-haemolytic transfusion reactions. *Vox Sang.*, **46**: 277–285.
16 Chambers, L.A., Knustall, D.G., Pacini, D.G. and Donovan, L.M. (1990) Febrile transfusion reactions after platelet transfusion: the effect of single versus multiple donors. *Transfusion*, **30**: 219–221.
17 Avoy, D.R. (1981) Delayed serum sickness-like transfusion reactions in a multiply transfused patient. *Vox Sang.*, **41**: 239–244.
18 Popovsky, M.A., Chaplin, H.C. and Moore, S.B. (1992) Transfusion-related acute lung injury: a neglected, serious complication of hemotherapy. *Transfusion*, **32**: 589–592.
19 Levy, G.J., Shabot, M.M., Hart, M.E., Mya, W.W. and Goldfinger, D. (1986) Transfusion-

associated noncardiogenic pulmonary edema: report of a case and a warning regarding treatment. *Transfusion*, **26**: 278–281.

20 de Rie, M.A., van der Plas-van Dalen, C.M., Engelfriet, C.P. and von dem Borne, A.E.G. Kr. (1985) The serology of febrile transfusion reactions. *Vox Sang.*, **49**: 126–134.

21 Ozawa, N., Shimizu, M., Imai, M., Miyakawa, Y. and Mayumi, M. (1986) Selective absence of immunoglobulin A1 or A2 amongst blood donors and hospital patients. *Transfusion*, **26**: 73–76.

22 Pineda, A.A. and Taswell, H.F. (1975) Transfusion reactions associated with anti-IgA antibodies: report of four cases and review of the literature. *Transfusion*, **15**: 10–15.

23 Branigan, E.F., Stevenson, M.M. and Charles, D. (1983) Blood transfusion reaction in a patient with immunoglobulin A deficiency. *Obstet. Gynecol.*, **61**: 47S–49S.

24 Laschinger, C., Gauthier, D., Valet, J.P. and Naylor, D.H. (1984) Fluctuating levels of serum IgA in individuals with selective IgA deficiency. *Vox Sang.*, **47**: 60–67.

25 Yap, P.L., Pryde, E.A.D. and McLelland, D.B.L. (1982) IgA contents of frozen-thawed-washed red blood cells and blood products measured by radioimmunoassay. *Transfusion*, **22**: 36–38.

26 Cunningham-Rundles, C., Wong, S., Bjorkander, J. and Hanson, L.A. (1986) Use of an IgA-depleted intravenous immunoglobulin in a patient with an anti-IgA antibody. *Clin. Immunol. Immunopathol.*, **38**: 141–149.

27 Strauss, R.A., Gloster, E.S., Schanfield, M.S., Kittinger, S.P. and Morgan, B.B. (1983) Anaphylactic transfusion reaction associated with a possible anti-A2m(1). *Clin. Lab. Haematol.*, **5**: 371–377.

28 Lambin, P., Le Pennec, P.Y., Hauptmann, G., Desaint, O., Habibi, B. and Salmon, Ch. (1984) Adverse transfusion reactions associated with a precipitating anti-C4 antibody of anti-Rodgers specificity. *Vox Sang.*, **47**: 242–249.

29 Muylle, L., Joos, M., Wouters, E., DeBock, R. and Peeterman, M.E. (1993) Increased tumour necrosis factor α(TNFα), interleukin 1, and interleukin 6 (IL-6) levels in the plasma of stored platelet concentrates: relationship between TNFα and IL-6 levels and febrile transfusion reactions. *Transfusion*, **33**: 195–199.

30 Muylle, L., Wouters, E., DeBock, R. and Peetermans, M.E. (1992) Reactions to platelet transfusion: the effect of the storage time of the concentrate. *Transfusion*, **2**: 289–293.

31 Frewin, D.B., Jonsson, J.R., Frewin, C.R. *et al.* (1989) Influence of blood storage time and plasma histamine levels on the pattern of transfusion reactions. *Vox Sang.*, **56**: 243–246.

32 Anderson, K.C. and Weinstein, H.J. (1990) Transfusion-associated graft-versus-host-disease. *N. Engl. J. Med.*, **323**: 315–321.

33 McMilin, K.D. and Johnson, R.L. (1993) HLA homozygosity and the risk of related-donor transfusion-associated graft-versus-host disease. *Transfusion Med. Rev.*, **8**: 37–41.

34 Otsuka, S., Kunieda, K., Kitamura, F. *et al.* (1991) The critical role of blood from HLA-homozygous donors in fatal transfusion-associated graft-versus-host disease in immuno-competent patients. *Transfusion*, **31**: 260–264.

35 Kanter, M.H. (1992) Transfusion-associated graft-versus-host disease: do transfusions from second-degree relatives pose a greater risk than those from first-degree relatives? *Transfusion*, **32**: 323–327.

36 Funkhouser, A.W., Vogelsang, G., Zehnbauer, B. *et al.* (1991) Graft versus-host-disease after blood transfusion in a premature infant. *Pediatrics*, **87**: 247–249.

37 Sanders, M.R. and Graeber, J.E. (1990) Post-transfusion graft-versus-host disease in infancy. *J. Pediatr.*, **117**: 159–163.

38 Brubaker, D.B. (1983) Human posttransfusion graft-versus-host disease. *Vox. Sang.*, **45**: 401–420.

39 Nikoskelainen, J., Soderstrom, K.-O., Rajamaki, A. *et al.* (1983) Graft-versus-host reaction in 3 adult leukaemia patients after transfusion of blood cell products. *Scand. J. Haematol.*, **31**: 403–409.

40 Linden, J.V. and Pisciotto, P.T. (1992) Transfusion-associated graft-versus-host-disease and blood irradiation. *Transfusion Med. Rev.*, **6**: 116–123.

41 Spitzer, T.R., Cahill, R., Cottler-Fox, M., Treat, J., Sacher, R. and Deeg, H.J. (1990) Trans-
    fusion-induced graft-versus-host-disease in patients with malignant lymphoma: a case
    report and review of the literature. *Cancer*, **66**: 2346–2349.
42 DeCoste, S.D., Boudreaux, C. and Dover, J.S. (1990) Transfusion-associated graft-versus-
    host-disease in patients with malignancies: report of two cases and review of the litera-
    ture. *Arch. Dermatol.*, **126**: 1324–1329.
43 Kunstmann, E., Bocker, T., Roewer, L., Sauer, H., Memple, W. and Epplen, J.T. (1992)
    Diagnosis of transfusion-associated graft-versus-host disease by genetic fingerprinting
    and polymerase chain reaction. *Transfusion*, **32**: 766–770.
44 Hayakawa, S., Chishima, F., Sakata, H. *et al.* (1993) A rapid molecular diagnosis of post-
    transfusion graft-versus-host-disease by polymerase chain reaction. *Transfusion*, **33**:
    413–417.
45 Moroff, G. and Luban, N.L.C. (1992) Prevention of transfusion-associated graft-versus-
    host-disease. *Transfusion*, **32**: 102–103.
46 Brugnara, C. and Churchill, W.H. (1992) Effect of irradiation on red cell cation content
    and transport. *Transfusion*, **32**: 246–252.
47 Dinning, G., Doughty, R.W., Reid, M.M. and Lloyd, H.L. (1991) Potassium concentra-
    tions in irradiated blood. *Br. Med. J.*, **303**: 1110.
48 Vogelsang, G., Kickler, T.S. and Bell, W.R. (1986) Post-transfusion purpura: a report of
    five patients and a review of the pathogenesis and management. *Am. J. Hematol.*, **21**:
    259–267.
49 Mueller-Eckhardt, C. (1986) Post transfusion purpura. *Br. J. Hematol.*, **64**: 419–424.
50 Ballem, P.J., Buskard, N.A., Decary, F. and Doubroff, P. (1987) Post-transfusion purpura
    secondary to passive transfer of anti-P1A1 by blood transfusion. *Br. J. Hematol.*, **66**:
    113–114.
51 Tartter, P.I., Steinberg, B., Barron, D.M. and Martinelli, G. (1989) Transfusion history T
    cell subsets and natural killer cytotoxicity in patients with colorectal cancer. *Vox Sang.*,
    56: 80–84.
52 Schot, J.D.L. and Schuurman, R.K.B. (1986) Blood transfusion suppresses cutaneous cell-
    mediated immunity. *Clin. Exp. Immunol.*, **65**: 336–344.
53 Sibrowski, W., Wegner, W. and Kuhnl, P. (1992) Immunomodulatory activity of differ-
    ent blood products on the mitogen-induced human lymphocyte transformation. *Transfu-
    sion Med.*, **2**: 215–221.
54 Tartter, P.I., Quintero, S. and Barron, D.M. (1986) Perioperative blood transfusion
    associated with infectious complications after colorectal cancer operations. *Am. J. Surg.*,
    152: 479–482.
55 Pinto, V., Baldonedo, R., Nicolas, C., Barez, A., Perez, A. and Aza, J. (1991) Relationship
    of transfusion and infectious complications after gastric carcinoma operations. *Transfu-
    sion*, **31**: 114–118.
56 George, C.D. and Morello, P.J. (1986) Immunologic effects of blood transfusion upon
    renal transplantation, tumour operations, and bacterial infections. *Am. J. Surg.*, **152**:
    329–337.
57 Agarwal, N., Murphy, J.G., Cayten, C.G. and Stahl, W.M. (1993) Blood transfusion
    increases the risk of infection after trauma. *Arch. Surg.*, **128**: 171–177.
58 Triulzi, D.J., Vanek, K., Ryan, D.H. and Blumberg, N. (1992) A clinical and immunologic
    study of blood transfusion and postoperative bacterial infection in spinal surgery. *Trans-
    fusion*, **32**: 517–524.
59 Manyonda, I.T., Shaw, D.E., Foulkes, A. and Osborne, D.E. (1986) Renal cell carcinoma:
    blood transfusion and survival. *Br. Med. J.*, **293**: 537–538.
60 Kaneda, M., Horimi, T., Ninomiya, M. *et al.* (1987) Adverse affect of blood transfusions
    on survival of patients with gastric cancer. *Transfusion*, **27**: 375–377.
61 Stephenson, K.R., Steinberg, S.M., Hughes, K.S., Vetto, J.T., Sugarbaker, P.H. and Chang,
    A.E. (1988) Perioperative blood transfusions are associated with decreased time to recur-
    rence and decreased survival after resection of colorectal liver metastases. *Ann. Surg.*,
    208: 679–687.
62 Parrott, N.R., Lennard, T.W.J., Taylor, R.M.R., Proud, G., Shenton, B.K. and Johnston,

I.D.A. (1986) Effect of perioperative blood transfusion on recurrence of colorectal cancer. *Br. J. Surg.*, **73**: 970–973.

63 Blumberg, N., Heal, J., Chuang, C., Murphy, P. and Agarwal, M. (1988) Further evidence supporting a cause and effect relationship between blood transfusion and earlier cancer recurrence. *Ann. Surg.*, **207**: 410–415.

64 Tartter, P.I. (1988) Blood transfusion history in colorectal cancer patients and cancer-free controls. *Transfusion*, **28**: 593–596.

65 Kieckbusch, M.E., O'Fallon, J.R., Ahmann, D.L. and Moore, S.B. (1989) Blood transfusion exposure does not influence survival in patients with carcinoma of the breast. *Transfusion*, **29**: 500–504.

66 Frankish, P.D., McNee, R.K., Alley, P.G. and Woodfield, D.G. (1985) Relationship between cancer of the colon and blood transfusion. *Br. Med. J.*, **290**: 1827.

67 Blumberg, N., Heal, J.M., Murphy, P., Agarwal, M.M. and Chuang, C. (1986) Association between transfusion of whole blood and recurrence of cancer. *Br. Med. J.*, **293**: 530–533.

68 Busch, O.R.C., Hop, W.C.J.M, Hoynck van Papendrecht, M.A.W., Marquet, R.L. and Jeekel, J. (1993) Blood transfusions and prognosis in colorectal cancer. *N. Engl. J. Med.*, **328**: 1372–1376.

69 Linden, J.V. and Kaplan, H.S. (1994) Transfusion errors: causes and effects. *Transfusion Med. Rev.*, **3**: 169–183.

24

Infections Transmissible by Transfusion

1 INTRODUCTION

The advent of blood transfusion provided an excellent opportunity for those pathogenic microorganisms either present in or transmitted via blood to gain access to new hosts. Throughout the world a great variety of parasitic infections are potentially transmissible in this way. The relative importance of each infection as a transfusion problem depends on its endemic frequency and the presence of natural immunity. Modern blood transfusion has become relatively safe as a consequence of the reduction of immunological, metabolic and organizational risks, with the result that the risk of transmitted infection has now emerged as the area of greatest concern. This is particularly true with regard to the use of labile blood components which cannot be subjected to sterilization or virucidal procedures.

Prevention of transmissible infection requires:

(1) Knowledge of the microorganisms causing transfusion-transmissible infections as well as information about their life-cycles.
(2) Recognition and reporting of all post-transfusion infections.
(3) Identification of 'high risk' donors by serological screening or by clinical means.
(4) Identification of categories of susceptible recipients.
(5) Knowledge of the viability of infective agents in blood and blood products.
(6) Recognition of the relative risk of various blood products.
(7) Development of the means of destruction of microorganisms in blood components or products.

Transmission of the hepatitis B and C viruses, cytomegalovirus (CMV) and the infective agent of acquired immunodeficiency syndrome (AIDS), i.e. human immunodeficiency virus (HIV), constitutes the major transfusion hazards. A large number of other agents can and do cause disease following transfusion of infective blood. Some of the most important are listed in Table 1.

2 POST-TRANSFUSION HEPATITIS

Jaundice and liver damage, occasionally with fatal consequences, soon came to be recognized as an unfortunate sequel to the rapid expansion of blood transfusion

Table 1 Infectious agents transmitted by blood transfusion

Pathogen	Transmitted illness
Hepatitis B virus (HBV) Hepatitis C virus (HCV)	Post-transfusion hepatitis
Cytomegalovirus (CMV)	Hepatitis, pneumonitis etc.
Human immunodeficiency virus (HIV)	Acquired immunodeficiency syndrome (AIDS)
Human T lymphotropic virus (HTLV1/2)	T cell leukaemia Myelopathy, spastic paraparesis
Treponema pallidum	Syphilis
Plasmodium spp.	Malaria
Trypanosoma cruzi	Chagas' disease
Various bacterial species	Bacteraemic shock

practice. Plasma was the vector and jaundice (serum hepatitis) was seen to follow episodes in which blood from carriers of hepatitis virus was transfused or inadvertently inoculated into susceptible recipients. From such observations stemmed much of the present-day insistence on hygienic clinical and laboratory practices for the handling of used syringes, needles and samples of blood and other pathological material.

Several viral species can cause post-transfusion hepatitis but the first to be recognized, and the most severe form, followed transmission of *hepatitis B virus (HBV)* (as distinct from the common and clinically similar hepatitis A virus which is virtually never transmitted by transfusion). Hepatitis B virus causes classical serum (post-transfusion) hepatitis. Post-transfusion hepatitis that could not be shown to be due to HBV or to other identifiable agents was designated *non-A non-B (NANB) hepatitis*. There is now good evidence that this mystery has been resolved with the discovery that most such episodes are due to infection with the recently identified hepatitis C virus (HCV).

2.1 Hepatitis Risk of Blood Components and Products

The risk of contracting post-transfusion hepatitis depends on several factors:

(1) The prevalence of hepatitis in the donor population.
(2) The number of donors contributing to the transfusion.
(3) The sensitivity of serological screening tests.
(4) The efficiency of virus inactivation procedures applied to blood products.

The incidences of hepatitis that have been reported following transfusion of blood or plasma vary according to the geographical population studied, the diagnostic criteria, the assiduousness of investigation of asymptomatic cases and, as a consequence of improving donor selection procedures, the date of the study. The most universally agreed criterion for diagnosis of post-transfusion hepatitis is the demonstration of otherwise unexplained elevations of hepatic enzyme (alanine transferase, ALT) between 2 and 20 weeks following transfusion.

The large pools of donations formerly used to prepare dried plasma were soon recognized to be highly dangerous with regard to hepatitis B transmission. The introduction of more rigorous donor selection, serological screening and adoption of smaller pool sizes greatly reduced this danger. Prior to the introduction of virucidal procedures and the very recent development of high-purity products it was the *coagulation factor concentrates* (Factors VIII and IX) prepared from the pooled plasma of several thousand donors that provided the greatest risk of hepatitis transmission.

Factors VIII and IX concentrate treatment programmes were estimated to carry almost a 100% chance of NANB infection. Around 10% acquired chronic HBV infection. A proportion of these patients (around 15–20%) developed persistent liver disease, in most cases presumably due to HCV infection.[1,2]

HBV infection may still remain a threat to haemophilia patients receiving concentrate therapy, and HBV vaccination is advised. The fact that hepatitis so frequently followed coagulation factor replacement was a major setback to the prospects of haemophilia sufferers offered a nearly normal life-style by modern treatment. However, the evidence is now encouraging that the combined effect of rigorous donor screening, improved virus removal and HBV vaccination will provide much welcome safety assurance to patients receiving regular coagulation factor support.

Hepatitis following transfusion of red cells and other blood components remains a possibility although the actual risks following transfusion are not easy to calculate. The more rigorous donor selection criteria, improved HBV and HCV screening and generally improved transfusion centre quality assurance must have very substantially reduced the risks below those formerly experienced. Risks have been estimated as ranging from 0.002, 0.1 and 0.9% per transfused unit in the UK, USA and Japan respectively,[3] and almost certainly relate most closely with virus prevalence rates in the community.

Table 2 Virus transmission risk of blood products

Absent risk
  Albumin
  Immunoglobulin for intramuscular use
  (apparently effective virucidal manufacturing process)

Very slight, but possible risk
  Pooled plasma products, e.g. fibrinogen, fibrin sealant (HBV)
  Factor VIII and IX concentrates (HBV, B19 parvovirus)
  Intravenous immunoglobulin (HCV)
  (ascribed to failure to maintain 100% manufacturing virucidal efficacy)

Low but finite risk
  Red cells, platelets, granulocytes, plasma and cryoprecipitate (HBV, HCV, HIV etc.),
  proportional to community incidence of recently acquired but seronegative infections

---

Blood products that are free from HBV and probably also HCV include *albumin derivatives* (as a result of heat treatment for 10 hours at 60 °C) and conventional intramuscular *immunoglobulin preparations*. Immunoglobulin preparations are purified by a part of the Cohn fractionation process that renders them free of infective HBV and probably also of HCV virus. Additionally they usually have anti-HBsAg activity as well as their normal antibody content. The position with regard to intravenous immunoglobulin is less clear; post-transfusion heptitis (PTH) transmission has been observed with isolated batches from several manufacturers' products using production methods previously thought to be safe.[4,5]

3 HEPATITIS B

Typical symptoms of this condition include *jaundice, malaise, gastrointestinal disturbances, abdominal pain, pale stools and dark urine.* These may last for 3–6 weeks before spontaneous resolution. The clinical symptoms and biochemical abnormalities are due to virus invasion and destruction of hepatic parenchymal cells. Hospital infection may follow transfusion of contaminated blood and blood products, injuries from needles or from splashes or aerosols of patients' body fluids reaching mucous membranes or small skin injuries. Natural spread is probably dependent on faeco-oral transmission, sexual contact or maternofetal infection during parturition; other possibilities such as shared toothbrushes or razors may play a role in intrafamily transmission. These factors are pertinent to the counselling of carriers (see section 6.2). The incubation period varies from 6 weeks up to 6 months.

The severity of post-transfusion hepatitis varies; the size of the infecting virus dose and the recipient susceptibility are probably important.

The majority of infections pass without symptoms and can be revealed only by liver function tests or serological tests. Of symptomatic cases 1% or so undergo a fulminant course, the mortality of which has been reported as 30–80%. Around 5% of all HBV infections may harbour the virus for prolonged periods (carrier status) and, in some, persistent liver damage is evident. A common but long delayed sequel to hepatitis B infections, where these are endemic, is development of *hepatocellular carcinoma*.

3.1 Laboratory Diagnosis of Hepatitis B

HBV has proved a recalcitrant laboratory captive and cannot be coaxed to grow in tissue culture systems. As a result virus culture and isolation cannot be used to aid diagnosis.

Virus particles can, however, be seen during electron microscopic examination of suitably prepared blood samples, but the technique is neither practicable nor necessary for routine diagnosis, for which various serological procedures are now available.

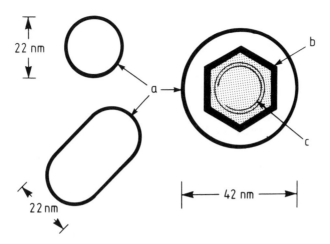

Figure 1 Diagram of hepatitis B virus particles. The antigenic structure of the complete virus comprises: (a) surface antigen (HBsAg) comprising the virus envelope; (b) core antigens (HBcAg and HBeAg) associated with the nucleocapsid; and (c) the inner circular largely double-stranded DNA. Also shown are the circular and cylindrical virus envelope particles which constitute the major part of serum HBsAg activity

Three types of particles may be distinguished by electron microscopy (Figure 1):

(1) The complete infective particle appears as a 42 nm sphere. The outer layer contains *hepatitis B surface antigen (HBsAg)* which is highly immunogenic and provokes the production of the corresponding *hepatitis B surface antibody (anti-HBs)*. In the centre of the sphere is a 27 nm core of *hepatitis B core antigen (HBcAg)* which induces *hepatitis B core antibody (anti-HBc)*. Contained within the core is the double-stranded circular viral DNA, part of which codes for surface antigen, and also a DNA polymerase. This enzyme is closely associated with another antigenic product, *e antigen (HBeAg)*, stimulating its own antibody *(anti-HBe)*. There are thus three principal pairs of serological markers for HBV infection.
(2) Smaller and much more abundant circular (22 nm diameter) particles.
(3) Cylindrical (22 nm diameter) particles.

Both these smaller particles consist mainly of surface antigen (HBsAg). They provide the source of the surface antigen detected by immunoassays, which form the basis of the principal diagnostic test. HBV DNA can be detected using DNA polymerase chain reaction (PCR) techniques in body fluids from a proportion of infected individuals. This presumably identifies only those that are currently infectious. DNA analysis is valuable as a research procedure in the investigation of the infectivity of individuals when the results of serological assays are inconclusive and may also be useful for HBV strain identification in epidemiological studies.

3.2   Serological Changes During Hepatitis B Infection

The antigenicity of HBV and the resulting antibodies have proved invaluable in both detection of infection and establishing the likely stage of the disease process. In addition, the most easily detectable antigen (HBsAg) shows at least four serologically detectable subtypes, designated adw, adr, ayw and ayr, which show differing geographical prevalences.

In typical HBV infection the various virus antigenic markers emerge in sequence then vanish, each to be followed by the appearance of their complementary antibodies. When, in the final stages, antibodies alone remain it is presumed that successful recovery and a state of immunity has supervened.

A simplified scheme of the serological changes occurring during progress of this disease is as follows:

(1) *Infection, pre-symptomatic and early incubation phase* (up to 6 months following exposure): there may be no detectable antigenic markers but blood is developing infectivity. Sometimes HBsAg is present in the later stages.
(2) *Onset of clinical and biochemical hepatitis*: serum HBsAg appears first and its presence may often parallel the duration of liver damage.

   With resolution of disease and convalescence (generally after 6 months) surface antigen disappears and is succeeded, after a variable period of up to 20 weeks, by *surface antibody (anti-HBs)*. This antibody can persist for years.

   In a few cases HBsAg has already disappeared by the time of the symptomatic phase; this can be diagnostically misleading!

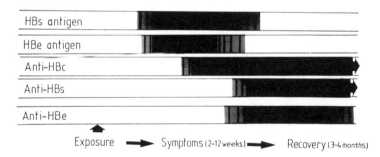

Figure 2   Serological changes during the course of hepatitis B virus infection and recovery

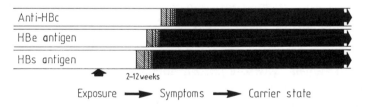

Figure 3   Serological profile typical of hepatitis B infection during progression to the chronic carrier state

Shortly after the appearance of surface antigen during acute infection a rising titre of *core antibody (anti-HBc)* is seen. Interestingly, the corresponding *core antigen*, the major nucleocapsid antigen, does not appear in serum and is therefore not useful as a diagnostic marker. Detection of core antibody is useful for several reasons:

(a) It is present throughout the interval between loss of surface antigen and appearance of surface antibody when the diagnosis might otherwise be missed.

(b) IgM anti-HBc is found in acute illness; IgG anti-HBc reflects convalescence or complete recovery.

(c) In a few people with chronic HBV infection, HBsAg is undetectable and anti-HBc may be the only indicator of infectivity. *HBeAg*, a soluble constituent of the nucleocapsid possibly derived from HBcAg, also appears during acute infection and later disappears to be replaced by anti-HBe.

(3) *Convalescent phase*: typical convalescence serum will contain anti-HBc, anti-HBs and anti-HBe. The corresponding viral antigens are not detectable. At this stage the blood is no longer infective.

(4) *Persistent HBV infections*: chronic HBV carriers with or without overt liver damage show persistence of HBsAg and often, but not always, HBeAg. Anti-HBs, anti-HBc and anti-HBe may also be present but such blood is still regarded as potentially infective.

The serological patterns described above are those typically found but some cases are not classified so easily. Expert help and study of sequential specimens will be needed on such occasions.

3.3 Routine Serological Methods

Detection of *HBsAg* is the routine diagnostic procedure. Enzyme linked immunoassays are now almost universally used for routine donation screening. Reverse passive haemagglutination assays are less sensitive but cheaper. They are convenient for rapid assay of small number of samples and can be used where enzyme-linked immunosorbent assay (ELISA) instrumentation is not available. Modern ELISA methods can reliably detect 0.5 IU HBsAg per millilitre and are much more sensitive than the early immunodiffusion and haemagglutination assays used when screening was first introduced. However, this increased sensitivity detects only about 2% more infective donors, as most positive donors in fact have fairly substantial antigenaemia, probably in excess of 20 IU/ml.[6] Unfortunately, a small number of infective donors, probably those who are at the stage of pre-symptomatic acute infections, seem to possess antigen concentrations undetectable by even the most sensitive tests available. Relatively recently it has been recognized that on rare occasions HBsAg can be entirely absent even in fulminant cases of infection. In some such cases HBV DNA analysis has revealed mutations in the precore region of the viral genome that prevent surface antigen synthesis and excretion.[7,8]

The principle of ELISA for HBsAg is shown in Figure 4. These assays depend

COLOUR DEVELOPMENT

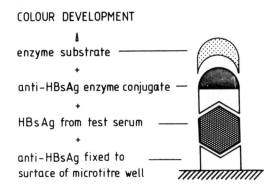

enzyme substrate

+

anti-HBsAg enzyme conjugate

+

HBsAg from test serum

+

anti-HBsAg fixed to
surface of microtitre well

Figure 4 Principle of enzyme-linked immunosorbent assay (ELISA) for hepatitis B surface antigen in serum. HBsAg in test serum is captured by immobilized HBsAg antibody. The presence of bound virus antigen is revealed by the addition of enzyme-conjugated anti-HBsAg and enzyme substrate. Final colour development is proportional to the concentration of HBsAg in the test sample

on solid phase-bound antibody which captures HBsAg in the serum sample. The second antibody in the sandwich is coupled to an enzyme, e.g. horseradish peroxidase, which catalyses a colourless substrate to form a coloured product. The resulting colour is proportional to the serum HBsAg concentration and can be measured photometrically. The specificity of positive results may be confirmed by repeating the test procedure after neutralization of any HBsAg in the sample with added anti-HBs. A negative result should be obtained with samples containing, HBsAg, whereas false positives will be unaffected.

ELISA methods are rapid and convenient and relatively straightforward. The assays should be controlled by including samples of known HBsAg concentration to confirm that sensitivity is being routinely maintained. Assays should also be examined for specificity performance by inclusion of panels of known positive and negative samples, including samples carrying the common HBsAg subtypes.

Various other constituents of the HBV can sometimes be detected in serum. During active viral replication, when HBe antigen is detectable, so also is HBV DNA (by molecular hybridization) and the corresponding HBV DNA polymerase. HBcAg is found in hepatocytes but is not free in serum. These virus components disappear with the resolution of the acute infection. The necessary virological studies can only be carried out by specialized laboratories.

3.4   Prophylaxis Against HBV Infection

Prophylactic therapy may be required when:

(1) Patients are transfused with blood products from which the risk of HBV transmission may not be completely eliminated.

(2) When staff become accidentally contaminated, either through needle injuries, splashes onto mucous membranes or damaged skin.
(3) When infectious donors who may provide a risk to members of their immediate family are discovered.

Two approaches are now possible: *passive immunization* can be provided by *immune serum globulin* and *active immunization* by *hepatitis B vaccines.*

Hepatitis immunoglobulin

The use of this material has been reviewed, but firm[9] conclusions cannot yet be made regarding efficacy. The reported trials used different HBs immunoglobulin, different time intervals from exposure to administration and the circumstances of the exposures also varied. Truly controlled trials have not been performed.

Reduction in the incidence of hepatitis B probably does occur[10] but protection is not complete,[11] and there is some evidence that use of immunoglobulin retards rather than actually prevents hepatitis.

The present state of knowledge suggests that hepatitis B immunoglobulin should be used where a clear episode of exposure has occurred. A protocol would be as follows:

(1) Administer anti-HBs as soon as practicable. Dosage is dependent on the preparation available; a repeat dose is advised after 1 month.
(2) The *infectivity of the inoculum* should be assessed by means of assay for HBsAg, HBeAg and anti-HBe. Small inocula of HBeAg-negative blood are unlikely to be very infectious.
(3) The *vulnerability of the recipient* should be assessed by assay for the presence of HbsAg and anti-HBs. These tests and also liver function tests should be repeated at intervals up to 1 year post exposure.

Treatment should not be held up unless the results of (2) and (3) can be rapidly available.

Active immunization (see below) should probably be given as well. There appears to be no interference with effectiveness of the vaccine.[12]

Hepatitis B vaccine[13]

Several effective and safe vaccines are now available. The first vaccines were prepared from purified HBsAg in the form of 22 nm particles from the blood of human HBsAg carriers. These were subject to a rigorous purification procedure designed to inactivate any possibility of live virus transmission.

Plasma-derived vaccines have now been superseded by those utilizing antigens prepared using recombinant DNA techniques. Analysis of the HBV genome and the subsequent transfer and expression principally of the S gene (HBsAg) and sometimes the adjacent pre-S region to either bacteria or yeasts have enabled industrial synthesis of antigen.

The success of vaccination is usually assessed after a course of three doses. Poor responders, i.e. those with antibody levels below 100 IU, are assumed to have incomplete protection and should be given a further booster dose.

Synthetic antigen vaccines are becoming less expensive and becoming more widely available. Their use is best targeted at those with a significantly enhanced risk of HBV infection. Within the context of blood transfusion practice, vaccination should be offered to newly diagnosed haemophilic patients, staff attending haemophilic patients, laboratory workers handling high-risk specimens and family members of *acutely* infectious donors.

4   HEPATITIS C

For many years a form of PTH that was not due to HAV, HBV, cytomegalovirus, Epstein–Barr virus or any other serologically diagnosable infection was designated non-A non-B (NANB) hepatitis. This has now been ascribed to infection by a newly recognized virus, hepatitis C virus (HCV), thus re-establishing the name originally utilized for the putative agent causing non-A non-B viral hepatitis. The HCV virion is now recognized to be an encapsulated single-stranded RNA molecule the transcription products of which can be detected in post-infection blood samples.

Clinically HCV hepatitis differs from that caused by HBV: most cases are not jaundiced but are revealed only by *hepatic enzyme elevation*. This condition was in fact defined by the occurrence of two consecutive two-fold elevations in serum ALT in patients either with or without jaundice, during the time interval of 2–26 weeks after transfusion. Fatal acute hepatitis probably does not occur. *Chronic hepatitis* occurs more frequently than with HBV infections; 40–50% of cases progress to this complication compared with around 5% following hepatitis B. Despite the high HCV transmission rate the clinical significance of HCV for routine transfusion recipients, i.e. those receiving single episodes of relatively modest amounts of blood, is uncertain. While occasional patients will experience serious morbidity, for the large majority the disease progresses extremely slowly and may not increase overall mortality[14]

Epidemiologically there are similarities with HBV in that both parenteral (by transfusion) and non-parenteral modes of transmission appear to occur. The risks of HCV hepatitis following transfusion have already been described (section 2.1). Following reduction of the incidence of HBV infection as a result of donor screening, HCV continued for many years to cause the majority of cases of PTH. The risk was by far the greatest for recipients of coagulation factor concentrates prepared from large pools of donor plasma. The long-term effects of the chronic hepatitis that has become apparent in these patients are a worrying concern.

4.1   Surrogate Tests

Prior to virus identification, a number of surrogate tests were proposed for identification of risky donors.[15]

Alanine transferase (ALT) measurements which reflect hepatic cell injury have been used most widely, although it was recognized that the tests lacks diagnostic accuracy, excluded many non-infective donors and resulted in only modest reduction of the incidence of PTH.[16]

Detection of *HBV core antibody* was also shown to eliminate some potentially infectious donations, possibly because of the frequent coincidence of both infections in certain high-risk sections of the population.

4.2 Laboratory Diagnosis

An important diagnostic advance was made in 1988. Viral RNA extracted from infectious chimpanzee plasma was transcribed into cDNA which was then inserted into a bacterial expression vector. Expressed protein products from the resulting clones were then examined for evidence of immune reactivity against samples of patients' serum presumed to contain antibodies against the putative viral agent. The antigen so identified was later recognized to be a non-structural

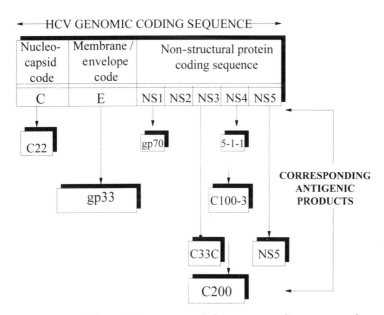

Figure 5 Organization of the HCV genome and the corresponding expressed proteins used for HCV antibody detection

protein of the newly identified HCV. This antigen (designated C100-3) could be shown to react against the sera of most 'NANB'-infected patients. The basis for the first diagnostic ELISA was thus established and it soon became clear that a high proportion of donors implicated in PTH transmission could be identified and that seroconversion could also be observed in the majority of recently infected patients. An accompanying radioimmunoblotting procedure (RIBA) utilizing the same viral antigen was designed as a confirmation of specificity. Confirmed positive results with HCV antibody assays seem indicative of infection and infectivity, but definitive proof depends on the use of the polymerase chain reaction (PCR) (by using a cDNA reverse transcriptase) to amplify any HCV RNA genome present in blood samples. The early (first-generation) HCV antibody assays proved remarkably effective at enabling specific diagnosis of HCV infections but were subject to a high false positive rate. This did little to reduce their value as a diagnostic aid, but was a severe problem in blood donor screening, particularly in a low-prevalence area such as the UK. (Only about 10% of the 1/200 initially reactive donations were confirmed as true infections by PCR examination.) Improvements on the tests in current use, both ELISA and the confirmatory RIBA, utilize an expanded repertoire of expressed HCV proteins. These include usually the non-structural C100-3 and an additional non-structural antigen C33 (both of which may be expressed together as a single polypeptide, C200). These are also included in the new 'four-antigen' RIBA assays, together with the '5-1-1' peptide sequence as well as the C22c structural core antigen (see Figures 5 and 6).

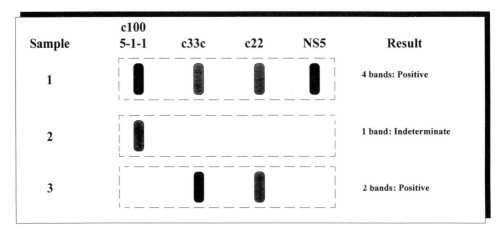

Figure 6 RIBA (immunoblot assay) for HCV antigens, e.g. c33c, NS5, c100, 5-1-1 and c22 (which may be recombinant or synthetic peptides), which are immobilized on the membrane. These bind any HCV antibodies present in test serum; bound antibody is disclosed by sequential application of enzyme-labelled anti-human IgG and enzyme substrate

'Four-antigen' RIBA results are regarded as 'positive' when there are two or more reactive bands and 'indeterminate' when antibody to only one band is demonstrable. These second-generation assays perform substantially better than their predecessors, both in terms of diagnostic sensitivity (earlier detection) and specificity. The majority of infective donations (80–90%) can therefore now be identified[17].

First-generation screening assays have been claimed to reduce NANB (HCV) transmission by approximately 67% and the more sensitive current assays are likely to be substantially better. Positive four-antigen RIBA test results show virtually complete concordance with PCR viral RNA detection. The significance of indeterminate four-antigen RIBA results is less certain. A small number are PCR

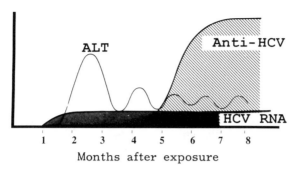

Figure 7   Sequence of appearance of markers for HCV infection

positive;[18] sequential studies have shown some to represent early infection although most remain unchanged and are presumed not to be indicative of infectivity.

Problems of specificity, although improved, still remain. Typically with 'second-generation' tests, 0.3% of British donors are initially reactive and 0.1% repeatedly so. Of these 10–15% appear to be RIBA positive, the remainder being negative or indeterminate.

Post-infection HCV antibody response[19]

Generally, peak ALT elevation and, when it occurs, clinical hepatitis precede seroconversion (see Figure 7). Using ELISA most post-transfusion infection seroconversions occur by 6 months (mean 3 months),[18,19] RIBA reactions sometimes being delayed or indeterminate in comparison with ELISA.[20]

The relative rate of appearance of specific reactivity to each of the four RIBA antigens is highly variable but it seems that increasing the variety of antigens expressed maximizes the chance of early detection. The finding of ELISA seroconversion before development of four-antigen RIBA positivity can cause some difficulties in interpretation during donor screening. This phenomenon is, however, likely to be rather rare because most members of the public bearing HCV markers are likely to be chronic carriers and not in the acute infection stage.

For management of seropositive donors see section 6.2.

5   OTHER VIRUSES CAUSING HEPATITIS

5.1   Hepatitis A Virus

Infection with this virus is probably the commonest cause of a 'history of jaundice' in donors. The viraemic period is short and, since the prospective donor is also likely to feel unwell, transmission via blood transfusion is vanishingly rare. A very few cases have, however, been reported. Previous infection leaves evidence in the form of anti-HAV antibody which can be found in 50–60% of healthy donors.

A recent surprising finding is the appearance of several as yet unexplained clusters of apparent HAV transmission with the use of solvent detergent-treated and chromatographically purified Factor VIII preparation.[21,22]

5.2 Delta Agent Hepatitis

An antigenic constituent in the blood of some patients with hepatitis B, initially thought to be part of the HBV structure, has now been recognized as being a marker for a separate viral entity known as delta agent. Delta agent is only found coexisting with HBV infections, and the superinfection appears to be an ominous occurrence greatly increasing the risk of fulminant hepatitis, or progression to a chronic active course. Although serological procedures have been devised for detection of delta agent, in practice sensitive screening for hepatitis B will also exclude blood infective for this virus.

6 SCREENING OF BLOOD DONORS: DONOR HISTORY AND LABORATORY TESTS

The incidence of the various hepatitis virus infections and the level of natural immunity varies considerably throughout the world. Accordingly conclusions regarding the chances that a blood donor with a history of jaundice will transmit hepatitis should not be applied beyond the confines of the population studied.

Protection of blood recipients by means of the elimination of potentially infectious donations is easiest to manage in Caucasian populations where the natural prevalence of hepatitis B infections is very low. In countries where the overwhelming majority of the population possess HBV markers it has been stated that screening, and the consequent elimination of a high proportion of donations, is unjustified.[23–25]

Resources may be conserved more prudently by restricting screening to blood provided for susceptible recipients; these usually comprise only the younger children. Even this practice is only rational when combined with a vaccination programme to curtail natural infection. The problem is particularly difficult where a sizeable potentially infective population coexists with a large number of susceptible recipients who should be protected.[26] In these instances an accurate assessment of post-transfusion HBV morbidity is necessary and containment measures must be considered in conjunction with those applicable to control of HBV infection in the general population.

6.1 Criteria for Donor Screening

Donors implicated in post-transfusion hepatitis

Before the development of laboratory screening measures the most effective and practicable measure for the control of post-transfusion hepatitis was the rejection of donors implicated in transmission of the condition. The introduction of this practice almost certainly started the decline in the incidence of PTH due to HBV. The problem was less straightforward for NANB (HCV) post-transfusion hepatitis since the condition is usually subclinical and less conclusively diagnosed.

History of jaundice

In areas such as the UK where hepatitis B and C are uncommon, a history of jaundice is generally due to previous hepatitis A infection and serological markers for HBV and HCV show no increase in frequency in these donors. In these populations HBV- and HCV-seropositive donors are no more liable than seronegative donors to have a past history of jaundice. Under these circumstances there is, therefore, no justification for excluding donors with a jaundice history for fear that they may carry an increased risk of hepatitis transmission. Donors who have a history of jaundice, but who lack serological markers of either hepatitis A, B or C, may have been infected with other viruses capable of causing jaundice, such as *Epstein–Barr virus, CMV, adenovirus and Coxsackie virus*. Rejection of these donors does not help to prevent PTH and indeed a history of jaundice is *not* a feature of those donors who are implicated in transmission of those few remaining instances of PTH.

In the USA the opposite view is held and prospective donors with a history of hepatitis or jaundice are still not accepted.[27] Support for this approach depends on a demonstration that HBV (carrier status) and transmission of NANB infections *have* occurred in a dominant proportion of such donors. It is also accepted that there is a need for better evidence for the efficacy of HCV screening in reducing residual PTH before refusal on the basis of hepatitis history can be abandoned. Indeed paid donors are well known to have a higher incidence of a previous hepatitis history and of HBV serological markers.

A history of receiving blood transfusions

This has not been found to be helpful in identifying risky donors but as a precaution donors are deferred for 12 months (in the UK), by which time any transfused virus should have declared its presence.

Hepatitis serological markers in donors

(1) Hepatitis A virus antibody (anti-HAV) is the commonest serological marker, being found in almost 60% of random donors. The incidence of anti-HAV is not greater in donors retrospectively found to transmit PTH, thus confirming that HAV is not the cause of PTH.
(2) HBsAg is found in less than 0.7% of volunteer North American and 0.15% of Western European donors. A higher frequency, reaching almost 20%, is found in Eastern Europe, the littoral Mediterranean and in the Far East. In East

Africa (Somalia) only 26% of the population are free of markers of HBV infection.

Blood from HBsAg-positive donors has been shown to have a very high likelihood of transmitting PTH; in Japan a risk of 80% has been observed which may reflect the increased incidence of the HBe antigen found in HBsAg-positive Japanese donors.

Fortunately, rejection of HBsAg-positive donors has resulted in a conspicuous decrease in the incidence of PTH in the UK. In the USA the overall reduction in PTH was not so striking, but the proportion due to HBV infection dropped from 60% to around 10%. Regrettably, some infective donations are still transfused, presumably because these have undetectable levels of HBsAg.

(3) Screening for anti-HBc (in addition to HBsAg and anti-HBs) is used in some countries as a surrogate marker for HIV and for NANB (HCV) hepatitis or as an aid to elimination of residual HBV transmission.[3,28]

Undoubtedly transmission of HBV can occur from HBsAg-negative, anti-HBc-positive donations particularly when the latter antibody is of high titre[29] and not accompanied by significant titres of HBs antibody. In some such instances high-titre anti-HBc presence has been correlated with the presence of HBV DNA.[30]

(4) *HCV antibody* (RIBA-positive) donations have been shown to have an approximately 50% chance of transmitting infection. A small proportion of RIBA-indeterminate samples (approx. 6%) may also do so.[31]

Hepatic enzyme estimations as a means of detecting donors with viral hepatitis

In some countries, principally the USA, serum ALT determination has been used, together with HBc antibody as a surrogate marker for NANB hepatitis infection. Retrospective studies have shown donors with such markers to have up to three times greater capacity to transmit PTH. However, elimination of such donors achieved only modest (approx. 30%)[32] reduction in NANB PTH. The recognition of HCV and the demonstrated value of HCV antibody assays in the reduction of PTH has largely removed the need for surrogate testing and countries (such as the UK) which had not introduced such screening will now have little reason to do so. However, serum ALT increases appear as an early sign of infection in the pre-seroconversion phase (see Figure 7) and retention of ALT screening may be

Table 3 Prevention of post-transfusion hepatitis: donor selection requirements

---

Rejection of donors:
    With a history of jaundice (USA)
    With a recent history of transfusion
    Following acupuncture, tattooing, ear piercing
    Who have been implicated in causing PTH
    With a history of intravenous drug abuse

---

argued whenever HCV prevalence is high, and where HCV PTH remains a significant problem.

6.2 Management of Seropositive Donors

It is unfortunate that altruistically motivated blood donors who are found to be seropositive for hepatitis viral markers sometimes find themselves placed in a position of distressing uncertainty with regard to their own health, that of their family and close contacts and of their acceptability to receive normal medical, surgical and dental care. Regrettably, these same uncertainties may be present in those members of the medical or dental profession in the closest position to give advice. It is therefore incumbent on those responsible for transfusion services to ensure that such donors receive accurate diagnosis of their medical status and informed and sympathetic advice.

HBV carriers

HBsAg-positive donors are usually chronic carriers but a minority will be undergoing acute infections. The serological characteristics of these states are discussed in section 3.2. *Acute infections* should be monitored by means of repeat samples. Family contacts should be offered vaccination. The donor should be advised as to when recovery (and possibly immunity) has occurred. Advice regarding hygienic precautions, bearing in mind the various possible modes of transmission, is necessary.

Chronic carriers with high levels of HBe antigen and lacking anti-HBe provide the greatest risk and should be advised to provide advance warning to medical attendants when medical and dental treatment is required. Special local arrangements will generally be in existence, e.g. designated dental clinics for treatment of HBV carriers. Vaccination of sexual partners may be unnecessary, where ample opportunity for transmission has already occurred. Common-sense advice should be given about not sharing razors, toothbrushes and about removal of blood contamination as soon as it occurs. In general, there will be no risks to colleagues at work. However, special consideration should be given to certain groups of health care workers; these should not participate in surgical or invasive procedures involving any risk of transmission of infection. It should be pointed out that blood-borne contamination appears considerably more infectious than other possible routes of transmission. Chronic carriers who are patients should therefore be placed on the end of operative session lists after which full theatre cleansing would normally be undertaken. Principles governing nursing and the collection, handling and analysis of blood samples from such patients have been described.[33]

Chronic HBsAg carriers without HBe antigen or with low titres of HBe probably constitute an insignificant risk if opportunities for blood-borne transmission are denied. Apart from notification to medical attendants, so as to allow particular attention to hygienic precautions, no special measures are indicated. It should be borne in mind that around 0.1% of all dental and medical patients in the UK are carrying HBsAg and are given medical and dental treatment with all parties unaware of the circumstances. Therefore routine surgical hygiene should always be carried out with this risk in mind.[34-36]

Management of HCV seropositive donors

All blood donors with positive or indeterminate HBC RIBA results will need counselling. Those with RIBA-positive results require specialized investigation and management although ideas on what should be done do vary.

Donors with RIBA-indeterminate results need the significance of this explained; although usually not indicative of infection the continued finding of such results precludes continued blood donation.

Specialist advice is necessary for donors with RIBA-positive results. Further investigation in the form of hepatic enzyme (ALT) studies and PCR examination for HCV RNA is usual and some hepatologists will advise liver biopsy in order to determine the presence of chronic active hepatitis or cirrhosis. Antiviral therapy, principally interferon α (INF-α) is under study and appears to alleviate hepatitis at least on a temporary basis. Donors will need advice about life-style changes; this should include information that HCV is not regarded as a sexually transmitted illness. However, as for HBV and HIV avoidance of blood-borne transmission opportunities is important as well as advice about limitation of alcohol intake.

7   CYTOMEGALOVIRUS INFECTION

Cytomegalovirus (CMV) infections are endemic throughout most populations. The majority of infections produce either no symptoms or are hardly noticeable. In a few patients, infectious mononucleosis-like symptoms occur, comprising *fever, malaise, atypical lymphocytosis, hepatitis and splenomegaly*. The incubation period is about 2–6 weeks. In contrast to infectious mononucleosis, lymphadenopathy and pharyngitis do not usually occur. The presence of CMV antibody in donors reveals evidence of past infection but, unlike hepatitis B, blood from many such individuals remains potentially infectious. It appears that during infection the virus genome becomes inserted into that of host leucocytes, where it persists indefinitely. Transfusion of these intact leucocytes provides the vehicle for infection of blood recipients.

The overall importance of transfusion-related CMV infection has been extremely difficult to determine. Undoubtedly severe, sometimes fatal cases have occurred, for example in *susceptible bone marrow transplant recipients and immunologically deficient neonates*. The role played by transfusion is not always clear as the possibility of reactivation of latent infections or infection from other sources must also be considered before conclusions can be drawn. Whether the observed morbidity and mortality of CMV infection in various clinical circumstances in which risk has been reported justifies the expenditure of the considerable resources required for preventative measures remains largely a matter for further critical study.

Table 4 Cytomegalovirus infection from transfusion

Vulnerable recipients
    Seronegative bone marrow transplant recipients
    Seronegative renal transplant recipients
    Premature neonates of seronegative mothers
    Fetuses receiving intrauterine transfusions

Risky blood components
    CMV antibody-positive cellular components, unless leucocyte depleted

7.1 Infectivity of Blood Components

The CMV antibody status of the donor

CMV antibody-negative donors are not infectious. However, over 50% of most Caucasian populations are CMV antibody positive and a small but unidentifiable proportion appear to carry latent infection. The proportion of seropositive donors rises with age and males have a higher incidence than females. The possession of IgM antibody which is found in around 5% of donors may be indicative of more recent infection and greater infectivity, but this supposition is not proven.

The leucocyte content of the blood

Leucocyte-free blood components, including those prepared by leucocyte filtration, appear not to transmit infection.

Effect of storage

Contrary to a prevalent belief it appears that storing blood does not remove its infectivity.

7.2 Susceptible Recipients

These include:

(1) *Transplant recipients*: recipients of *renal transplants* show a high incidence of infection; reactivation will be responsible in many instances, and blood transfusion probably plays a relatively minor role. The transplanted kidney, or its associated blood, may be the vehicle. Containment of the problem requires serological screening of the recipients and the kidney donors as well as any transfused blood. Fortunately, clinically symptomatic CMV infection only appears to be a serious problem in a minority of cases. There is evidence,

however, that primary CMV infection may provoke or accelerate renal graft rejection even for recipients of well-matched kidneys. For this reason some transplant centres place importance on CMV matching of grafts for seronegative recipients.

CMV infection is a substantial risk for bone marrow transplant recipients for whom, prior to the availability of seronegative transfusion support, CMV infection was probably the commonest cause of death. Acute graft-versus-host disease appears to increase the likelihood of overt CMV infection both in seropositive recipients in whom reactivation occurs and in seronegative recipients of potentially infective blood transfusions.[37] If the transplanted marrow, or any of the transfused blood or components, are from seropositive donors transmitted infection is highly likely. A serious and sometimes life-threatening complication of infection in these patients is *interstitial pneumonitis*. Other effects of CMV infection include *pneumonia, hepatitis, thrombocytopenia and haemolytic anaemia*. CMV infection may also cause *immune depression* and later opportunistic infection with bacteria, fungi or other viruses. Deranged immune functions such as reduced concanavalin A response and increased numbers of suppressor T cells have been described.[38]

(2) *Transfused neonates*: incidences of 13% to nearly 30%[39,40] have been reported in early studies of transfused infants of seronegative mothers who received seropositive blood. These morbidity risks appear to have diminished in more recent studies; although unproven it has been speculated that current donor-screening procedures introduced primarily for HIV containment have eliminated the most infectious categories of donors. Serious infections are, however, probably confined to those who are *premature and of very low birth weight* (below 1500 g), probably as a consequence of their relatively undeveloped immune system. The precise degree of risk for this group is not yet clear, but it would probably be advisable to use either CMV antibody-negative blood or blood depleted of leucocytes by filtration[40] when transfusing premature and very low birth weight infants of seronegative mothers. The fetuses of seronegative women may also be placed at risk through intrauterine infection and for this reason CMV-negative blood should be used for transfusion of seronegative pregnant women. Intrauterine infections are an important cause of mental retardation and morbidity.

(3) *Patients with immunodeficiency states*, both natural and acquired, including patients with HIV infection.

(4) *Recipients of large amounts of blood*: this was well described in some transfused *cardiac surgical patients* who showed a condition known as post-perfusion syndrome with symptoms and signs similar to those of naturally acquired infection. Most infections are asymptomatic, revealed only by rising antibody levels; serious illness is unusual. The condition is seen most frequently but not exclusively in seronegative patients. Severe CMV infection has also been described in patients who have been both transfused and splenectomized during resuscitation after trauma.[41]

However, transfusion-associated CMV infection is not a significant clinical problem for the vast majority of blood transfusion recipients and preventative measures are therefore not justified.

7.3 Mode of Transmission

(1) Infection usually appears to follow *transfusion of leucocytes from seropositive donors*. The intact virus does not seem to be present; the infective unit seems to be the viral genome which has become incorporated into leucocyte DNA (Trojan horse entry). In view of their long life-cycle, lymphocytes seem to be the most likely carrier cells.

   The relatively large numbers of blood units that are seropositive and appear to be infective suggests that a chronic carrier state is common. It seems extremely unlikely that all such donors are undergoing asymptomatic acute infections.

(2) Probably in some cases apparent transmission is due to *reactivation of latent CMV* in recipient leucocytes. This may be the explanation for CMV infections appearing when only seronegative blood has been used. The mechanism is unknown, but it may be that the recipient's lymphocytes, stimulated by the alloantigenic challenge of transfusion, allow escape of their contained CMV.

7.4 Diagnosis of CMV Infection

This depends on the following:

(1) Awareness of the symptoms of CMV infection and of the susceptible groups of patients.
(2) Appearance of *rising titres* of CMV antibody.
(3) *Culture of virus*: virus from urine, buffy coats or throat swabs can be grown in fibroblast cultures, which are then observed for cytopathic effects. These are slow to appear and may take up to 6–8 weeks. Multiple samples are often necessary.
(4) *Histological diagnosis* is possible because of the unusual cytological effects shown by infected cells. These become giant cells with refractile, apparently vacuolated, cytoplasm and the nuclei may contain eosinophilic inclusions (hence the name cytomegalovirus).
(5) *Polymerase chain reaction (PCR)* techniques can be used to detect viral presence. DNA sequence analysis can be helpful in showing whether reactivation of endogenous infection or acquired new strain infection has occurred in seropositive patients.

7.5 Prevention of Transfusion-related CMV Infection

This depends largely on avoiding transfusion of potentially infectious products into susceptible patients. *Donor screening for CMV antibodies* can be performed by several methods, and commercially produced passive haemagglutination and ELISA techniques are now available.

Leucocyte filtration to below 10^6 leucocytes per transfusion has been shown to be effective in removing infectivity from unscreened or seropositive products[42,43] and can be used as an alternative when seronegative products are unavailable.

8   EPSTEIN–BARR VIRUS INFECTION

Epstein–Barr virus (EBV) infections producing infectious mononucleosis (glandular fever) affect most people at some stage of their life. As a result, only a minority of adults will have escaped exposure and therefore be susceptible to post-transfusion infection. EBV behaves similarly to CMV in that viral DNA becomes incorporated into the nuclei of host lymphocytes. Since after infection the virus remains indefinitely in a latent form in lymphocytes, most donor blood has the theoretical capacity to transmit EBV, although infectivity is probably higher during acute illness. Transmission during transfusion causing symptomatic illness is uncommon, though well documented. Post-transfusion EBV infection as a cause of overt hepatitis is probably even less frequent. Symptoms generally follow 5–7 weeks post exposure.

Post-transfusion EBV infection probably shows itself most typically as the so-called post-perfusion syndrome (fever and mononucleosis similar to that following CMV infection) in recipients of large amounts of blood.[44] Although the condition has been clearly observed in cardiac surgery patients, it occurs with equal frequency in other similarly transfused patients.

Even when post-transfusion EBV infection does occur it does not seem to constitute a significant clinical problem. Most concern surrounds the consequence of infection in immunosuppressed individuals, but the importance of this still remains uncertain.

In the UK, donors are excluded for 2 years following infectious mononucleosis, based on an assumption that by that time the latent viraemia has declined to acceptable levels. In view of the ubiquitous nature of this agent in the donor population screening procedures would be impracticable and, on the basis of present information, unwarranted. Since EBV is predominantly intracellular, it is presumed, as with CMV, that the transfusion risk is greatest with blood products containing intact leucocytes.

9   ACQUIRED IMMUNODEFICIENCY SYNDROME

The sudden and epidemic arrival during the early 1980s of this previously unknown disease has presented a major challenge to modern medicine. Infections due to what is now known to be the causative virus have been shown to be transmitted predominantly via the sexual route, promiscuous homosexuals forming by far the most vulnerable group. Infection presumably results from inoculation of virus carried in the blood, semen or saliva through areas of mucosal injury and in this respect the virus appears to follow the pattern of HBV transmission. It was not long, however, before transmission through blood transfusion was shown to be possible—a fact which placed this disease firmly in the position of the most important problem to be faced by blood transfusion services.[45,46]

Now that an *infective agent* has been isolated, a *diagnostic serological response* has been recognized in infected subjects and high-risk groups have been identified within the potential blood donor community, the prospects for containment of AIDS as a transfusion-related problem have greatly improved.

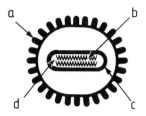

Figure 8 HIV diagrammatic structure. (a) Virus envelope (location of gp41 and gp120/gp160 glycoprotein antigens (*env* gene products)). (b) Coiled RNA comprising viral genome. (c) Nucleocapsid (p17/p24 core protein antigens, *gag* gene products). (d) Location of reverse transcriptase (*pol* gene product, p64)

9.1 Human Immunodeficiency Virus

It is now abundantly clear from work almost simultaneously completed by French[47] and American workers[48] that AIDS is one clinical form of infection by a lymphocytopathic retrovirus which has now become known as human immunodeficiency virus (HIV). A second closely related but so far much less common variant has been recognized. The viruses are now designated HIV-I and HIV-II in order of their recognition.

Retroviruses are so named because their genetic material is carried in the form of RNA and not DNA. They contain, therefore, an enzyme known as reverse transcriptase, which enables construction of the complementary viral DNA sequence once infection within the target cells is accomplished. The newly assembled viral DNA then utilizes the cellular synthetic machinery and directs production of further RNA copies together with the reverse transcriptase and capsule proteins necessary for construction of a new generation of infective virus particles. HIV has specific predilection for the helper subset of T lymphocytes characterized in the laboratory by OKT4 antisera; it has a *cytopathic* effect in these cells in culture and causes depletion of their numbers in infected subjects. In clinical terms this results in *depression* of many facets of *cell-mediated immunity* coupled with an unusual *susceptibility to infections*.

9.2 HIV Infection[49]

The initial discovery of what appeared to be a rising epidemic of disease characterized by acquired impairment of cell-mediated immunity and infections due to various unusual opportunistic microorganisms, of which *Pneumocystis carinii* was a front runner, was highly alarming. Clinically recognized cases had a high mortality rate and neither the underlying condition nor the opportunistic infection appeared to be amenable to treatment. It is now appreciated that the progress of HIV infection may take a variable time course. Asymptomatic infections predominate in the early phase; however, the disease typically progresses inexorably to become clinically overt.

The principal forms of infection include the following:

(1) *Early asymptomatic infections*: this is the phase in which infected individuals, many of which may be unaware of their infectious status, pose the greatest threat as potential blood donors or as a source of infection in the community. Although in the early months seroconversion may not have occurred, these infections can normally be identified by the presence of anti-HIV antibodies in the blood (see below).

(2) *Persistent generalized lymphadenopathy (PGL)*, also known as extended lympha-denopathy syndrome, AIDS-related complex: this condition is probably the most usual form of chronic HIV infection and may sometimes, but not always, progress to full-blown AIDS.[50] Symptoms include *lymphadenopathy and spleno-megaly, fatigue, fever, night sweats, weight loss, jaundice, diarrhoea and thrush*. Laboratory features may show leucopenia, thrombocytopenia, hypergamma-globulinaemia, reduced numbers of OKT4 (T helper cells) and greatly reduced helper/suppressor T cell ratios (OKT4/OKT8 ratios).

(3) *AIDS*: This represents the most serious form of infection. The diagnosis depends on exclusion of other forms of cellular immunodeficiency together with the demonstration of serological evidence of HIV infection or (for cases of unusual difficulty) virus culture samples of pathological material.

It may be that not all infected subjects develop the full clinical syndrome of AIDS, although it is important to realize that clinically apparent disease may take as long as 2–5 years to appear.

The pathological events follow as a result of a severe helper T cell (OKT4) deficiency. The clinical features vary but appear to arise from defective cellular immunity causing predisposition to severe infection by a range of organisms not otherwise noted for potent pathogenicity. The full clinical syndrome includes symptoms of *persistent generalized lymphadenopathy* together with those directly related to particular infections. These infections include most commonly:

(a) Protozoal diseases: *Pneumocystis carinii* pneumonia (the most frequent pathogen), *Entamoeba histolytica* enteritis.

(b) *Toxoplasma* infections.

(c) Fungal infections due to *Cryptococcus neoformans* and *Candida albicans*.

(d) Bacterial infections: for example, *Mycobacterium avium intracellulare*.

(e) Viral infections such as those due to CMV and herpes hominus.

(f) The rare Kaposi's sarcoma, a cutaneous tumour of vascular tissue origin, appears in nearly 40% of AIDS sufferers.

(4) The symptoms of *acute HIV infection* have been documented following obser-vations of the rare episodes of needlestick transmission[51] and also prospective studies of high-risk groups.[52] An infective mononucleosis-like syndrome appears 1–2 weeks following infection by the virus. The symptoms include generalized lymphadenopathy, fever, arthralgia, headaches, sore throat, night sweats, diarrhoea and a macular erythematous skin rash. Seroconversion is usually observed 3–8 weeks after the onset of symptoms.

9.3   Laboratory Diagnosis of HIV Infection

Screening procedures

The demonstration that *antibodies to HIV* can be found in virtually all patients with AIDS and progressive generalized lymphadenopathy has permitted accurate clinical diagnosis and also the identification of potentially infective blood donations.[53]

Commercially produced *enzyme-linked immunoassay* test kits for HIV antibody are now universally used. These use immobilized HIV antigen, derived either from disrupted whole virus particles or prepared by recombinant DNA techniques, as a means of detecting serum or plasma antibodies and have proved extremely effective for initial diagnostic and screening purposes (Figure 9). Although HIV-II is exceptionally rare in Western Europe and North America, it poses an emergent threat to the security of the blood supply and assays are now available combining both HIV-I and HIV-II antigens in a single screening test. All screening procedures suffer from a small proportion of false positive results, probably reflecting non-specific activity with one or more of the viral antigens incorporated into the test system. Positive screening tests therefore require confirmation that the serological activity reflects genuine specificity for identified antigenic components of the virus.

Confirmatory assays

The availability of reliable tests for confirming the results of HIV screen test procedures is obviously of outstanding importance for transfusion services faced with the task of caring for the interests of blood donors.

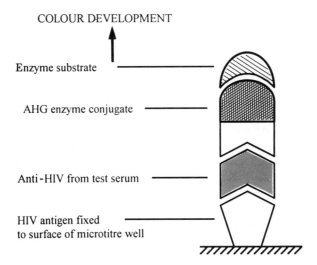

COLOUR DEVELOPMENT

Enzyme substrate

AHG enzyme conjugate

Anti-HIV from test serum

HIV antigen fixed
to surface of microtitre well

Figure 9   ELISA for HIV antibody

(1) The most widely accepted procedure for confirmation has been the *Western blot technique* (virus strip assay). In this rather complex technique, disrupted virus antigenic constituents are separated by electrophoresis so that their individual reactions with any antibodies that may be present in the sera of infected patients can be analysed (see Figure 10).

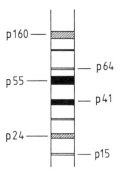

Figure 10 Diagram of immunoblotting analysis of an HIV antibody-positive serum sample. Electrophoretically separated viral antigens, e.g. p15 (15 kDa proteins), can be used to reveal specific components of the HIV antibody response

Several of the HIV proteins provoke an antibody response which can be useful diagnostically. These include 17 and 24 kDa proteins derived from the core of the virus (p17, p24), and larger reverse transcriptase proteins (e.g. p64) and a range of glycoproteins (gp41 to gp160) which form part of the virus envelope. If sera containing HIV antibodies are allowed to react with these separated antigenic components, a more precise and specific analysis of the antibody response is possible. It appears so far that antibodies to p24 and gp41 are markers for early seroconversion, while antibodies to gp126/160 are not so reliably found in the early stages of infection but are present in most cases of clinical disease. Only a minority (around 20%) of repeatedly reactive ELISA-positive donor samples can be confirmed positive by Western blot assay. A positive result requires the presence of at least two bands, one being in the p24, gp41 area and the other should be in the gp120–gp160 area. Single bands, or band patterns that do not meet the above criteria, are labelled indeterminate.[54] The significance of indeterminate Western blot assays has not yet been fully resolved. A relatively small number, e.g. those with p24 reactivity alone, may be in the earliest stages of seroconversion and samples collected later will then provide a more typical positive antibody profile. Most indeterminate results, however, appear to reflect the presence of a variety of false positive cross-reactivities, e.g. for antigens in the lysate of the virus antigen expression vector.[54]

(2) *Use of an alternative ELISA system*: the specificity of modern enzyme immunoassays is now extremely high and use can be made of the fact that *true positive* samples will react with alternative test systems.[55]

The second test system should obviously utilize a different source of virus antigen to minimize recurrence of the same phenomenon of false positivity.

Competitive ELISA systems in which the test sample antibodies are detected by their capacity to compete for HIV antigen binding with reagent anti-HIV are particularly suitable for confirming the true specificity of reactions.

Donations giving what are concluded to be false positive reactions can be accepted for transfusion purposes. The usual procedure is to re-examine further donations and if the apparent initial abnormal findings cannot be repeated at 6 and 12 months following the initial donation, reinstatement to the panel is possible.

Diagnosis of early infection

Serological diagnosis using the HIV antibodies which result from viral infection have proved a highly effective measure for identification of risky donations. Sero-conversion has been observed as early as 4 weeks following exposure but, more significantly as far as donor screening for transfusion services is concerned, in many instances 6 months or so may pass before antibody responses are demonstrable. It has now been clearly shown that, as with many other viral illnesses, early infection is associated with a phase of viraemia that precedes the appearance of antibodies. HIV p24 antigen typically appears early in the bloodstream following infection[56] and assays for p24 have been proposed for donor screening to cover this silent period of covert infectivity. In practice, however, it has been found that antigenaemic seronegative subjects are extremely rare, being probably less than 5% of the numbers of seropositive people. Accordingly, HIV p24 antigen screening has been generally considered not worthwhile for transfusion services in Western Europe and North America,[57,58] although the argument may be more persuasive for populations with a higher HIV infection prevalence rate.[59] In this regard it must also be recognized that the substantial improvements in sensitivity of ELISA screening assay have narrowed the potential diagnostic advantage of HIV p24 antigen assays.

Although detection of anti-HIV antibodies represents the only logistically feasible means of routinely confirming viral infection, there are a number of alternative methods for studying pathological material believed to harbour viable virus. Peripheral blood mononuclear cells collected from patients and co-cultured with their normal counterparts may demonstrate a phase of virus replication that can be detected by p24 antigen assays or by virus transcriptase assays. Viral RNA can also be revealed by PCR and this technique can be useful for studying the early events following infection.[60,61]

9.4 HIV Antibodies: Clinical Significance

These antibodies are *not* neutralizing and unfortunately are not indicative of a state of immunity. In this respect HIV infection resembles CMV infection, where antibody-positive donations are infectious, and differ from hepatitis B, where the presence of anti-HBs signifies a state of immunity and convalescence. The presence of HIV antibodies is indicative of exposure to the virus and is presumed also to reflect potential infectivity due to the possible persistence of the virus in lymphocytes or body fluids. It has been recently shown that the viral envelope proteins from different strains show considerable variability and this suggests the occurrence of a high mutation rate within the viral genome. It is possibly for this reason that HIV appears to be able to escape from the neutralizing effects of circulating antibodies. Antibodies have been found in patients with AIDS, PGL and also in fit asymptomatic people and do not, therefore, carry prognostic or diagnostic significance beyond confirming viral infection.

9.5 Immunological Effects of HIV Infection

HIV exhibits a particular tropism for OKT4 helper lymphocytes. Virus replication in these cells has marked cytopathic effects, the clinical consequences of which are reduction of absolute numbers of OKT4 lymphocytes, reduction of T4/T8 ratios and overall depression of cell-mediated immunity. Thus impaired responses to mitogens such as phytohaemagglutinin and *Candida* and to allogeneic cells represent the most conspicuous immunological defects, and these are associated with inability to resist invasion by a range of microorganisms that are not normally pathogenic.

Humoral immunity is less disrupted; in fact, polyclonal hypergammaglobulinaemia is usual, the serum antibody changes mirroring the protracted battles against subacute and chronic microbial invasions.

Autoimmune thrombocytopenia is seen unusually frequently in AIDS and PGL; a postulated but unproven mechanism involves immune complex injury to platelets arising from virus–antiviral antibody interactions.

9.6 Epidemiology and High-risk Donor Categories

AIDS was recognized from the outset of its arrival in the Western world to show a particular propensity to affect *promiscuous homosexuals,* and somewhat later but to an increasing extent *intravenous drug abusers.* Natural transmission has now spread to heterosexual partners, and infants born to affected mothers have also developed AIDS. Progressive lymphadenopathy syndrome and the asymptomatic HIV carrier state have also become prevalent within the same behavioural patterns. These sections of the population must, therefore, be strongly discouraged from offering their services as blood donors. Those unfortunate episodes of transfusion-associated AIDS have almost invariably been traced back to the donors who, though apparently healthy at the time, were members of these high-risk donor groups, and have subsequently developed clinical manifestations of AIDS of progressive lymphadenopathy. The possible future extension of HIV infections to the wider community will obviously present a major problem, not least to transfusion services, since serological screening procedures will always be vulnerable during early infection before seroconversion has occurred. The incidence of HIV seropositivity amongst blood donors appears substantially lower than estimates for the population as a whole, which provides comforting evidence of the successful operation of donor selection procedures (see section 9.8). In the UK in 1988, only 0.004% of new donors and 0.002% of established donors were found to be seropositive. In most cases further interviews with seropositive blood donors have shown them to belong to high-risk categories,[62,63] most having not fully understood the application of the exclusion criteria. These findings point to scope for improvements in donor-interviewing screening procedures. Reported figures from Africa highlight the problem of controlling transfusion-related HIV,[64] with around 11% of donors being HIV antibody positive. A seroconversion rate of 2.1% within the donor panel and an incidence of almost 1% of transfusing a sero-logically silent HIV infective donation was calculated.

The geographical distribution of the virus has now become apparent although its origin is obscure. HIV infection seems to be widespread in certain Central African countries, where its spread appears to be by largely heterosexual transmission rather than the behavioural activities recognized as hazardous in other parts of the world. It probably spread as a sexually transmitted disease to north America and Europe and to an increasing extent to other parts of the world. Persons from endemic Central African countries and their sexual partners are now also regarded as 'at-risk' donors in Europe and north America and have been added to the list of excluded donor categories.

9.7 HIV Infection Transmitted via Transfusion

Prior to the introduction of preventative measures the unequivocal evidence that HIV infection was being transmitted via infected clotting factor concentrates and by blood donations was one of the more alarming features of the emergent epidemic.

(1) Patients with *haemophilia* have formed by far the most susceptible group.[65] Sufficient HIV-contaminated Factor VIII and Factor IX preparations have been administered to ensure that a large proportion of patients had already been exposed before laboratory screening of blood donation and virus inactivation of blood products could be introduced. The many infected patients progressing inexorably through to more severe clinical disease present a demanding challenge to haemophiliac services. In haemophiliacs (as in other patients) HIV antibodies indicate viral exposure alone, but reduced OKT4/T8 ratios due to reduced T4 cells suggest progression to a clinically more serious state of infection.

(2) Although many hundreds of *blood transfusion-related* cases of AIDS have occurred in the early years of the HIV epidemic, virus transmission has now been reduced in many countries of the industrialized world to become a rare event. The transmission rates depend very much on natural prevalence rates and hence the frequency of infection from pre-seroconversion donations. However, when this is considered against the massive scale of transfusion practice in the developed world, the incidence remains exceptionally small. Infectivity risk levels of the order of one per 60 000 (for a high prevalance area)[66] or substantially lower (one per 250 000 to one per 1 000 000) have been

reported for the USA.[67] However, in one high-prevalence West African country a residual risk, even after screening, has been estimated to approach 1% per donation transfused.[64] In Britain the incidence appears so far to be less than one per million. Transfusion-associated AIDS, like naturally acquired illness, is slow in its manifestation. Symptoms usually take around 4–9 months to appear in neonates and up to 7 years in adults, although seroconversion will be seen considerably sooner. Follow-up of patients who received blood from anti-HIV-positive donors suggests that almost all will show serological evidence of infection and will eventually become symptomatic.

9.8 Reducing the Risk from Transfusion

(1) Donor selection programmes now take account of *high-risk groups* (see Table 5) and actively debar donations. Sexual partners of patients with haemophilia who were formerly encouraged to donate blood have now unfortunately been brought into this category.
(2) With the introduction of *HIV antibody screening* all donations of blood are being tested prior to transfusion. Positive results require confirmation by means of an independent test system (see section 9.3).
(3) Virus inactivation stages are now incorporated into production of all blood products. Clotting factor concentrates, e.g. Factors VIII and IX, are now *heat treated* or subject to chemical virus inactivation procedures or further purification stages to remove virus infectivity (see chapter 3, section 3.4).
(4) All unnecessary transfusions must be avoided. Autologous or other alternatives to conventional transfusions should be considered when appropriate (see chapter 15).

9.9 The Infectivity of HIV Antibody-positive Patients and their Blood Samples

Despite the rapid arrival and spread of AIDS it seems that HIV is in fact an organism of relatively low natural infectivity other than by means of sexual intercourse between members of high-risk groups. This lack of infectivity has been

Table 5 Prevention of HIV transmission: donor selection requirements (UK 1994)

Exclusion of high-risk donors
    Men who have had sex with other men
    Intravenous drug abusers
    People who have worked as prostitutes
    Those who have had sex with residents of HIV endemic areas
    Patients with haemophilia
    Those who are HIV positive or think they could be
    And sexual partners of all the above

---

clearly shown by the fact that even house contacts assisting in the home treatment of antibody-positive haemophilia patients have shown no evidence of seroconversion. It seems most appropriate that, as far as hospitals and laboratories are concerned, the advice and containment measures for hepatitis B antigen carriers should be applied. Preventative measures should concentrate on protection against *inoculation* injury, since the risk from aerosol contamination has not been demonstrated.

9.10   HTLV-I Infection and Blood Transfusion

The discovery of the HTLV-I retrovirus preceded that of HIV (formerly designated HTLV-III) by several years and it was the first of the human retroviruses to be shown conclusively to have oncogenic activity.[68]

Its initial name, *adult T cell leukaemia virus* or *human T cell leukaemia virus*, conveyed an indication of its most clearly recognized pathogenic activity. Later, following the discovery of the genetically similar HTLV-II and HIV retroviruses, which have differing biological effects, the names became changed to the more generically apt *human T cell lymphotropic virus*. Whereas HIV is cytopathic for T cells, the effect of HTLV-I is the reverse; proliferation is stimulated and in a minority of cases malignant T cell transformation is induced which has led to overt leukaemia. HTLV-I infection is also associated with tropical spastic paraparesis (TSP). Both adult T cell leukaemia (ATL) and TSP are exceptionally rare consequences of infection; a lifetime risk of ATL appearance has been estimated at 4%.[69] Coupled with this the incubation time of overt illness appears very lengthy, probably measured in decades, making the significance of virus infection in the blood transfusion context very problematic.

The HTLV-I carrier status is widespread amongst many areas of Africa, the Caribbean and Japan (where its potential to cause T cell leukaemia was first recognized) and it is also present in a small proportion of immigrants from these countries. Parenteral infection and vertical infection appear to be the means of virus spread throughout the population. There is little evidence to date that transfusion of blood containing HTLV-I causes more than a small risk of disease transmission; a few cases of transfusion-associated myelopathy have been reported.[70]

However, seroconversion frequently does occur[71] and is prevented by serological screening of donations. Seroconversion seems to be limited to recipients of cellular products alone; cell-free fresh frozen plasma products appear to be free from transmission risk.

Donor screening has been introduced in those countries, e.g. Japan and the USA, where either the virus prevalence rate or its frequency amongst immigrant populations is sufficiently high that blood transfusions might provide an additional means of viral spread. Pilot donor-screening results in the UK indicate a seropositive prevalence rate of below 0.5 per 10 000 and at this figure the expected clinical level of post-transfusion morbidity is likely to be very small. In the USA donations are screened using ELISA and repeatable positive samples examined by Western blot assay or radioimmunoprecipitation for evidence of core protein antibodies (p19, p24) or envelope protein antibodies (gp46, gp61/68). Current tests do not allow distinction between infection with HTLV-I or the closely related HTLV-II, which has never been associated with human disease. This problem clearly makes the task of advising and counselling infected donors much more difficult. Clear evidence has been obtained from Japan that blood donation screening has virtually eliminated transfusion-transmitted HTLV-I infection.

10 MISCELLANEOUS VIRUSES TRANSMISSIBLE BY TRANSFUSION

A number of tropical viral illnesses are associated with a viraemic phase that makes them transmissible by blood transfusion. These include Dengue, Marburg virus, lassa fever virus, Rift Valley fever virus and Ebola virus infections. The customary regulations regarding exclusion of donors for 6 months following return from tropical areas to prevent malaria transmission also reduce the probability of these viruses being transmitted through blood transfusion in non-tropical areas. Practical measures to prevent transfusion-associated infection are more difficult where these viral diseases are endemic although, in some instances, a high frequency of pre-existing immunity obtains in the population.

Blood from patients with *Creutzfeldt–Jakob* disease is regarded as potentially infectious and people in whom this disease is suspected should not be donors. No cases of proven blood-borne transmission are known to have occurred but,[72] since human pituitary-derived growth hormone had been found to be infectious, exclusion of affected donors seems prudent. Although no supportive evidence exists for risk, the same caution should be exercised when dealing with multiple sclerosis.

B19 parvovirus, a ubiquitous but for most infected people a relatively innocuous organism, has been shown to be a common contaminant of coagulation and factor concentrates. B19 parvovirus has a protein rather than lipid envelope and is highly resistant to virus inactivation procedures. Seroconversion has been shown to occur in most recipients of intermediate-purity Factor VIII concentrates, but infections appear to be asymptomatic and have not been shown to be harmful. B19 infection is typically associated with erythematous rashes in children, together with arthropathy in adults. More seriously, infections in pregnancy cause fetal loss or hydrops. B19 infections can also cause aplastic crises in patients with haemolytic anaemia. These have not been recognized so far as transfusion-transmitted infections.

11 SYPHILIS: *TREPONEMA PALLIDUM* INFECTION

In the early years of transfusion practice transmission of syphilis was recognized as a serious and not infrequent complication of blood transfusion. The risk declined as a result of:

(1) Reduction in the incidence of syphilis in the community.
(2) Introduction of serological tests for screening donors.

(3) Routine use of blood which had been refrigerated, thus resulting in death of the parasite.

The risk had been considered recently to be so small that the need to continue any form of routine serological screening of donor blood has been seriously questioned.[73] Most transfusion services have not, however, abandoned donor screening. The use of fresh and unrefrigerated blood products, such as whole blood, platelet and granulocyte preparations, has also increased and these may amount to up to 50% of all donations collected by some transfusion centres. There may therefore be some justification for continuing serological screening for donations from which these products are made.

11.1 Infectivity of Donors

Unfortunately, spirochaetes may be found in the blood in the pre-symptomatic incubation phase of disease and also before any serological tests are positive. Blood is also infectious in primary syphilis and is assumed, but not firmly proven to be so, in secondary and tertiary disease. It is, however, the donor in the incubation phase, unaware of any impending illness, who might present a risk as far as transfusion is concerned.

11.2 Laboratory Testing of Donors for Syphilis

(1) Tests for *reaginic antibody* (Wasserman reaction, VDRL tests) are designed to detect an antibody, appearing during syphilitic infections, which fortuitously was found to react with a purified component of beef heart known as cardiolipin. The antibody is not a specific antitreponemal antibody and occasional false positive reactions occur. Test procedures are cheap, rapid, simple and, until recently, provided the mainstay of screening and diagnosis. A commonly performed test procedure was the VDRL (Venereal Disease Reference Laboratory) flocculation test, which could be adapted for use by automated blood-grouping apparatus. Well-performed cardiolipin tests are claimed to detect 78% (or miss 22%) of primary syphilis and 98% of secondary disease.

(2) *Passive haemagglutination* and ELISA are available for detection of specific antitreponemal antibodies. The procedures are more expensive and slower than reaginic tests for cardiolipin antibody but their use may be justified as they appear to give positive results earlier during the development of the disease. These procedures have largely replaced cardiolipin tests for routine screening of blood donations. However, even taking into account the increased gain in sensitivity, it must be appreciated that some donors with early infections will still be missed. Where other treponemal infections such as yaws are endemic, the majority of positive results amongst blood donors will reflect those infections rather than the presence of syphilis.

(3) *Fluorescent antibody* tests are highly specific and are used to confirm positive results obtained during screening procedures.

11.3 Transfusion-transmitted Syphilis

Symptoms of syphilis arising from blood transfusion appear after 1–3 months and consist of fever, enlarged lymph nodes and skin rashes. If untreated this would progress to entail central nervous system and cardiovascular damage.

12 PROTOZOAL INFECTIONS TRANSMITTED BY BLOOD TRANSFUSION

12.1 Malaria: *Plasmodium* Infection[74]

Transfusion-transmitted malaria is a frequent and constant risk in endemic areas. In other countries the source of infection is provided by donors, usually tourists or even service personnel, returning from malarious areas. Their blood may be dangerous even if their stay has been short. In the absence of widely available suitable screening tests for evidence of malarial infection in donors, control of transfusion malaria depends largely on avoidance of blood donation until sufficient time has elapsed for infectivity to disappear. This practice unfortunately excludes many donors who in fact are perfectly safe. The incidence of transfusion malaria in 'non-malarious' areas is less than one per million transfused units but is liable to increase if increased numbers of travellers return home having unknowingly become infected overseas.

The parasite in infective blood

Infection is transmitted by the ring-shaped trophozoites residing within the red cells. These reproduce asexually forming multinucleate schizonts; later red cell rupture releases these as merozoites ready to invade further red cells and grow into the next generation of trophozoites. The Duffy antigen site appears to be essential for parasite attachment—a fact which seems to have led to the natural selection of a high proportion of Fy(a– b–) individuals in some malarious areas.

Symptoms of post-transfusion malaria

These may appear at any time from 1 week to 3 months following parasite introduction. Their appearance is influenced by:

(1) The size of the inoculum of infused parasites.
(2) The state of pre-existing immunity (if any) of the patient.
(3) Coincidental administration of antimalarial drugs.

Symptoms can be highly variable but the cyclic episodes of intravascular lysis of red cells causes *anaemia*; the release of toxic products causes *paroxysmal chills and fever, toxaemia, vomiting, diarrhoea, shock, oedema and hepatosplenomegaly. Plasmodium falciparum* causes the most severe illness. *Fatalities* are much more likely with malaria gained through transfusion, and up to 20% mortality may occur. This is largely because of lack of awareness of the problem, which in turn leads to delayed diagnosis and treatment.

Patients at risk

(1) *Premature babies* and *neonates* receiving exchange transfusions.[75,76]
(2) *Splenectomized patients* are more vulnerable because the spleen is an important organ for maintaining immunity and defence against malaria.[77]
(3) Patients with *immunodeficiency*.

Most transfusion recipients in non-endemic areas lack any naturally acquired immunity.

Diagnosis of post-transfusion malaria

This depends on awareness of the risk and recognition of suspicious symptoms. The diagnosis is confirmed by careful blood film examination; blood samples should be taken 8-hourly for 2–3 days and thick and thin films examined. Thin films enable identification of the malaria species and selection of the appropriate therapy.

Measures for control of transfusion-associated malaria

(1) *Recognition of malarial areas*: this is aided by the lists of countries and maps available from the World Health Organization.
(2) Public health *surveillance of the incidence and sources of imported malaria*, as this provides forewarning of a risk of malaria as a transfusion hazard.
(3) *Avoidance of blood collection from travellers returning from malarious areas*: in practice most infections will have shown up within 12 months after return and donors may then safely give blood. This forms the basis of restrictions in many countries.
(4) Donors who have had malaria or are native or long-stay residents in malaria countries are excluded for 3 years (USA) or are used only for plasma fractions (UK). The 3-year exclusion is based on the observation that the majority of people are parasite free well within this time. An exception is *Plasmodium malariae* infection in which parasitaemia may, on occasions, persist indefinitely. It is *P. malariae* infections that are therefore transmitted (although rarely) by donors many years after malaria exposure.
(5) More satisfactory donor selection may be possible shortly by means of testing for malaria antibodies by sandwich-type indirect immunofluorescence tests[78] or by enzyme-linked immunoassay.[79] This will allow many of the potential donors currently rejected, through travel or residence in malarious areas but who are in fact safe to give blood.

In countries where malaria is endemic, possible approaches include the establishment of a *screened pool of negative donations* to be reserved for the most susceptible recipients, *pre-treatment of donors* with chloroquine or *prophylactic treatment of recipients* with chloroquine 600 mg of base followed by 300 mg at 6, 24 and 48 hours.[80]

Infective blood components

These include all red cell preparations and probably also other cellular components by virtue of their red cell contamination. Storage at 4 °C does not remove infectivity. Transfusion has also occurred with fresh frozen plasma and cryoprecipitate but stable blood products (e.g. albumin, coagulation concentrates) are safe.

Antimalarial therapy

It is most important to avoid under-treatment of malarial infection and the reader is advised to consult up-to-date reference sources.

(1) Donors should have completed the routine malaria prophylaxis for travellers; e.g. Mefloquine is advised particularly for visits to highly endemic areas where chloroquine resistance is known, or alternatively chloroquine is taken weekly and for 6 weeks after return.[81]

(2) Treatment of transfusion malaria:[82] if adequate reference sources are not immediately available, if the type of malaria is in doubt or if chloroquine-resistant falciparum malaria is a possibility, give quinine either orally or intravenously. Oral Fansidar (sulphadoxine and pyrimethamine) or deoxycycline have also been found to be effective. For other malarial infections it will be sufficient to start with chloroquine until more expert guidance is available. These recommendations are based on the need to give prompt treatment to the most severe possible conditions. i.e, chloroquine-resistant falciparum malaria. Exchange transfusion has been used for severe falciparum infection with in excess of 10% red cell parasitaemia.

12.2 Trypanosomiasis, Toxoplasmosis and Other Protozoal Infections

In South America transmission of trypanasomiasis (Chagas' disease) is a major risk of blood transfusion.[83] The organism, *Trypanosoma cruzi*, is clearly present in the blood of asymptomatic carriers as evidenced by the incidence of seroconversion or rising antibody titres in transfusion recipients. It appears that both frozen plasma and blood transfusion transmit the organism, and transfusion transmission provides a high proportion of all infections in endemic areas served by under-developed transfusion services. Natural transmission is largely through insect bites. Symptoms appearing after 1–2 weeks include fever, lymphadeno-pathy, hepatosplenomegaly and skin rashes. On occasions myocardial and neuro-logical involvement occur, causing arrhythmias, lassitude or fits. Long-delayed chronic disease may also occur, affecting the myocardium and autonomic nervous system. Simple reliable diagnostic methods suitable for screening are being actively developed. Various immunological procedures, e.g. complement fixation, haemagglutination and ELISA, are available and may prove suitable for screening donors in endemic areas. In view of the very high percentage of sero-positive donors in such regions, additives such as crystal violet (0.4% solution) have been added to blood before transfusion in order to inactivate the trypano-some. Because of the increasing scale of immigration of people from endemic areas into countries where Chagas' disease is not recognized as a health problem, the risk of sporadic transfusion transmission is becoming a serious concern. Several cases have already been recognized in North America and the true numbers may be greater since not all instances are accompanied by immediate clinical symptoms. The most practicable approach, where the risk is recognized may be to combine the use of a risk assessment questionnaire[84] with serological screening for *T. Cruzi* antibodies.

Toxoplasmosis

Toxoplasma gondii is an obligate intracellular parasite capable of causing an infec-tious mononucleosis-like syndrome. Severe illness is unusual but is more likely in patients with immunodeficiency. A high proportion of adults show low-titre antibody levels as evidence of past infection but clearly do not appear to be infectious as far as most recipients are concerned. It seems reasonable to exclude donors with recent infections as confirmed by high titres of antibodies (in parti-cular IgM antibodies). The organisms appear to be conveyed in leucocytes. As with CMV and EBV there exists a latent and persistent potential for transmission of infection, and there may be a risk to neonates and those with impaired immune function.

Miscellaneous parasitic infections that may be transmissible by blood

These include babesiosis, microfilariasis and leishmaniasis. They do not, however, appear to constitute significant transfusion problems.

13 BACTERIAL CONTAMINATION OF BLOOD

Fortunately, significant bacterial contamination of blood for transfusion is now rare. Its occurrence in the past, usually attended by dramatic, often fatal con-sequences, has led to the definition of rigorous standards of hygienic practice that must be applied during the collection, storage and transfusion of blood. The present-day freedom from such events should not allow vigilance to lapse. The introduction of closed plastic bag systems and disposable administration sets has also played a major part in ensuring this aspect of safety in transfusion.

13.1 The Causative Organisms and their Origin[85-87]

(1) Cold-growing bacteria may be introduced into damaged packs through minor injuries to the plastic wall. These include *Serratia* species and *Pseudomonas* species, both widely found on dirty or soil-contaminated surfaces. These organisms have on occasions been found to contaminate local anaesthetic solutions or blood pack anticoagulants through failures of manufacturing sterile procedures. The organisms grow slowly and steadily in the cold but less well at body temperatures. A relatively recent problem has been the emergence of *Yersinia enterocolitica* as a recognized human gastrointestinal pathogen.[88]

   Donations collected during or following recent infections have been implicated in severe, sometimes fatal transfusion reactions and it is presumed that donors have asymptomatic bacteraemia at the time of donation.

(2) Familiar pathogenic strains of Gram-negative bacteria, e.g. *Pseudomonas* species, produce lipopolysaccharide endotoxin when introduced into blood packs. This results in acute and dramatic shock in transfused recipients.

(3) Gram-positive bacteria (especially staphylococci and diphtheroids) rarely cause problems. Both groups are liable to be introduced into the packs through faulty skin cleansing or poor aseptic sampling techniques. Sources of contamination include donor skin, and small skin fragments collected into the needle and pack, as well as the hands and respiratory system of attendant staff.

It must be appreciated that absolutely aseptic blood collection is probably not possible; low levels of microbial contamination of blood at the time of collection are not infrequent and, fortunately, do not result in viable bacterial growth or clinical consequences. Low-level bacteraemia in the donor is probably not of major importance. Short-lived bacteraemias are common consequences of everyday activity; their occurrence is not solely confined to traumatic events such as dental extractions. However, following extractions an interval of 24 hours is generally advised before donation is sanctioned.

13.2 Donor Selection and Blood Collection

(1) Donor selection criteria are designed to exclude those with active infection or any recent dental treatment liable to be associated with significant bacteraemia. The recognition of *Yersinia enterocolitica* as a cause of contaminated transfusions sometimes linked to gastrointestinal symptoms in blood donors has prompted greater vigilance in donor assessment for evidence of recent infections. However, mild gastrointestinal upsets are relatively common and do not usually reflect *Yersinia* infection. Rejection of all such donors, unless symptomatic at the time, has not been judged to be practicable.[89]

(2) Aseptic techniques are essential. These entail a rigorous approach to skin cleansing,[90,91] which should be monitored to confirm efficacy.

Donors who have had brucellosis

Brucella bacteraemia in infected subjects may be persistent and the blood of donors who have had brucellosis has been known to transmit infection.

13.3 Storage of Blood after Collection

The citrate and glucose and anticoagulant preservative solutions are ready-made energy sources for bacteria. It is fortunate, as far as the practice of transfusion is concerned, that blood has a natural bactericidal capacity. This property, which is probably dependent on the presence of leucocytes,[92] is enhanced by a period of delay in refrigeration after collection. Unrefrigerated storage of up to 8 hours and probably even 24 hours (while leucocytes are still viable) presents no danger, although with more prolonged storage refrigeration becomes desirable. The universal practice of refrigeration inhibits growth of the great majority of both pathogenic strains and the normal commensal flora. This is not the case for certain other bacterial species, many of which grow easily in blood at 4 °C as well as at ambient temperature.

If these bacteria are allowed to contaminate the contents of blood packs they may cause haemolysis and their proliferation also results in accumulation of often fatal quantities of toxic bacterial metabolic products.

Despite this optimal requirement for refrigeration, limited storage of platelet concentrates at 20–24 °C is now commonplace and apparently devoid of perceptibly increased risk. This is particularly noteworthy since many of the recipients of platelet concentrate therapy have neutropenia and deficient immune function. A recent estimate of the risk of bacterial contamination of components has provided figures of 0.03% for apheresis platelets, 0.014% for pooled random donor platelet concentrates,[93] and 0.003% for red cells. Since clinical reactions are very rare, it seems likely that in most instances significant bacterial proliferation does not occur.

Rewarming of blood after a period of refrigeration is most definitely not advised (unless during infusion); the natural antibacterial capacity by this time is absent and dangerous microbial proliferation is possible. Serious transfusion reactions due to infected blood components are now a rarity, but the risk is by no means abolished, and the continued publication of details of transfusion disasters due to this cause should serve as a reminder to maintain vigilance.

13.4 Prevention of Bacterial Contamination

(1) Use of closed plastic bag systems for blood collection and processing: where re-usable equipment is unavoidable steam autoclaving or ethylene oxide dry sterilization should be used.

(2) Blood components prepared by procedures which entail exposure to the environment should be manipulated using sterile handling procedures and in a filtered air environment. A shelf life of 24 hours is probably the maximum permissible. This is clearly an arbitrarily selected time interval, and the exact risk will depend on the degree of microbiological contamination inherent in the particular manipulation.

(3) Blood units should be administered within 4–6 hours following removal from refrigeration. After this time, units that have been allowed to rewarm should neither be transfused nor returned for re-use.

(4) Blood administration sets should be changed at least every 24 hours to remove the risk of microbial proliferation.

(5) Procedures for processing and administration of blood should be designed to prevent growth of any organisms that have been inadvertently introduced and prevent any additional risks of contamination due to damage or exposure to dirty environmental conditions.

(6) The appearance of blood units should always be inspected before administration. Infected units may show haemolysis and sometimes purplish discoloration, particularly when compared with blood in segments of the donor line.[94]

13.5 Consequences of Transfusion of Blood Contaminated by Bacteria

Symptoms following transfusion of contaminated blood

The nature and severity of symptoms depend on the numbers and type of organisms infused. Consequences range from relatively *mild pyrexias* to *chills, fevers, headache, back pain, severe gastrointestinal upset, circulatory collapse and death*. These are rapid in onset and fatalities generally occur within 24–48 hours. Symptoms may be due to endotoxic shock, septicaemia or disseminated intravascular coagulation.

Treatment and investigation of suspected cases

Circulatory collapse is due to vasodilation. Plasma expanders, pressor agents, steroids and parenteral broad-spectrum antibacterial therapy should be given without delay until the nature of the organism is known.

Laboratory investigation of suspected reactions is liable to give rise to misleading false positive conclusions unless meticulous care is taken to ensure aseptic collection of samples for culture.

The residue of the blood unit should be inspected for haemolysis as well as discoloration of red cells, which indicates the formation of methaemoglobin due to bacterial contamination. Gram-stained films prepared from the residue will show bacteria only if the organism count at the time of sampling exceeds around 10 000 per millilitre. Cultures taken from the remaining contents of the blood packs some hours after transfusion may well reflect bacteria introduced at the time of setting up the transfusion and not the presence of organisms in the transfused blood.

The following action is advised:

(1) Inspect remaining contents of the blood pack.
(2) Prepare Gram-stained films of the blood.
(3) After aseptic sampling, culture blood from the residue and also from any closed segments of plastic tube and from the patient's blood.

Incubation should be performed at 4 °C, room temperature (nutrient agar) and 37 °C (blood agar) for 3 weeks, 1 week and 48 hours, respectively. Recovery of anaerobic organisms is assisted by preparing cultures in thioglycolate broth; a quantitative estimate of the bacterial count per unit volume of blood is helpful. Negative cultures throughout exclude the presence of significant bacterial contamination of the unit. Positive cultures from blood pack residues alone but not elsewhere (e.g. tubing segments), especially when organism counts are low, provide only weak evidence for significant contamination.

Investigation of the incident

Transfusion of an infected blood component must be regarded as an extremely serious event and all possible causes for its occurrence should be investigated in the hope that further recurrences will be prevented.

(1) *At the hospital*:
   (a) Records of blood administration should be inspected to confirm that the correct procedures were in place and that pre-transfusion examination of the blood pack appearance (red cell units usually show discoloration) could have taken place.
   (b) The storage history of blood units should be examined. Were the units cross-matched for other patients and held out of controlled refrigeration at any time? Attention should be paid to the quality and cleanliness of storage and transport arrangements and it should be checked that relevant temperature records are satisfactory.
   (c) The age of the blood pack should be recorded.
(2) *At the transfusion centre*: in addition to the above, consideration should be paid to:
   (a) Component-processing arrangements. Are conditions hygienic and safe for blood pack manipulation? Results of microbial monitoring of environmental conditions should be inspected and for certain contaminants, e.g. *Pseudomonas*, a search should be made for the same organism throughout the blood component-processing pathway.
   (b) Attention should be paid to collection arrangements, in particular records of donor arm-cleansing efficacy should confirm that secure aseptic procedures are in place. The possibility of contaminated equipment should be considered; microbial contamination of blood packs, local anaesthetic etc.

have been implicated in the past. Batch numbers should be noted and the episode reported to the parent institution and the manufacturer in the hope that any simultaneous recurrences can lead to identification of common causes.

(c) The donor history may be relevant, e.g. evidence of recent infection. In the case of *Yersinia*, serum samples collected over a few weeks may show a rising antibody titre to confirm previous infection.

(d) Samples of the organism should be retained so that strain typing, either serologically or by DNA techniques, can be performed and any epidemiological links established.

REFERENCES

1 Aledort, L.M., Levine, P.H., Hilgartner, M. *et al.* (1985) A study of liver biopsies and liver disease among haemophiliacs. *Blood*, **66**: 367–372.
2 Stevens, R.F., Cuthbert, A.C., Piyaseeli, R.P. *et al.* (1983) Liver disease in haemophiliacs: an overstated problem? *Br. J. Haematol.*, **55**: 649–655.
3 Reesink, H.W., Nydegger, U.E., Tegtmeier, G.E. *et al.* (1992) Blood donor screening or 'over-screening': how far to go in avoiding transmission of infectious agents? (Editorial.) *Vox Sang.*, **63**: 59–69.
4 Rousell, R.H., Budinger, M.D., Pirofsky, B. and Schiff, R.I. (1991) Prospective study on the hepatitis safety of intravenous immunoglobulin, pH4.25. *Vox Sang.*, **60**: 65.
5 Webster, A.D.B. and Lever, A.M.L. (1986) Non-A, non-B hepatitis after intravenous gammaglobulin. *Lancet*, 322.
6 Nath, N., Fang, C.T., Berberian, L.F. *et al.* (1980) Hepatitis-associated markers in the American Red Cross volunteer blood donor population. *Vox Sang.*, **39**: 73–78.
7 Kojima, M., Shimizu, M., Tsuchimochi, T. *et al.* (1991) Post transfusion fulminant hepatitis B associated with precore-defective HBV mutants. *Vox Sang.*, **60**: 34–39.
8 Harrison, T.J. and Zuckerman, A.J. (1992) Variants of hepatitis B virus. *Vox Sang.*, **63**: 161–167.
9 Working Party on the Clinical Use of Specific Immunoglobulin in Hepatitis B (1982) Use of immunoglobulin with high content of antibody to hepatitis B surface antigen (anti-HBs). *Br. Med. J.*, **285**: 951–953.
10 A combined Medical Research Council and Public Health Laboratory Service Report (1980) The incidence of hepatitis B infection after accidental exposure and anti-HBs immunoglobulin prophylaxis. *Lancet*, i: 6–7.
11 Frosner, G.G., Frosner, H.R., Dienhardt, F., Haussman, W. and Knabe, U.H. (1977) Failure of hyperimmune serum globulin, given several days after exposure, to protect against hepatitis B. *Lancet*, ii: 1023.
12 Szmuness, W., Oleszko, W.R., Stevens, C.E. and Goodman, A. (1981) Passive–active immunisation against hepatitis B: immunogenicity studies in adult Americans. *Lancet*, i: 575–577.
13 Eddleston, A. (1990) Modern vaccines: hepatitis. *Lancet*, **335**: 1142–1144.
14 Seeff, L.B., Buskell-Bales, A., Wright, E.C. *et al.* (1992) Long-term mortality after transfusion-associated non-A, non-B hepatitis. *N. Engl. J. Med.*, **327**: 1906–1911.
15 Alter, H.J. (1984) Indirect tests to detect the non-A, non-B hepatitis carrier state. *Ann. Intern. Med.*, **101**: 859–861.
16 Report of the ad hoc committee on ALT testing (1982) *Transfusion*, **22**: 4–5.
17 Larsen, J., Skaug, K. and Maeland, A. (1992) Second-generation anti-HCV tests predict infectivity. *Vox Sang.*, **63**: 39.
18 Bresters, D., Cuypers, H.T.M., Reesink, H.W. *et al.* (1992) Enhanced sensitivity of a second generation ELISA for antibody to hepatitis C virus. *Vox Sang.*, **62**: 213–217.

19 Van der Peol, C.L., Bresters, D., Reesink, H.W. *et al.* (1992) Early anti hepatitis C virus response with second-generation C200/C22 ELISA. *Vox Sang.,* **62**: 208–212.
20 Wang, J.T., Wang, T.H., Lin, J.T., Sheu, J.C., Lee, C.Z. and Chen, D.S. (1992) Improved serodiagnosis of post transfusion hepatitis C virus infection by a second-generation immunoassay based on multiple recombinant antigens. *Vox Sang.,* **62**: 21–24.
21 Mannucci, P.M. (1992) Outbreak of hepatitis A among Italian patients with haemophilia. *Lancet,* **339**: 819.
22 Robinson, S.M., Schwinn, H. and Smith, A. (1992) Clotting factors and hepatitis A. *Lancet,* **340**: 1465.
23 Ryder, R.W., Wojjecowsky, T., Baker, B.A. *et al.* (1984) Screening for hepatitis B virus markers is not justified in West African transfusion centres. *Lancet,* **ii**: 449–452.
24 Bowry, T.R. and Shah, M.V. (1983) A pilot study of hepatitis B viral markers in volunteer blood donors in Kenya, East Africa. *Vox Sang.,* **44**: 385–389.
25 Ndumbe, P.M. and Nyouma, E. (1990) Transmission of hepatitis B virus by blood transfusion in Yaounde, Cameroon. *Br. Med. J.,* **301**: 523–524.
26 Brunengo, J.F., Morier, F., Pecarrere, J.L. *et al.* (1988) Cost of preventing transfusion of hepatitis B virus in hyperendemic areas. *Lancet,* **i**: 1105.
27 *Council of Community Blood Centres Newsletter* (1992) (25/9/92).
28 Dodd, R.Y., Popovsky, M.A. and the Members of the Scientific Section Coordinating Committee (1991) Antibodies to hepatitis B core antigen and the infectivity of the blood supply. *Transfusion,* **31**: 443–449.
29 Hoofnagle, J.H. (1990) Post transfusion hepatitis B. *Transfusion,* **30**: 384–386.
30 Iizuka, H., Ohmura, K., Ishijima, A. *et al.* (1992) Correlation between anti-HBc titers and HBV DNA in blood units without detectable HBsAg. *Vox Sang.,* **63**: 107–111.
31 Kolho, E., Naukkarinen, R. and Krusius, T. (1992) Transmission of HCV infection by RIBA indeterminate and positive blood units. *Transfusion Med.,* **2**: 243–248.
32 Stevens, C.E., Aach, R.D., Hollinger, F.B. *et al.* (1984) Hepatitis B virus antibody in blood donors and the occurrence of non-A, non-B hepatitis in transfusion recipients. *Ann. Intern. Med.,* **101**: 733–738.
33 Tedder, R.S. (1980) Hepatitis B in hospitals. *Br. J. Hosp. Med.,* **23**: 266–269.
34 Leading article (1983) The Hepatitis B carrier in hospital. *Lancet,* **ii**: 1285–1286.
35 Leading article (1980) Hepatitis B virus infection among surgeons. *Lancet,* **ii**: 300.
36 Callender, M.E., White, Y. and Williams, R. (1982) Hepatitis B virus infection in medical and health care personnel. *Br. Med. J.,* **284**: 324–326.
37 Meyers, J.D., Flournoy, N. and Thomas, E.D. (1986) Risk factors for cytomegalovirus infection after human marrow transplantation. *J. Infect. Dis.,* **153**: 478–488.
38 Verdonck, L.F. and DeGast, G.C. (1984) Is cytomegalovirus infection a major cause of T cell alterations after (autologous) bone-marrow transplantation? *Lancet,* **i**: 932–935.
39 Yeager, A., Grumet, F.C., Hafleigh, E., Arvin, A., Bradley, J.S. and Prober, C.G. (1981) Prevention of transfusion-acquired cytomegalovirus infections in newborn infants. *J. Pediatr.,* **98**: 281–287.
40 Adler, S.P., Lawrence, L.T., Baggett, J., Biro, V. and Sharp, D.E. (1984) Prevention of transfusion-associated cytomegalovirus infection in very low-birthweight infants using frozen blood and donors seronegative for cytomegalovirus. *Transfusion,* **24**: 333–335.
41 Baumgartner, J.D., Burgo-Black, A.L., Pyndiah, N., Glauser, M.P., Black, R.D. and Chiolero, R. (1982) Severe cytomegalovirus infection in multiply transfused, splenectomised, trauma patients. *Lancet,* **ii**: 63–65.
42 Gilbert, G.L., Hudson, I.L., Hayes, K., James, J. and the Neonatal Cytomegalovirus Infection Study Group (1989) Prevention of transfusion-acquired cytomegalovirus infection in infants by blood filtration to remove leucocytes. *Lancet,* **i**: 1228–1231.
43 de Graan-Hentzen, Y.C.E., Gratama, J.W., Mudde, G.C. *et al.* (1989) Prevention of primary cytomegalovirus infection in patients with hematologic malignancies by intensive white cell depletion of blood products. *Transfusion,* **29**: 757–760.
44 McMonigal, K., Horwitz, C.A., Henle, W. *et al.* (1983) Post-perfusion syndrome due to Epstein–Barr virus. *Transfusion,* **23**: 331–335.

45 Peterman, T.A., Jaffe, H.W., Feorino, P.M. *et al.* (1985) Transfusion-associated acquired immunodeficiency syndrome in the United States. *JAMA*, **254**: 2913–2917.

46 Melief, C.J.M. and Goundsmit, J. (1986) Transmission of lymphotropic retroviruses (HTLV-I and LAV/HTLV-III) by blood transfusion and blood products. *Vox Sang.*, **50**: 1–11.

47 Vilmer, E., Rouzioux, C., Brun, F.V. *et al.* (1984) Isolation of new lymphotropic retrovirus from two siblings with haemophilia B, one with AIDS. *Lancet*, i: 753–757.

48 Popovic, M., Sarngadharan, M.G., Read, E. and Gallo, R.C. (1984) Detection, isolation and continuous production of cytopathic retroviruses (HTLV-III) from patients with AIDS and pre-AIDS. *Science*, **224**: 497–500.

49 Pantaleo, G., Graziosi, C. and Fauci, A.S. (1993) The immunopathogenesis of human immunodeficiency virus infection. *N. Engl. J. Med.*, **328**: 327–334.

50 Mathur-Wagh, U., Spigland, I., Sacks, H.S. *et al.* (1984) Longitudinal study of persistent generalised lymphadenopathy in homosexual men: relation to acquired immunodeficiency syndrome. *Lancet*, i: 1033–1038.

51 Needlestick transmission of HTLV-III from a patient infected in Africa (1984) *Lancet*, ii: 1376–1377.

52 McEvoy, M., Porter, K., Mortimer, P., Simmons, N. and Shanson, D. (1987) Prospective study of clinical, laboratory, and ancillary staff with accidental exposures to blood or body fluids from patients infected with HIV. *Br. Med. J.*, **294**: 1595–1597.

53 McDougal, J.S., Jaffe, H.W., Cabridilla, C.D. *et al.* (1985) Screening tests for blood donors presumed to have transmitted the acquired immunodeficiency syndrome. *Blood*, **65**: 772–775.

54 Jackson, J.B. (1992) Human immunodeficiency virus (HIV)-indeterminate Western blots and latent HIV infection. *Transfusion*, **32**: 497–499.

55 Mortimer, P.P. (1991) The fallibility of HIV western blot. *Lancet*, **337**: 286–287.

56 von Sydow, M., Gaines, H., Sonnerborg, A., Forsgren, M., Pehrson, P.O. and Strannegard, O. (1988). Antigen detection in primary HIV infection. *Br. Med. J.*, **296**: 238–240.

57 Eble, B.E., Busch, M.P., Khayam-Bashi, H., Nason, M.A., Samson, S. and Vyas, G.N. (1992) Resolution of infection status of human immunodeficiency virus (HIV)-sero-indeterminate donors and high-risk seronegative individuals with polymerase chain reaction and virus culture: absence of persistent silent HIV type 1 infection in a high-prevalence area. *Transfusion*, **32**: 503–508.

58 Busch, M., Eble, B., Heilbron, D. and Vyas, G. (1990) Risk associated with transfusion of HIV-antibody-negative blood (letter). *N. Engl. J. Med.*, **322**: 850–851.

59 Nuchprayoon, C., Tanprasert, S. and Chumnijarakij, T. (1992) Is routine p24 HIV antigen screening justified in Thai blood donors? *Lancet*, **340**: 1041.

60 Hart, C., Spira, T., Moore, J. *et al.* (1988) Direct detection of HIV RNA expression in seropositive subjects. *Lancet*, ii: 596–599.

61 Soriano, V., Hewlett, I., Gutierrez, M. *et al.* (1992) Significance of positive polymerase chain reaction results in HIV-seronegative individuals. *Vox Sang.*, **63**: 287–288.

62 Lefrere, J.J., Elghouzzi, M.H., Paquez, F., N'Dalla, J. and Nubel, L. (1992) Interviews with anti-HIV-positive individuals detected through the systematic screening of blood donations: consequences on predonation medical interview. *Vox Sang.*, **62**: 25–28.

63 Gunson, H.H. and Rawlinson, V.I. (1988) HIV antibody screening of blood donations in the United Kingdom. *Vox Sang.*, **54**: 34–38.

64 Savarit, D., De Cock, K.M., Schutz, R., Konate, S., Lackritz, E. and Bondurand, A. (1992) Risk of HIV infection from transfusion with blood negative for HIV antibody in a West African city. *Br. Med. J.*, **305**: 498–502.

65 Ragni, M.V., Winklestein, A., Kingsley, L., Spero, J.A. and Lewis, J.H. (1987) 1986 update of HIV seroprevalence, seroconversion, AIDS incidence, and immunologic correlates of HIV infection in patients with hemophilia A and B. *Blood*, **70**: 786–790.

66 Busch, M.P., Eble, B.E., Khayam-Bashi, H. *et al.* (1991) Evaluation of screened blood donations for human immunodeficiency virus type 1 infection by culture and DNA amplification of pooled cells. *N. Engl. J. Med.*, **325**: 1–5.

67 Strauss, R.G. (1994) Paid cytapheresis sellers, not donors. (Letter.) *Transfusion*, **34**: 836.

68 Wong-Staal, F. and Gallo, R.C. (1985) The family of human T-lymphotropic leukemia viruses: HTLV-I as the cause of adult T cell leukemia and HTLV-III as the cause of acquired immunodeficiency syndrome. *J. Am. Soc. Hematol.*, **65**: 253–263.

69 Levine, P.H. and Manns, A. (1993) Transfusion transmission of human T-lymphotropic virus types I and II: lessons to be learned from look-back investigations and implications for patient counseling. *Transfusion*, **33**: 4–5.

70 Osame, M., Izumo, S., Igata, A. *et al.* (1986) Blood transfusion and HTLV-I associated myelopathy. *Lancet*, **ii**: 104–105.

71 Kleinman, S., Swanson, P., Allain, J.P. and Lee, H. (1993) Transfusion transmission of human T-lymphotropic virus types I and II: serologic and polymerase chain reaction results in recipients identified through look-back investigations. *Transfusion*, **31**: 14–18.

72 Esmonde, T.F.G., Slattery, J.M. *et al.* (1993) Creutzfeldt–Jakob disease and blood transfusion. *Lancet*, **341**: 205–207.

73 International Forum (1981) Does it make sense for blood transfusion services to continue the time-honoured syphilis screening with cardiolipin antigen? *Vox Sang.*, **41**: 183–192.

74 Bruce-Chwatt, L.J. (1982) Transfusion malaria revisited. *Trop. Dis. Bull.*, **79**: 179–186.

75 Shulman, I.A., Saxena, S., Nelson, J.M. and Furmanski, M. (1984) Neonatal exchange transfusions complicated by transfusion-induced malaria. *Pediatrics*, **73**: 330–332.

76 Piccoli, D.A., Perlman, S. and Ephros, M. (1983) Transfusion acquired *Plasmodium malariae* infection in two premature infants. *Pediatrics*, **72**: 560–563.

77 Joishy, S.K. and Lopez, C.G. (1980) Transfusion-induced malaria in a splenectomized β-thalassemia major patient and review of blood donor screening methods. *Am. J. Hematol.*, **8**: 221–229.

78 Deroff, P., Reuger, M., Simitzis, A.M., Boudon, A. and Saleun, J.P. (1983) Screening blood donors for *Plasmodium falciparum* malaria: application of ready-to-use homologous antigens. *Vox Sang.*, **45**: 392–396.

79 Wells, L. and Ala, F.A. (1985) Malaria and blood transfusion. *Lancet*, **i**: 1317–1318.

80 Camazine, B. (1985) Transfusion-associated malaria. *Lancet*, **ii**: 37.

81 *Communicable Disease Report Weekly* (1993) Prevention of malaria in travellers from the United Kingdom. **3**: 99.

82 Molyneux, M. and Fox, R. (1993) Diagnosis and treatment of malaria in Britain. *Br. Med. J.*, **306**: 1175–1180.

83 Wendel, S. and Gonzaga, L. (1993) Chagas' disease and blood transfusion: a New World problem? *Vox Sang.*, **64**: 1–12.

84 Appleman, M.D., Shulman, I.A., Saxena, S. and Kirchhoff, L.V. (1993) Use of a questionnaire to identify potential blood donors at risk for infection with *Trypanosoma cruzi*. *Transfusion*, **33**: 61–64.

85 Tipple, M.A., Bland, L.A., Murphy, J.J. *et al.* (1990) Sepsis associated with transfusion of red cells contaminated with *Yersinia entercolitica*. *Transfusion*, **30**: 207–213.

86 Murray, A.E., Bartzokas, C.A., Shepherd, A.J.N. and Roberts, F.M. (1987) Blood transfusion-associated *Pseudomonas fluorescens* septicemia: is this an increasing problem? *J. Hosp. Infect.*, **9**: 243–248.

87 Heltberg, O., Skov, F., Gerner-Smidt, P. *et al.* (1993) Nosocomial epidemic of *Serratia marcescens* septicemia ascribed to contaminated blood transfusion bags. *Transfusion*, **33**: 221–227.

88 Prentice, M. (1992) Transfusing *Yersinia enterocolitica*: rare but deadly. (Editorial.) *Br. Med. J.*, **305**: 663–664.

89 Hoppe, P.A. (1992) Interim measures for detection of bacterially contaminated red cell components. (Editorial.) *Transfusion*, **32**: 200–201.

90 Puckett, A., Davison, G., Entwistle, C.C. and Barbara, J.A.J. (1992) Post transfusion septicaemia 1980–1989: importance of donor arm cleansing. *J. Clin. Pathol.*, **45**: 155–157.

91 Stenhouse, M.A.E. and Milner, L.V. (1992) A survey of cold-growing Gram-negative organisms isolated from the skin of prospective blood donors. *Transfusion Med.*, **2**: 235–237.

92 Hogman, C.F., Gong, J., Eriksson, L., Hambraeus, A. and Johansson, C.S. (1991) White cells protect donor blood against bacterial contamination. *Transfusion*, **31**: 620–626.
93 Anderson, K.C. (1993) Current trends: evolving concepts in transfusion medicine. Bacterial contamination of platelets. *Transfusion Sci.*, **14**: 159–162.
94 Kim, D.M., Brecher, M.E., Bland, L.A., Estes, T.J., Carmen, R.A. and Nelson, E.J. (1992) Visual identification of bacterially contaminated red cells. *Transfusion*, **32**: 221–225.

Part H
ORGANIZATION AND MANAGEMENT

25

Organization and Management of Transfusion Practice

1 ORGANIZATION OF TRANSFUSION WITHIN HOSPITALS

Blood transfusion is an important and highly effective part of medical practice. It is, however, associated with significant hazards and must therefore be carried out following procedures and standards that are designed to minimize risks. Blood transfusion laboratories and transfusion activities within a hospital must be supervised by suitably qualified medical personnel. In the UK this will be carried out by consultant haematologists holding the MRCPath qualification. In the USA the blood transfusion subspecialty examination of the American Board of Pathologists will usually be required. Comparable requirements have been defined in many other countries. This person carries prime responsibility for the safety of transfusion procedures. He or she must ensure:

(1) Appropriate liaison with other hospital staff.
(2) That rules and guidance for transfusion procedures exist.
(3) That the transfusion laboratory is staffed adequately by suitably trained personnel.

Laboratories maintaining high standards of professional practice will be inspected for accreditation purposes where this is available (e.g. Clinical Pathology Accreditation UK). These inspections examine all key aspects of laboratory organization as identified in guides to good laboratory practice[1] and ensure that quality-assurance procedures[2] are in place as well as appropriate participation in externally organized laboratory proficiency assessment schemes.[3]

Liaison with hospital staff

This must principally involve other medical practitioners, nursing and laboratory staff involved in transfusion matters. *The Hospital Transfusion Committee*[4] can provide an excellent means for facilitating the interplay between the Clinical Transfusion Service and its users. The Hospital Transfusion Committee can assist with:

(1) Promulgation of education and guidance in the use of blood and blood products and in rules and procedures for their administration; these can include nationally produced guidelines, consensus statements and user handbooks for clinical staff.
(2) Review of transfusion practices against locally or nationally agreed audit criteria: this can also include investigation into errors, misuse of blood products and wastage. Review of the performance of the Clinical Transfusion Service in terms of users' expectations is also important.
(3) Consideration of the legal aspects of transfusion, for example, consent and product liability.
(4) Arrangements for training of medical and nursing staff in blood transfusion procedures.

Staff involved in any aspect of transfusion must be trained and qualified to perform the task concerned. This is particularly important during the collection and labelling of blood specimens for transfusion purposes and also for the correct completion of the blood transfusion request form. The same requirements also apply to administration of blood as this is the point at which probably the greatest number of fatal errors occur. All staff must be conversant with and comply with laid-down blood transfusion procedures (see section 3). In this regard the practice in some hospitals in the USA of establishing trained intra-venous therapy teams has much to commend it.

Transportation of blood by porters from banks to wards or theatres carries a potential safety risk and it is advised that such staff, who are not trained to carry out the required identity checks, take no direct responsibility other than for the physical transportation. Confirmation that the units of blood are those intended for the patient concerned should be performed by trained staff both at the point of issue and at reception in wards or theatres.

Rules and guidelines for transfusion procedures

The person responsible for the hospital transfusion laboratory and clinical trans-fusion service should devise and promulgate local rules governing blood transfu-sion procedures (see section 3) whenever necessary.

Staffing of the transfusion laboratory

It is important that those who have day-to-day charge of blood transfusion laboratories are experienced staff. In the UK they will require academic qualifica-tions adequate for registration with the Council of Professions Supplementary to Medicine. Comparable requirements exist in other countries.

Staff in training who lack these qualifications should be closely supervised by fully trained personnel. It is important to ensure adequate manning levels of transfusion laboratories. This must to some extent be a matter of judgement but some guidance can be obtained by a study of workload statistics, such as those obtained from the College of American Pathologists. These provide an indication of the manpower required for a given amount of specified laboratory work.

2   ROUTINE RED CELL TRANSFUSION SEROLOGY

Routine blood bank serological tests are designed to *prevent* overt *haemolytic trans-fusion reactions* and to ensure as far as possible that transfused red cells have a *normal survival* in the recipient. While the first aim should always be achieved, a variety of reasons may make the second goal less easy to secure with certainty. There are three principal phases to serological testing:

(1) *ABO and Rh D grouping of donations* (performed by the blood collection centre) and also of the *recipient* (performed by the hospital laboratory): donations of identical ABO and Rh D group are usually selected for transfusion but on occasions it may be necessary to select 'compatible' ABO groups, e.g. group O blood for group B recipients.
(2) *Antibody screening of the recipient (patient's serum)* to search for unexpected antibodies that may complicate the transfusion.
(3) *Cross-match testing* (cross-matching) to demonstrate the absence of any anti-

bodies in the patient's serum that react specifically with the chosen donor red cells.

2.1 Selection of Donor Blood

Donor blood packs held by a hospital transfusion service will be prelabelled showing:

- *ABO and Rh D group.*
- A unique *donation number* assigned by the blood collection centre.
- *Withdrawal* and *expiry* dates.

There may also be other supplementary details regarding the donation, for example the probable *Rh genotype* or more detailed *red cell typing* information. More extensively phenotyped blood is sometimes provided for certain transfusion recipients (e.g. children with haemoglobinopathies—see chapter 4) in order to forestall red cell alloimmunization.[5]

The blood collection (transfusion) centre will therefore have performed the following tests:

- ABO grouping.
- Rh C, D, E grouping.
- Irregular antibody screening.
- Mandatory microbiology screening (see chapter 24).

Larger blood collection centres will have utilized automated blood-grouping and data-processing apparatus which ensure blood pack labelling with an exceptionally high degree of accuracy. Even with such arrangements, however, it is unwise to assume that errors can never occur. A more complete description of transfusion centre procedures is given below (section 2.8).

2.2 Blood Grouping Tests on the Recipient

Essential test procedures

It is recommended that the recipient's red cells, as a 3–5% suspension in saline, be tested against:

- Anti-A.
- Anti-B.
- Anti-D.

These reagents, formerly derived from human serum, have now largely been replaced by blends of monoclonal antibodies.

The recipient's serum should be tested against the following red cell suspensions:

- A_1rr.
- Brr.

Additional tests

(1) Testing red cells against anti-A,B is advised. It provides confirmation of the accuracy of results with either anti-A or anti-B, provided that a suitable blend of monoclonal antibodies has been used. A or B subgroups or weakened antigens should also be more easily detected. In these cases, however, transfusion of group O blood is perfectly acceptable. Group O red cells should always be transfused when the ABO group is in doubt.

(2) Some laboratories also test the recipient's red cells against anti-A_1 and the recipient's serum against A_2 cells. (This latter practice assists recognition of weak A_2B blood groups, especially those in which an anti-A_1 is present; these might otherwise be grouped as B.) Most, however, would regard group A subgrouping on a routine basis as unnecessary.

(3) Testing the patient's serum against group O cells is also useful. Negative results give confidence that the positive results seen against A or B reagent cells are correct and are not due to cold agglutinins or other irregular antibodies. Positive results obviously require further investigation.

(4) False positive errors are a serious concern during Rh D grouping of patients. *It is therefore safer practice to routinely use two D grouping reagents* before a definitive Rh positive group is assigned. For Rh D grouping of recipients, use of reagents unreactive with D^{VI} cells (see chapter 2) ensures these rarities, who could form anti-D, are treated as Rh D negative. In some laboratories negative results obtained during Rh grouping are confirmed by an antiglobulin D typing procedure, in order to detect D^u groups. This practice is unnecessary and is a major source of D grouping errors.

Decisions as to whether to perform tests additional to the minimum indicated above depend on judgements such as the clinical significance of a given possible error (e.g. typing Ax red cells as group O) against the extra work that would be routinely involved. Mistyping of hospital D^u patients as D negative is quite unimportant It is far more important to be absolutely certain that the Rh-positive groups are correct!

Causes of error in ABO grouping

Incorrect ABO groups can arise as a result of *transposition* of specimens, incorrect *interpretation* of results or following *transcription errors*. These are the commonest and potentially most serious form of blood bank errors. For their avoidance see section 3.

Technical problems can, however, also be important causes of incorrect results:

(1) Tube techniques for ABO grouping are more reliable that tile methods.

(2) If unwashed red cells are used for grouping the remaining plasma may contain enough complement to cause cell lysis. This may be reported as no agglutination or 'negative' results. ABO group-specific substances in the plasma can also neutralize grouping reagents if the latter are of poor quality. A 3–5% saline washed cell suspension is preferred.

(3) *Cold agglutinins* may give misleading false positive serum group results (with A and B cells) but should be easily identified because they also cause agglutination of group O test cells.
(4) *Weak subgroups* of A may give such weak results with anti-A sera that they appear to be negative unless examined microscopically. Apparent negative reactions should therefore always be examined under magnification.

Various other serological anomalies may also complicate ABO grouping; these are discussed in chapter 2.

Principal causes of Rh D grouping errors

(1) False positive errors can arise during D typing of cells with a positive direct antiglobulin test due to immunoglobulin coating. This is a particular problem when D typing is performed using the antiglobulin test (a procedure which is not recommended) or when using reagents containing high protein concentrations as potentiators. In these latter instances a suitable diluent control, lacking anti-D, is essential. Use of chemically modified anti-D reagents not requiring the presence of high-protein media gives more reliable D grouping results but diluent controls may still be necessary.
(2) Red cells that are C+, D− may react with the anti-C (or anti-G) that may occasionally remain in serum-based anti-D grouping reagents. This type of problem is particularly likely when reagents are used in methods which differ from those recommended by the manufacturer.
(3) Human-based D grouping reagents have been known to have unsuspected contaminants (e.g. anti-Bg).
(4) Weak D (D^U) can present problems (see chapter 2).

2.3 Procedures for Detection of Irregular Antibodies

These procedures are designed to disclose the presence of *antibodies in the recipient's (patient's) serum* which can react against either the reagent antibody-screening cells or against *red cells of the intended donor*. Not all antibodies so detected have the ability to cause destruction of transfused red cells. Conversely, premature red cell destruction may occur even when scrupulous pre-transfusion testing has given negative results. Re-stimulation by transfusion of latent antibodies arising from previous transfusions or pregnancies is a cause of delayed haemolysis.

An increasing choice of serological techniques has developed for the purposes for antibody detection. However, the trend towards a search for every conceivable antibody irrespective of clinical relevance has now begun to give way to realization that the time and expense may well be unjustified in terms of the contribution towards safety for the recipient. The goal is therefore to select methods for detection of only those antibodies likely to cause haemolysis of transfused cells.

Saline agglutination tests

Certain antibodies, principally those of the IgM class, are capable of direct agglutination of a saline suspension of red cells. IgM antibodies are large enough to be capable of bridging the gap between adjacent red cells in suspension. These red cells are normally held apart by their mutually repulsive electronegative surface charges. This process of agglutination is facilitated by the presence of a high density of antigen sites on the red cell surface. Agglutination is often most pronounced during reactions at room temperature (18–22 °C) or below. However, antibodies detected only by saline agglutination tests at room temperature are clinically unimportant and such tests are unnecessary for routine compatibility testing.[6,7]

The use of 37 °C saline agglutination tests served primarily to elucidate the problems disclosed by room temperature tests and are in consequence of little value.

Albumin tests

Addition of concentrated albumin (as 20–30% solutions) as an additive for enhancing agglutination tests has proved valuable in the detection of incomplete antibodies. Albumin appears to exert its effect by shielding the negative surface charges of the red cells, thereby reducing their mutual repulsion and allowing them to settle in closer proximity. This allows IgG antibodies, which have a smaller reach between their binding sites than IgM antibodies, to cross-link adjacent red cells. Albumin tests should not in theory detect antibodies which cannot now be found better by other means,[8] and their continued use during routine screening or compatibility testing would therefore seem inappropriate. However, albumin techniques are convenient and can certainly be valuable for red cell typing purposes.

Enzyme methods

Treatment of red cells with proteolytic enzymes removes some negatively charged surface glycoproteins and as a result may allow antibody molecules stereochemical access to antigen sites otherwise inaccessible. Some red cell antigens are, however, destroyed as a result of such treatment (see chapter 2, section 6), a fact which may facilitate the analysis of sera containing mixtures of antibodies. Enzyme-pre-treated cells are more sensitive for antibody detection than one-step sedimentation or mixing enzyme techniques. They are undoubtedly highly sensitive for Rh antibody detection and will detect some antibodies that are not found by antiglobulin tests. However, there seems little evidence that most such antibodies are clinically significant. It is evident from proficiency test surveys that some allegedly 'enzyme-only antibodies' detected by laboratories should have reacted by the antiglobulin test had the latter been adequately performed. Enzyme tests are particularly suitable and convenient for antibody screening but are not generally recommended for the 'cross-match' phase.

The indirect antiglobulin test

The discovery that red cells coated, but not agglutinated, by antibodies could be made to agglutinate by addition of a second anti-immunoglobulin antibody (*anti-human IgG* is the important component) directed against the first antibody provided an enormous impetus to red cell serology. The introduction of the 'anti-globulin' test utilizing this principle (Figure 1) facilitated the discovery and under-standing of a series of new blood group systems, foremost of which was the Rh system. The indirect antiglobulin test is the single most valuable technique for both screening and cross-match testing. When low ionic strength saline (LISS) is used in place of normal saline for the initial red cell suspension both the speed of reaction and the sensitivity of the test for most antibodies are improved.

It appears that normal saline solutions have a high density of charged ions interfering with the electrostatically charged areas attracting antibodies to antigens. The reduced ionic concentrations of LISS solutions reduces this impedi-

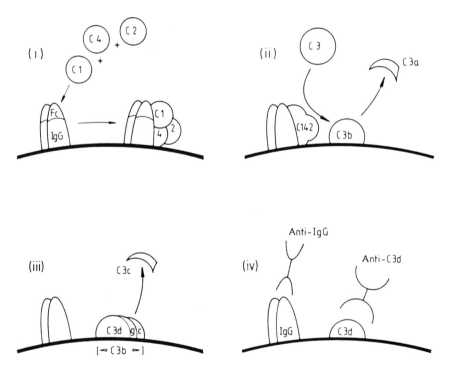

Figure 1 Detection of red cell-bound IgG and complement during the antiglobulin test. The binding of antibody to the red cell surface reactions is followed by conformational changes in the immunoglobulin Fc region. This creates a receptor site for C1 (the first com-plement component) and later also for C4 and C2 (i). The C142 complex (C3 convertase) activates C3 leaving a free portion (C3a) and a cell-bound portion, C3b (ii). C3b comprises further subcomponents which include C3c and C3g (iii), both lost by degradation of the parent molecule, to leave C3d as the final residue on the red cell surface (iv). C3d is the component detected during the *direct* antiglobulin test. The detection of C3b or C3c is more important when *in vitro* reactions are studied during the *indirect* test

ment and vastly speeds antibody uptake rates. A troublesome difficulty is the undoubted enhancement of some clinically insignificant cold antibodies such as anti-I and -P_1 that may produce positive reactions by LISS antiglobulin techniques, whereas with normal saline their reactions might have been confined to the room-temperature agglutination phase alone. LISS solutions do not enhance detection of all IgG antibodies. Anti-E reactions may not be improved; certainly anti-K uptake may be less strong in LISS[9,10] and it has been claimed that haemolytic examples of anti-K can be missed.[11] These episodes do not, however, detract from the overall benefits of using LISS solutions for antibody detection. Even the difficulties of anti-K detection can be overcome by ensuring that sufficiently high serum cell ratios are used in the incubation mixtures.[12]

There has been a debate as to the need for *anti-complement* as well as anti-IgG activity in the antiglobulin sera for pre-transfusion testing. Some antibodies, e.g. anti-Fy^a, and anti-Jk^a, have clearly been shown to be best detected when anti-complement is present,[13-15] and the same may also be true of some examples of anti-K.[13] Antiglobulin reagents for compatibility testing should be standardized and shown to contain optimal amounts of anti-human IgG, anti-C3c and anti-C3d.[16] The C3d antigen is exposed and potentially reactive on all cell-bound forms of C3, i.e. C3b, C3c and C3g.

Anti-IgM is not required since IgM antibodies do not usually remain on the red cells during 37 °C testing; those that are clinically important sensitize the red cell to complement, which should be detected.

Errors can occur during performance of this important test. Inadequate washing of the red cell suspension may cause unbound immunoglobulin to remain and neutralize the antiglobulin reagent, preventing it from agglutinating the sensitized red cells. This can be shown by addition of a control suspension of weakly sensitized red cells to all apparent negative results.[17] If washing has been inadequate these sensitized cells will not be agglutinated.

If positive results are obtained during antiglobulin testing a *direct antiglobulin test*, i.e. washed red cells and antiglobulin reagent, must be performed on the cells. Positive results indicate that *in vivo* sensitization is occurring in the circulation of the red cell *donor*.

Variations in the detailed performance of antiglobulin test, e.g. use of high cell serum ratios, use of microscopic reading, avoidance of excessive agitation of agglutinates, have all been shown to be important in maximizing sensitivity of the procedure.

2.4 Antibody Screening

Antibody screening entails the testing of patients' serum against two or more red cell suspensions containing the most frequently occurring and important blood group antigens in order to detect unsuspected antibodies. The practice has become widely adopted as a supplement to the conventional cross-match during pre-transfusion compatibility testing. However, as laboratories get busier and resources apparently scarcer the need to retain both the screening and cross-match phases as part of routine pre-transfusion testing becomes increasingly questionable. It is argued that the risk of undetected incompatibilities after careful antibody screening is so small as to render the cross-match (compatibility test) redundant. It is, however, necessary to be clear that each of the procedures offers important and distinct benefits. The *advantages of antibody screening are*:

(1) Screening cells can be of selected and controlled antigenicity (including homozygous cells whenever possible) to maximize the chances of antibody detection.
(2) The screening procedure may forewarn of the presence of serological problems before compatibility testing is required.
(3) Screening can and should best be performed on freshly received serum to maximize the chances of detecting complement-enhanced reactions.
(4) A less comprehensive compatibility test protocol is required.
(5) Routine use of the antibody screen procedure alone in place of cross-matching for surgical procedures in which blood is rarely used reduces blood wastage (see section 6).

Many commercial suppliers and large transfusion centres prepare and distribute sets of antibody screening cells. Generally, two or three cell suspensions are provided in which homozygosity for the most clinically important antigens (e.g. D, C, c, Fy^a, Fy^b, Jk^a, Jk^b, S, s) is often sought.

Screening cells should also contain E, e, K, k, Le^a, Le^b, M, N, Js^b, Kp^b and P_1. Attention will also have to be paid to whether uncommon antigens such as C^w, Kp^a and Lu^a are present. Screening cell vials should preferably contain red cells from a single donor as this improves the sensitivity of antibody detection. Screening procedures must include the *indirect antiglobulin test* and for reasons discussed above an additional *two-stage enzyme technique* may be advantageous.

Because so very few of the 'enzyme only' antibodies are of clinical significance, the need to retain an enzyme screening phase has been disputed.[18] The decision to discontinue enzyme procedures should be supported by demonstrably high proficiency during antiglobulin test performance.

The direct *antiglobulin test* on the patient's cells or alternatively an *autocontrol test* (patient's cells plus patient's serum) is often examined as part of screening or cross-matching procedures. These tests can disclose an unsuspected autoimmune haemolytic state, or if the patient has been transfused recently may reveal the formation of alloantibodies against surviving donor red cells. It has been suggested that the routine performance of these tests is unproductive and that they should be reserved for patients transfused within the last 2 weeks or for those suspected of having relevant haematological or serological abnormalities.[19]

Transfusions repeated over a short period of time

Any transfusion carries the risk of stimulating or reactivating an immune response and because of this it is generally accepted, though not without some contention, that 3 days should be the maximum interval that a pre-transfusion serum can be used for further matching purposes.[20] This time limit represents a *practical* compromise, designed to optimize the chances of detecting *emergent immune responses*.

The change from the previous AABB requirement not to exceed a 48-hour interval has been estimated to carry some extra risk of *acute or delayed haemolytic transfusion reaction.*[21] Under these circumstances, performance of an auto-control cross-match (own cells/own serum) increases the chances of alloantibody detection, albeit directed against previously transfused cells.[22]

2.5 The Compatibility Test (Cross-match)

The testing of mixtures of donors' blood with that of the recipient conceptually provides a complete and secure test for compatibility. Historically a cross-match entailed:

- Recipient's serum plus donor red cells (major cross-match).
- Donor plasma plus recipient's red cells (minor cross-match).

Minor cross-matching is now regarded as unnecessary because:

(1) Donor blood is routinely screened by the collection centre for clinically significant antibodies.
(2) The post-transfusion dilution of donor plasma renders all except very high-titre donor antibodies unimportant with regard to damage to recipient red cells.
(3) Plasma-reduced red cell units are increasingly supplied from transfusion centres in place of whole blood. This trend will continue with the adoption of optimal additive red cell packs (chapter 3, section 1.4). Accordingly the presence of antibodies in the original donation becomes irrelevant.

Antibodies in donor plasma are important in a few circumstances. Group O plateletpheresis donations transfused to non-O recipients have been known to cause haemolytic transfusion reactions and should accordingly be screened for the presence of *high-titre haemolysins*. Where large amounts of donor plasma will be administered to neonates (e.g. during massive or exchange transfusion) a screen on donor plasma or equivalent sensitivity to that for patient screening should be employed (see chapter 20, section 2.1).

The *major cross-match* (usually referred to as the cross-match or compatibility test) provides:

(1) An important security against an ABO mismatch arising from mistyping and some, but not all, sample transposition errors.
(2) A test for the presence of antibodies against rare antigens on one of the donor cells but which may be lacking on the screening cells.
(3) A further chance of detecting antibodies that might have been missed during the screening procedure.

To secure the first objective an immediate saline spin procedure will suffice,[23] although rare false negative[24] and false positive reactions can be a problem.* If

---

* Immediate spin techniques do not reliably detect reaction between A_2B donor cells and group B recipients. In practice, however, it must be appreciated that the statistical chances of the occurrence of this error are extremely small.[27]

the benefits of (1) and (3) above are considered worthwhile, speed and safety can be achieved with the use of a low ionic strength antiglobulin test. The reactions can be usefully inspected for agglutination and lysis after an immediate spin and before proceeding to the antiglobulin phase.[25] Contrary to general belief the indirect antiglobulin test is at least as good if not better than saline tests for detection of ABO reactions.[26,27] Thus use of an additional saline room-temperature tube is unnecessary.

2.6 Is the Cross-match Necessary?[28–31]

The current pressures for cost containment have also led to questioning of the need to include a cross-match (donor red cell plus patient serum mixtures) in the search for alloantibodies when a negative screening test result has already been obtained. Despite the increasing evidence of safety of this approach, in many laboratories there has been considerable reluctance to accept any substantial reduction in the cross-match protocol. It must be remembered, however, that full compatibility testing entails:

(1) Examination of a patient's previous transfusion history.
(2) Testing and selection of appropriate ABO and Rh D groups.
(3) Antibody screening.
(4) The conventional cross-match procedure.

All these steps play a part in ensuring ultimate safety for the transfusion recipient.[32] Those who propose abolition of the conventional cross-match point out that if careful antibody screening has been performed both the theoretical and the observed chances of finding clinically significant antibodies during the direct matching is vanishingly low and few of the antibodies 'missed' during screening are potentially haemolytic.[33] Indeed, reliance on antibody screening alone for pre-transfusion testing has not been found to lead to an increased incidence of haemolytic transfusion reactions.[29,34] Incompatibilities due to antibodies against *low frequency antigens* are likely to be missed during screening but these, by definition, are excessively rare. The antigens would be found on one transfused donation alone and thus unlikely to cause serious harm. Cross-match testing, it is pointed out, leads to blood wastage, adds extra costs to the transfusion service and, on occasions, delays transfusion to the extent that patients' lives are sometimes endangered.

For this reason, provided that validated procedures are in place to prevent ABO incompatibility, computer-controlled release of ABO-compatible blood units (electronic cross-match) is now permitted in some countries.[35]

Regrettably serological risk factors assessed by highly motivated and skilled transfusion teams cannot be assumed to hold true of the blood-banking community at large. Nationwide proficiency testing of blood banks points to the presence of a substantial number of participants who have failed to detect the antibodies provided[36,37] and many of these antibodies were potent and of undoubted clinical significance. It might reasonably be expected that, where the patient's serum is examined on two occasions such as during screening and again during cross-match testing and that if two operators are involved, the final risk of error is greatly minimized. Even those in favour of dropping the cross-match do in fact perform an immediate spin procedure to prevent ABO mishaps. It seems a small step to proceed through to an antiglobulin test, thereby greatly enhancing the serological value.[38]

2.7 New Techniques in Serology

Currently available screening and compatibility testing procedures suffer from various imperfections:

(1) Reading and interpretation of test reactions is subjective rather than objective. Thus experience, training, fatigue and knowledge of results of previous tests are all factors which may adversely affect the recorded result.
(2) It is much more difficult to standardize and control the quality of manual procedures. Some degree of inconsistency is always liable to occur unless rigid adherence to standard operating instructions can be assured.
(3) There may be a need for increased sensitivity for the detection of clinically significant antibodies.
(4) Current compatibility test procedures are unable to distinguish between potentially haemolytic antibodies and those which are of no *in vivo* importance.

The introduction of automated blood-grouping and antibody-screening systems, suitable in size and capacity for hospital transfusion laboratories, coupled with blood bank computerization will be of considerable value in the search for improved safety and efficiency. Widespread adoption of, for example, sensitive automated antibody-screening systems could reduce the chances of a patient's serum containing irregular antibodies being presented for routine compatibility testing. Acceptable automated donor–recipient cross-matching systems have yet to be devised. Liquid-phase microplate-based adaptations of conventional tube tests are now becoming commonplace for red cell-grouping and antibody-screening procedures.[39]

Semi-automated serology techniques involving solid-phase reactions are readily applicable to antibody-screening procedures.[40,41] Photometric reading of red cell settling patterns or enzyme–substrate reactions arising from the use of enzyme-linked antiglobulin procedures allow objective reading of test results.

A technique gaining in popularity is that based on the use of microtubes filled with a semi-solid (e.g. Sephadex gel) medium to detect red cell agglutination reactions.[42] Red cell agglutinates become trapped on top of the gels, while free cells percolate towards the column base. The settling patterns of positive agglutinates can thus be readily distinguished from negative reactions. The technique can be adapted for red cell grouping, antiglobulin testing and antibody screening. Where applicable antisera or antiglobulin reagents will be incorporated within the gel matrix and cells overlaid above or, alternatively, cell–serum reactants are applied to the top of the column. Cassettes holding a set of microtubes are centrifuged to drive unagglutinated cells down through the column matrix, thereby allowing the reaction pattern to be recorded. The commercially available systems have so far been found to be at least comparable in sensitivity to conventional tube techniques.[43,44] The technique has the advantage of being relatively easy to standardize and to be less dependent upon high levels of operator skills.

2.8 Serological Tests on Donor Blood Performed at the Transfusion Centre

Blood grouping and antibody screening at the larger blood collection centres now use continuous-flow or discrete automated serology systems or semi-automated microtitre systems. Test results are read photometrically and patterns of reaction to various reagents are analysed by microprocessors which determine the blood group result and relate it to the donation number, which can also be read electronically and reliably from the blood sample tube label. Computers can be used to control both blood grouping and blood pack labelling procedures to ensure that only the correct blood group label can be applied. These systems depend on the use of machine-readable (e.g. bar-coded) labels for sample tubes, blood packs and blood group information. Where these procedures are in operation the relevant labels have bar-coded information adjacent to the conventional eye-readable numbers or blood group information. Information on the blood pack labels, for example donation identification numbers, ABO and Rh groups or blood product types, can therefore be read by machine as well as by eye.

Typically individual blood donations will be tested as below:

(1) Donor red cells against:
   - Anti-A.
   - Anti-A_1.
   - Anti-B.
   - Anti-A + B (O serum).
   - Anti-D ($\times 2$).
   - Cells may also be tested against anti-C+D and anti-D+E.
   Rh D typing will utilize at least one reagent designed to detect category D^{IV} and most weak D (D^U) cells.
(2) Donor plasma (or serum) will be tested against:
   - A_1 cells.
   - A_2 cells.
   - B cells.
   - Group O R_1R_2 cells $\left.\right\}$ for antibody screening.
   - Group O rr K+ cells
(3) 'Spare channels' may be used for other purposes such as syphilis serology or the determination of other red cell genotype results. Final Rh genotyping and resolution of any anomalies that have appeared during ABO typing will usually be resolved by repeating tests using manual procedures.

3   SAFE TRANSFUSION THROUGH ERROR AVOIDANCE (GETTING THE RIGHT BLOOD TO THE RIGHT PATIENT)[63]

Experience unfortunately shows that mistakes can and will, unless the utmost care is taken, occur at any step during the organization of blood transfusion. The following pages describe rules for transfusion procedures and the principles behind them that have been found to be reliable as a means to reduce errors. Many variations of these arrangements, conferring an equal measure of safety, will be found in other institutions. The basic principles should, however, be broadly similar. One rule that should obtain universally is that blood transfusion procedures should be clearly written down, should be brought to the attention of all staff concerned and must be enforced.

Accurate identification of *patient samples* is crucial, and rules and paper work for ensuring reliability should be clear and precise. Excessive cross-checking and complicated paperwork is counter-productive and may distract staff from focusing on the essential elements that ensure safety. Identity checks prevent mishaps; they should involve only the patient's information that does not alter during the current hospital stay (see below). Certain information related to patients such as the name of their ward or their attending physician may be convenient but does not contribute to accurate identification. Systems which require cross-checking of such information can be confusing and dangerous. Each step in the chain of events leading to transfusion of a unit of blood must be considered during the organization of blood transfusion in hospitals. These stages include:

(1) The procedure for collection of the blood-grouping and compatibility test sample from the intended recipient.
(2) Design of the specimen bottle label and the request form.
(3) The procedure for handling the blood sample and the request form within the laboratory during blood grouping and compatibility testing.
(4) Attachment of the compatibility labels to blood packs.
(5) Collection of blood packs from the transfusion laboratory.
(6) Administration of the blood pack to the patient.

3.1   Collection of Patients' Samples for Blood Transfusion Purposes

Identification of patients, their blood samples and request forms

Minimum acceptable details for patient identification should be agreed upon for transfusion purposes. In the UK the following identity details are required:[45]

- Patient's name and forenames.
- Sex.
- Date of birth.
- Case record number (assigned by the hospital).

Such a 'set' of information serves to identify the patient and all blood samples and associated paperwork. No less should be accepted except in extreme circumstances.

Local practice may require inclusion of alternative information, such as the patient's ward or attending physician. While there may be arguments in favour of their use as identification features, they are liable to change within the duration of any patient's stay in hospital and may therefore lead to errors.

Collection of blood samples

The *sequence* of events in the collection of labelling of samples is important. A brief instruction sheet as shown in Table 1 may be helpful.

Having obtained the patient's case notes and approached the patient who requires transfusion, it is of vital importance to confirm accurately his or her identity. This must be done by asking the patient to *volunteer* his or her name and other personal identification information as shown above. This information must be checked stepwise against that obtained from the patient's case notes. The patient should never be asked 'Are you . . . ?' etc. Patients who are sick, confused or hard of hearing may easily give an affirmative answer which could lead to a dangerous mistake.

When patients are *confused* or *unconscious* all these details must be obtained from a 'permanently affixed wrist band'. The case record number (or accident or casualty number) must also form part of the identification check and will be available on the above-mentioned wrist band. On admission to hospital, unconscious patients should be given at least a temporary wrist band bearing a casualty unit number which then serves as the key identifying feature until other information becomes available. It is most important to stress that information from wallets, handbags etc. cannot be relied upon as a means of identifying patients for transfusion purposes.

The above procedures are designed to ensure as far as possible that the *specimen* tube correctly contains all the required identification details and that these have been verified by comparison with those *volunteered* by the *patient* and obtained from the *wrist band*. All subsequent work in a transfusion laboratory

---

Table 1 Collection of blood samples for blood grouping and cross-matching[*]

1. Obtain case notes with summary sheet
2. Confirm patient's identity verbally or check wrist band
3. Collect the blood sample into an approved grouping and cross-matching bottle and then complete label with the following details from the case notes (or use pre-printed label):
   Patient's name and forenames
   Sex
   Date of birth
   Case record number (when available)
4. Check that identity details are correct by asking the patient to volunteer them (excluding case record number). For unconscious patients confirm with wrist band
5. Complete the request form using the specimen tube details or pre-printed labels
6. CROSS-CHECK SPECIMEN TUBE AND FORM

---

[*]These instructions could be printed on the reverse of the request form.

should utilize these details *from the specimen tube*. As an additional security, the person collecting the sample may wish to sign the tube, thereby vouching for the accuracy of the collection.

Patients who have recently been transfused or pregnant (e.g. within the last 3 months) are more likely to have emergent irregular antibodies which could cause delayed haemolytic transfusion reactions. For this reason samples for pre-transfusion testing should be collected no more than 3 days prior to the next planned transfusion.

The blood transfusion specimen bottle

Although plain clotted blood samples in any container will be adequate for transfusion purposes it is good practice to make use of a unique and specially designated sample container which is used for no other purpose. This should carry a label with spaces for the obligatory identification details. Unused specimen tubes that have completed or partly completed labels should be discarded to prevent inadvertent use for another patient.

The blood transfusion request form

Many satisfactory designs for these exist. It is necessary to have spaces for the obligatory patient identification details such as those listed above. In addition other pieces of information are required:

(1) The patient's physician. This name should be written legibly so that urgent enquiries are not impeded.
(2) Patient's ward.
(3) Reason for blood transfusion.
(4) The previous transfusion history (including the date of the last transfusion).
(5) Whether the patient has been pregnant and any known clinical history of serological relevance.
(6) Number and type of blood components required.
(7) Degree of urgency.
(8) Date and time required.
(9) Legible signature of medical officer requesting transfusion (to whom problems may in the first instance be referred).

Attention should be paid to the layout of the form. The eye should be led naturally in sequence through the areas of the form that require completion. In that way it will be easy to see when all the information requested has been provided. Spaces for laboratory entries should be clearly separated from those requiring completion by clinical staff. A badly designed request form encourages errors where no encouragement is needed. Carbon copies and card backing allow simultaneous dispatch of copies to ward or theatre, while the card backing can be retained for laboratory record purposes.

Table 2

STOP!

Before transfusing be sure this is
the right blood for this patient

1. If possible ask patient to VOLUNTEER:
   Full name; address; date of birth; and confirm these agree with compatibility label
2. Confirm that COMPATIBILITY LABEL details, including case record number, agree
   with WRIST BAND and CASE NOTES
3. If a BLOOD GROUP result is available in notes check this
4. Donation number on BLOOD PACK should agree with that on THIS LABEL
5. Check expiry date and inspect pack for leakage or unusual appearance
6. Sign compatibility label. Witness to this procedure should also sign

Following transfusion the blood pack should be sealed and retained on the ward for 24
hours until the chance of a serious reaction has passed.

Administration of the blood unit

Staff performing this task should be suitably instructed and possess appropriate
medical or nursing qualifications. It is suggested that two staff members cooperate
in this task; a recommended procedure (which could be detailed on the back of
the compatibility label) is shown in Table 2.

A well-designed compatibility label may facilitate these procedures. It is again
of the utmost importance that whenever possible the patient is *asked to volunteer*
his or her identity details. Confirmation that the blood pack has not passed its
expiry date and has no untoward appearance (e.g. haemolysis, presence of gas
bubbles) should have been performed in the transfusion laboratory but a further
check is necessary at the point of administration. The first 30 minutes of each
transfused unit may provide early warning of reactions (see chapter 4, section
1.4). These observations provide an *in vivo* compatibility test!

Collection and transportation of blood within the hospital

Hasty and careless collection of blood units from hospital blood banks for use in
theatres has on occasion begun a chain of errors leading to transfusion disasters.
Experience has shown a need to ensure accurate identity checks at each and
every stage on the route to administration. It is therefore recommended that
such blood is collected by suitably trained staff, who bring with them a form
containing all the identity details that require to be cross-checked with the blood
pack compatibility labels. There should be an *issues book* in the blood bank
showing the blood pack unit number and details of the intended recipient. The
person removing the pack should sign the appropriate entry in the book,
entering also the date and time. Untrained staff required to collect and transport
blood will be unable to accept any part of the responsibility for accurate patient
identification. They should, however, be equipped with a form showing this
information which may either be checked and completed by blood bank techni-

cal staff at the point of issue or by ward or theatre staff on receipt of the blood. In this latter case the form should be returned to the blood bank to allow the appropriate entry to be made in the blood bank issues book.

3.2 Laboratory Protocols: Handling of Samples for Grouping and Compatibility Testing Within the Laboratory.

Hospital blood transfusion laboratories usually evolve their own detailed procedures which prove to be most efficient and safe under the prevailing circumstances. This section will therefore only be concerned with the principal aspects likely to affect safety.

Since *most morbidities and fatalities follow ABO incompatibilities* the laboratory's greatest guarantee of safety is ensured by performing the compatibility test on serum that is taken directly from the original labelled specimen tube at the time of performing the test. This practice necessitates the storing of serum 'on the clot' which has the disadvantage of diminishing the chance of detection of antibodies requiring complement. These are, however, better detected by antibody screening as described above.

The following practices are suggested:

(1) Remove into labelled tubes (name, initials and case record number) cells and serum for grouping and antibody screening. Keep the clotted sample tube at 4 °C for compatibility testing later.

(2) Security of ABO and Rh D grouping is best ensured by one or more of the following:

 (a) Grouping performed on samples collected on two separate occasions.

 (b) Cell and serum groups performed by different operators (Rh D groups performed in duplicate using different reagents).

 (c) Two operators reading and recording the results independently and in ignorance of each other's findings. Laboratory work books can be specially designed to facilitate this procedure.

Computerization of the blood bank can facilitate cross-checking the information from any of the above procedures. Computers should also recall for comparison blood group information obtained on a previous occasion.

(3) Compatibility tests are best set up and read by one and the same member of staff. Each step of the test should be performed for only one patient at a time to reduce the risk of transposition of samples. At the start of compatibility testing the original specimen tube, being the source of the patient's serum, should be placed in the cross-match rack, from which it should not be removed until tests are fully completed and the compatibility labels have been prepared. This tube must be used as the source of identity details for preparation of compatibility labels. The blood transfusion request form should not be used for this purpose and is best kept apart from the compatibility testing rack. Test tubes containing the donor red cell suspensions should carry the appropriate blood pack donation numbers. Unless a computerized system is in use, labels for the compatibility packs should be made out adjacent to the

compatibility test rack, copying details from the *specimen tube* and the donor red cell suspension tubes. This operation should again be performed for only *one patient at a time*. Labels should be affixed to the correct blood packs immediately.

(4) The original blood transfusion request form may then be issued as a report to confirm that blood has been compatibility tested and is available. It is best that this is not issued simultaneously with the blood units as this encourages ward staff to cross-check details on the compatibility label with those on the request form—a procedure which is clearly illogical as far as the patient's safety is concerned. The practice confers no security and distracts attention from the main task, i.e. that of checking the compatibility label details with the patient's identity as volunteered verbally or on the patient's wrist band.

The *transfusion request* form should be retained in the patient's case notes as part of the legally required documentation. The records should indicate:

• The blood pack donation number.
• The names of persons checking the patient's identity at the time of blood administration.
• The blood group of the administered blood component.
• The type of component administered.

Compatibility labels can be designed so that the above information is contained on a detachable portion which can then be transferred to the patient's case notes. Other information pertaining to the transfusion should also be noted; these include records of pulse, blood pressure, urine output, volume of component administered and the time of beginning and ending the transfusion, together with any appropriate clinical observations.

4 EMERGENCY TRANSFUSION PROBLEMS

Patients requiring emergency transfusions are at a greater risk of receiving mismatched blood, largely as a direct consequence of procedural short-cuts. Patient identification rules must be adhered to at all times. Unconscious or incompletely identified persons must be given a number fixed to a wrist band as described above. Compatibility testing may have to be abbreviated as described in chapter 11.

Inadequately labelled samples

In most hospitals a continual state of vigilance is needed to ensure that blood transfusion samples arrive correctly identified. Where time allows, inadequately identified samples should be returned promptly to the sender. If this is too risky for the patient, it may be best to proceed with the request but a written statement that *responsibility for patient identification has been verbally accepted by the medical officer* should be attached to the request form. Recurrent episodes of this nature should be reported to the head of the clinical team involved.

5 MAJOR DISASTER ARRANGEMENTS

All large blood transfusion laboratories and regional blood collection centres should have updated and accessible instructions for responding to a demand for treatment of mass casualties.[46] Although fortunately rare, such events may happen at times when senior staff are not instantly available within the timescale of the response required. On-call blood transfusion staff should therefore be briefed as to the correct course of action.

A *regional blood collection centre* will require the following list of names and telephone numbers:

(1) Senior medical and laboratory staff who may be required to liaise and organize help.
(2) Administrative and transport staff to organize despatch of blood consignments and liaise with police or ambulance services. Telephone numbers of these services together with those of other emergency transportation facilities will also be required.
(3) Nearby blood transfusion centres in case assistance is required to meet overwhelming demands.
(4) Blood donor organization staff. It is not usually necessary to organize special emergency donor sessions. These tend to add to the difficulties because large amounts of blood from previously untyped and untested donors have to be processed. Liaison with the public via press and radio may, however, be required to handle an enthusiastic response to donate blood.

Reliable information concerning blood or plasma needs may be difficult to ascertain. Unrealistic panic demands may, however, be made which could overwhelm the resources of those attempting to cope with the situation. It may be prudent to select an emergency predetermined package of the common groups of blood and of albumin solution, so that this can be despatched promptly to the receiving hospitals as a holding operation until more precise information becomes available. This should be packed in specially labelled containers and the utmost care must be taken to ensure that it is stored correctly following receipt, otherwise vital stocks may be jeopardized during the disorganization which may occur.

Arrangements at a hospital or casualty blood bank

(1) Telephone numbers of senior staff must be available and kept up to date. Extra laboratory staff may be required during emergency hours and these should be organized by the most senior member of the laboratory staff available. Within the transfusion laboratory the following procedures may have to be considered.
(2) Samples (patient's) must be identified as a minimum by an *accident number*. This must be clearly written on the cross-match sample container.
(3) Specimens should be sorted on the basis of a clearly indicated clinical priority, so that the most urgent requests are dealt with first. This situation must be

clearly understood by clinical staff, who should alert the blood transfusion laboratory when clinical deterioration occurs in patients previously considered not to be at risk. Conversely, when a patient who is receiving massive transfusion support dies, the laboratory must also be notified promptly to prevent further expenditure of effort.

(4) For the sake of technical simplicity, it will be sufficient to perform ABO typing by cell grouping alone. Under conditions of extreme difficulty Rh D typing could be restricted to women of reproductive age.

(5) If staff and space permit, cross-matching areas for group O recipients and non-O recipients should be separated. As far as possible, cross-matching staff should be deployed so that patients are attended to on a one-to-one basis. It is probably most efficient to organize blood provision as described for treatment of acute blood loss (chapter 11, section 5.3). The compatibility label may show only the accident unit number pertaining to the patient concerned. It may well be counter-productive to attempt to add additional, possibly inaccurate, information.

   Blood stocks may be inadequate to cope with any substantial accident demand but an emergency human albumin solution (4.5% albumin in saline) should be kept by all blood banks at which any significant risk of receiving casualties exists. The arrangements operated by the regional blood collection centre for supply of blood under these circumstances should be clearly displayed.

Arrangements at resuscitation areas

Clinical aspects of resuscitation should follow the principles outlined in chapter 11. In general it is to be expected that casualties will be resuscitated with saline and colloid solutions until arrival at hospital. Blood transfusion at the site of the casualty area should be an uncommon events, with the exception of seriously bleeding subjects who are trapped in vehicles or buildings. Where transfusion must be undertaken under such circumstances, the patient must be identified as described above and blood samples collected before transfusion is attempted.

6   EFFICIENCY IN BLOOD BANKING

Efficiency in blood transfusion practice requires that:

(1) Patients receive therapy for the right reasons and in the right amounts.
(2) Unnecessary laboratory procedures are identified and eliminated.
(3) Stock control procedures are established in order to minimize wastage from outdating.

Wastage of red cell units through outdating is a common and conspicuous example of misuse of a scarce resource. The problem can be tackled in several ways.

Tariff lists for elective surgery

Analysis of retrospective blood use for surgical procedures can provide useful guidance for the establishment of future cross-matching practices. Where a given surgical procedure carries less than a 5% chance of requiring blood, or the average number of blood units used per case does not exceed 0.5, it is sufficient to perform blood grouping and antibody screening alone.[47] Cross-matching of blood for these procedures is only necessary for the occasional cases in which excessive bleeding occurs. Those surgical procedures in which blood transfusion is often required should be analysed in detail to show the actual amounts of blood used. A *tariff list* can be constructed from such an analysis which shows the numbers of blood units that would be sufficient to cover the blood transfusion needs of 90% of occasions in which the particular procedure is performed. This amount should be that recommended as the routine cross-match tariff. Tariff lists for elective surgery are sometimes referred to as *maximum blood order schedules*. Numerous examples of the successful operation of group and screen and maximum blood order schedules have been published.[48]

The need for clinical consultation over blood-ordering policies

The introduction of group and screen and tariff list arrangements requires the active participation, consultation and cooperation of all clinical staff concerned. The legitimate anxieties of theatre staff confronted by unexpected or excessive blood loss must be sympathetically understood. These colleagues require assurance that sudden emergency needs will be met by an appropriately prompt supply of adequately matched blood.

A careful combination of group and antibody screen policies together with tariff lists for surgical procedures can help to reduce unnecessary cross-matching. They should not, however, be applied too rigidly. Certain general clinical circumstances, e.g. *anaemic or debilitated patients, presence of cancer, previous radiotherapy to the operative site or repeat operative procedures,* are all associated with above-average blood loss and greater blood needs. As a specific example, actual blood use during Caesarean section has been analysed. A number of factors were shown to be predictive for high red cell use and these included 'disorders of placental implantation, pre-eclampsia, premature labour with tocolytic therapy, fetal distress and augmentation of dysfunctional labour'.[49] For reasons such as these, senior medical or surgical staff will need at times to override the tariff allocation for individual patients.

Cross-match/transfusion ratio analysis

If the total number of units of blood cross-matched for a given surgical procedure is divided by the total actually used, the cross-match transfusion ratio (C/T ratio) is obtained. This can be calculated for individual surgical procedures, for surgical specialties or alternatively a global figure for blood bank practice within a given hospital. A ratio above 2.5 is indicative of excessive cross-matching.[50]

High C/T ratios point to a need for education and discussion within the hospital concerned regarding the efficiency of transfusion practices.

Appropriateness of blood use

Despite the expanding literature in transfusion medicine and the publication of numerous consensus conference proceedings and guidelines of good transfusion practice, there is ample evidence that a significant majority of clinical transfusion practices continues uninfluenced by the considered deliberations of experts in the field.[51] Even accepting the necessity for clinical freedom, these divergences must be tempered by what is supportable on sound clinical practice. Studies have shown that energetic publicity of treatment protocols and establishment of audit criteria for good component use,[52,53] coupled with regular review, will improve the quality of transfusion practice. The hospital transfusion service should, using national or other generally accepted guidelines for component use, attempt to obtain general agreement about the implementation of locally agreed versions.[54] Blood component usage patterns should be included in the medical audit process[55,56] so that the validity of diversions from agreed criteria can be debated. It has been shown that prescribing practice can be improved by energetic review at the time of orders using computerized[57] or non-computerized systems.[58]

Avoidance of overstocking

It is generally agreed that the holding of excessive blood stock levels contributes to waste; certainly blood shortages and low stock levels stimulate economies in blood utilization. Blood consumption rates, the likelihood of casualty emergencies, delivery frequencies as well as the distance from the nearest blood collection centre must be taken into account in determining hospital blood bank stock levels.

Keeping blood stocks moving

Blood should be shipped from collection centres to hospitals with as long an expiry date as possible. Blood bank management policies should result in prompt cross-matching of blood received and prompt re-cross-matching of unused units.

Table 3 Aids to efficient use of blood

Group and screen and tariff lists for surgical procedures
Cross-match/transfusion (C/T) ratio analysis
Prompt issue of blood from regional centre, prompt cross-matching and re-cross-matching
Avoidance of excessive stock levels
Use of maximum permissible shelf life
Component use guidelines
Audit of blood use

If these practices are combined with low C/T ratios, the risk of red cells outdating will be minimized and it will also be found that the average age of red cell units transfused will be reduced so that patients will receive blood at its best condition. Clinical staff should be made aware that cross-matched blood units not used within a given time will automatically be returned to stock.

7   DIFFICULT TRANSFUSION RECIPIENTS

Patients who must be transfused but whose serum contains multiple antibodies, antibodies against high frequency (public) antigens or who possess a null-type blood group present some of the most taxing transfusion problems. Time is required for analysis of the problem but when this is at a premium clinical judgements as to the least risky course of action must be made. Several possibilities should be considered:

(1) *Is the antibody haemolytic?* Some antibodies to high-frequency antigens are of low affinity and lack haemolytic potential. Examples of antibodies which have on occasions been shown to be at worst only weakly haemolytic include anti-LW^a, anti-Lan, anti-Cr^a, anti-JMH, anti-Kn^a and anti-Hy^{a}.[59,60] It cannot, of course, be assumed that all examples of these antibodies will behave in the same way. The patient's life should, however, not be put at risk as a result of undue serological caution. If both time and facilities are available, a radio-isotope-labelled donor red cell survival study[59-61] can provide an indication as to whether severe haemolysis will occur. The results can, however, be misleading in that the post-transfusion survival of small volumes of transfused cells, such as would be used in these investigations, may well be substantially shorter than that of larger volumes of blood.[59] This approach is unlikely to be helpful for patients with null-type blood groups or those who have antibody mixtures. It is important to remember, however, that cold antibodies in antibody mixtures, e.g. anti-P, -Le^a, -Le^b, -M, -N, -A$_1$, can usually be disregarded and this may widen the choice of available red cell units.
(2) *Are there potential donors in the family?* Family studies, especially of siblings, may reveal a compatible donor where antibodies to high-frequency antigens are the problem. A young, fit, informed and willing family member may be able to provide two units within a week if circumstances make it desirable.
(3) *Are red cells absolutely necessary?* Provided oxygenation is good and blood volume is corrected with synthetic volume expanders or albumin solution, up to 3 l of blood can be lost in healthy non-anaemic adult subjects before haemodilution becomes dangerous. Starting at 14 g/dl, the haemoglobin after 3 l have been replaced by asanguineous fluids should be around 6 g/dl. Clearly this is not desirable but neither is it life-threatening. The patient's clinical condition and likelihood of other post-operative complications are important considerations. Iron therapy and erythropoietin (see chapter 15) will speed red cell regeneration.
(4) *Intra-operative blood salvage*: transport of a patient to a hospital unit where such equipment is available and where there are staff trained in its use may well be

better than reliance on blood from rare donor panels. Autologous transfusion is discussed in chapter 15.

(5) *Pre-operative blood collection* (see chapter 15): this is a relatively easy approach where time and the patient's clinical condition permit. Blood units can be stored frozen, in which case a more leisurely approach is allowed and the operation performed at any time after accumulation of the requisite number of blood units.

(6) *Banks of frozen rare donations* are generally set up on a regional, national or international basis (see Appendix A). Information should be held by major blood collection centres, who will arrange for the search for compatible donations and probably also coordinate transport arrangements. A major disadvantage exists in that such blood must be thawed and washed before use and, once prepared, a 24-hour expiry time is set. Frozen blood is most suitable when the timing of transfusion and the amount of blood required are reasonably certain. It is also necessary to have special laboratory facilities available for reconstitution of the frozen units. Where transfusion needs are difficult to predict this inflexibility is a major obstacle.

(7) *Panels of rare blood donors* will again be held on a regional, national or international basis as with frozen blood. These donors can be bled into adenine-supplemented packs and whole blood can be kept as long as 42 days. If necessary red cell regeneration can extend the life of the packs still further (see chapter 3, section 2.3). A transfusion service may well maintain a list of accessible donors compatible with known 'difficult' recipients. These people may be prepared to provide donations at relatively short notice to cover emergencies.

8 COLLECTION OF BLOOD FROM VOLUNTARY DONORS

The following brief notes are intended as a guide to blood collection from normal donors in places where this is not a routine activity. Regular blood collection centres evolve their own detailed guidelines for the selection and bleeding of donors which will be more comprehensive and may vary slightly from those described below.[62]

A cardinal principle is that the act of donation should not, as far as can be prevented, result in any harm either to the donor or to the prospective recipient. Blood collection from donors is only to be undertaken by staff trained in all aspects of the procedure and whose continued competence is regularly assessed. Where this does not happen it should be closely supervised by medical staff familiar with procedures.

8.1 Selection of Donors

Assessment of donors

This entails:

(1) An *interview* designed to disclose any relevant medical information.

(2) Some transfusion services include a brief *physical examination* to ensure that the pulse, blood pressure and temperature are normal.

(3) *Haemoglobin screening* to exclude anaemia: haemoglobin levels should exceed 13.5 g/dl and 12.5 g/dl for men and women, respectively.

The following requirements should apply:

(a) The donor's *age* should be between 18 years and 65 years.

(b) The *weight* should be over 50 kg.

(c) Donors should be fully fit and not requiring any form of prescribed medication or medical supervision. Many aspirin-related analgesics interfere with platelet function and platelet donations should not, therefore, be collected where these have been taken during the preceding 7 days.

(d) Use of oral contraceptives does not affect ability to donate.

(e) Occasional consumption of tranquillizers or sleeping tablets is also acceptable.

(f) It is customary to require an interval of 24 hours following minor dental treatment.

(g) Probably at least a week should be allowed after dental extractions, minor outpatient surgery, and after completing antibiotic treatment for acute infections. These intervals before donations are accepted, of course, subject to the discretion of the doctor concerned.

(h) At least 12 months should elapse following blood transfusion to reduce the risk of transmitted infection or after major surgery.

(i) Volunteers with a past history of malignancy, or chronic disorders such as rheumatoid arthritis or diabetes, cardiovascular illness and epilepsy, should not donate.

(j) The advent of acquired immunodeficiency syndrome (AIDS) has resulted in a need to identify and reject donors in at-risk groups (see chapter 24, section 9.8).

(k) To reduce the risk of hepatitis B transmission a 12-month period should elapse following tattooing, acupuncture, ear piercing or hair implants.

(l)   (i) At least 12 months should be allowed following return from areas where malaria is endemic (see chapter 24, section 12.1). Donors visiting South American areas where *Trypanosoma cruzi* is endemic are restricted to plasma donation alone.

(ii) A history of jaundice excludes donation in the USA but not in the UK (see chapter 24, section 6).

(iii) Previous history of infected illness may necessitate deferral: e.g. tuberculosis, 2 years after completion of therapy; sexually transmitted diseases require 12 month deferral. A period of 3 weeks is usually advised following recovery from chicken-pox, mumps, measles and herpes infections, and 3 months following rubella infection. After this time donations may be valuable for their content of immune plasma.

(m) An interval of 12 months is customary following pregnancy.

(n) Two to six months (according to local practice) should be allowed following earlier blood donations.

In the case of donors who are relatives, or donors providing unusually important donations, exceptions to these rules may at times be necessary. These should be decided on an individual basis by doctors who keep the donor's best interests in mind. This is clearly easier if they are not primarily engaged in the care of the prospective recipient.

8.2 Donation Technique

Venepuncture and blood collection

Blood is most easily collected from the antecubital veins. After skin cleansing, administration of local anaesthetic (not universally used) and venous occlusion to a pressure of around 50 mmHg, the donation needle is inserted and secured firmly to obtain a steady uninterrupted flow. The blood should be mixed with anticoagulant at intervals and an arrangement made for ensuring accurate collection of the required 450 ml of blood. It will be necessary to collect additional blood samples for blood grouping tests and microbiological screening tests.

Following donation

After donation is completed a rest of 20–30 minutes is advisable, following which refreshments should be offered and the donor encouraged to stay and relax for a while. During the post-donation period donors should be observed for signs of incipient faints or other medical problems.

Documentation

The donor must sign his or her informed consent to the procedure and should testify that, to the best of their knowledge, he or she is medically eligible to donate. A record must be made of the donation and all blood samples should be labelled in such a way that they can be linked to paperwork showing the full identification details of the donor.

General aspects

It is important to welcome, to reassure and to thank the prospective donor for volunteering to give blood in what may well be unfamiliar and intimidating surroundings. A general air of efficiency and professionalism is important. Donor reactions such as faints, falls, bruises, feelings of nausea or vomiting attacks must be anticipated and attended to promptly. The nature of the procedure should be explained to the donor, together with an indication (that is not too discouraging) of the possible adverse reactions following donation. This is particularly important for people who may be strenuously active or who have occupations where syncopal attacks could be unusually dangerous.

9 MEDICOLEGAL CONSIDERATIONS

Blood transfusion, as with all other forms of medical intervention, is inescapably associated with a certain amount of risk. There is a duty to take care and to exercise professional skills so that neither donors nor recipients are harmed as a result of collection or administration of blood. Sometimes injuries do occur which, because of the current limitations of scientific knowledge, could neither be foreseen nor prevented. More commonly, however, the possibility exists that an element of *negligence* contributes to the injury. It is the task of medicolegal experts to establish whether injury has occurred that can be attributed to the transfusion incident, and to resolve the question as to whether an element of negligence has been involved. Medicolegal practice varies considerably in different countries and may also change according to different circumstances and the natural evolution of legal attitudes. It is only possible, therefore, to make generalizations which might serve as a basis for handling various problems. Legal judgements, although taking previous similar cases into account, must of course be decided on an individual basis according to the particular circumstances of each case. It is therefore impossible to make confident predictions as to the likely outcome of the legal deliberations of any given event. Some of the more frequently encountered aspects are considered in the following discussion.

9.1 Consent

It is necessary to consider the need for some form of consent both from *donors* and from *recipients* of transfusion. In the UK it is assumed that voluntary donors attending a blood donor session have by virtue of their attendance and their acquiescence to the usual procedure given *implied consent* to blood donation. Formal written evidence for this consent is not necessary, the serious risks of routine donation being so exceptionally infrequent that it is deemed unnecessary to make a specific point of giving cautionary advice. It is nevertheless prudent particularly for first-time donors to ensure appropriate information is available covering potential problems, and giving advice on seeking help where appropriate. Where more elaborate or potentially hazardous procedures are considered, for example deliberate immunization of donors, or collection of single-donor platelet or granulocyte preparations, some discussion of the possible risks is necessary. For these procedures, written and witnessed evidence of informed consent, confirming that an explanation has been given, should always be obtained. In any event failure to explain the risks and obtain informed consent, where *significant risks are foreseeable,* is regarded as negligence for which a claim may be established if injury to the donor occurs. Unlike patients, these procedures are always elective, and no judgement has to be made between the risks of intervention and non-intervention. Accordingly, it is prudent to ensure donors are always made fully aware of the small but finite chances that complications may arise.

Minimum age of donors

In the UK donors of routine blood donations must be at least 18 years old. Under special circumstances donations may be given by those between 16 years and 18 years of age, but both their own consent and the written consent of one of their parents is necessary.

Mental health of potential donors

No form of consent either *implied* (by their attendance and acquiescence to the act of donation) or *expressed* (where consent is obtained in writing on a consent form, or by word of mouth) can have any validity if the potential donor can in any way be regarded as being mentally unfit to make the decision.

Legal status of consent

Consent of any form provides protection for medical staff and their assistants against accusations of assault and battery and consequential claims for damages arising from the procedure of donation. This, of course, only holds true provided the procedure is carried out in the usual way and according to normal professional standards. Compensation can only be claimed in respect of *injuries* sustained by the donor; these may be recoverable from the medical attendants if any element of negligence can be shown. There may, alternatively, be an apportionment of costs against both the hospital or health authority and the medical practitioner whose negligent actions led to the injury. Where there is negligence on the part of other staff in failing to carry out designated procedures, the responsibility is likely to be placed upon the hospital or health authority being vicariously liable for the correct action of its employees.

Consent for transfusion

Unless the patient expresses an explicit wish that blood transfusion should not be given, it is usually assumed in the UK that consent for transfusion is implied by voluntary admission to hospital, or that consent is included in the signed consent obtained before operative procedures are undertaken. As with the act of blood donation, the risks of accepting blood transfusion have been considered sufficiently small to justify this arrangement. The situation differs in the USA, where explanation and informed consent is usually obtained prior to all but emergency transfusions. This difference has probably arisen from the greater incidence of both litigation claims and of post-transfusion infection. The heightened perception of the risk of transfusion generally may cause reappraisal of the need to seek consent for transfusions in the UK. Even where explicit informed consent is not required patients should, where circumstances permit, be told of the need for transfusion. The opportunity should be taken to justify the decision and explain in a balanced way the possibility of post-transfusion problems, taking particular heed of any concerns that the patient may have. Where alternatives to conventional allogeneic blood transfusion (e.g. autologous transfusion) are appropriate and available this should be explained. Under certain circumstances consent for transfusion, or the lack of it, requires particular consideration:

(1) Jehovah's Witnesses may expressly refuse transfusion and this wish must be respected for adults who are conscious and able to make the decision and understand its implications.
(2) During emergencies and where the patient is in no fit state to make this decision it is, in the UK, permissible to transfuse to save life. Transfusion cannot be prohibited by relatives purporting to express what might be the patient's views.
(3) It is advisable to obtain a signed and witnessed statement that transfusions have been refused, thereby absolving the hospital and its staff from possible claims for negligence. This must be retained safely in the case notes. It is advisable that two doctors, each independently of the other, explain clearly the consequences of refusing transfusion treatment.
(4) Women who are pregnant, and by refusing transfusion threaten the life of unborn children, present a special problem. A court order should be sought to protect the life of the child. A more difficult problem is that of a parent whose death would leave children unprovided for. Again, it could be argued that this represents an act of irresponsibility that should not be acceded to.
(5) Transfusion of minors (under 18 years): the consent of the parent or guardian is normally obtained for children under 16. Between the ages of 16 and 18 children can give their own consent and that of their parents is not required. Neither can parents veto the consent of their children. It is again advisable that two doctors independently explain clearly the consequences of refusing transfusion treatment.

Life-saving transfusions, or those required to prevent permanent injury, for children of any age cannot be refused by parents irrespective of their religious objections. Where time permits, it should be explained to the parents that, if they continue refusal, the child may have to be removed by court order from their care to that of the local authority. The local authority may then sanction transfusion.

During emergencies transfusions should be given without delay. In the United Kingdom there is no likelihood of successful legal action, provided that the professional judgement was soundly based.

9.2 Negligence

This may be defined as failure to comply with accepted good standards of medical practice. Negligence has already been referred to with regard to failure to explain the risks of a procedure before informed consent is obtained. Claims for negligence in other areas are judged according to whether staff or their employing authorities have adequately fulfilled their professional duties. Where professional guidelines exist they are used in making an assessment of the validity of a claim for negligence. These professional guidelines may emanate from a variety of sources and cover all areas of transfusion activity from donor selection, blood collection, laboratory procedures for testing donations, for testing compatibility of blood for transfusion and for organizational procedures concerned with specimen identification, and blood transfusion administration. They will also cover the requirement for accurate record keeping and, not least, documentation of the need for transfusion and selection of the appropriate product. References to such published guidelines are given in the appendices.

Negligence can also arise where transfusion procedures are carried out in un-licensed institutions in countries where licensing arrangements for these are required. Blood banks, hospitals or blood collection centres operate within differ-ent legal frameworks in different countries. Granting of licences can be taken to indicate that staff are professionally qualified and that satisfactory equipment and organizational facilities exist. These requirements obviously apply even when formal licensing arrangements are not necessary. An important element of protec-tion against allegations of substandard laboratory practices can also be gained by participating and obtaining successful results in the available schemes for quality control and proficiency evaluation.

Claims for negligence can of course only be sustained where evidence exists that *injury* has resulted from the alleged negligent actions. As far as blood trans-fusion is concerned, however, some injuries follow unavoidable risks. Examples of these include some post-transfusion infections and certain transfusion reactions. In these cases it is only necessary to show that acceptable precautionary measures had been taken in order to refute the claim of negligence. ABO haemolytic trans-fusion reactions can, on the other hand, only happen as a result of negligent performance and form a classic example of *res ipsa loquitur* (the thing speaks for itself). The conclusion of guilt on the part of the defendant is virtually unavoid-able. The apportionment of blame and recovery of damages are, however, subject to court enquiry and discretion but would follow the principles discussed earlier (section 9.1). Under the worst circumstances where gross or wilful breaches of professional practice have taken place there may be grounds for considering the case one of criminal rather than the more usual civil negligence. This could apply, for example, where records are falsified in order to conceal the true facts of an ABO-incompatible transfusion reaction.

9.3 Product Liability

Injuries resulting from alleged deficiencies in the quality of transfused blood are very much a concern in modern blood transfusion practice. The activities of European blood transfusion services are now affected by the European Com-munity Directive on Product Liability, which requires producers of medicinal products to be *strictly liable* (i.e. be liable *without* proof of negligence) for death or injury arising from use of their products. Because of the scientific inability to ensure total absence of risk manufacturers may, though this remains to be clarified, be allowed to seek a 'state of the art' defence under certain circumstances. Manufacturers must be able to show that accepted standards with regard to product safety and efficacy had been achieved. If this cannot be done, they may in any case be held responsible for negligence. Where risks are foreseeable but unpredictable and unavoidable it is necessary for the defence to show that adequate *warning* of the possibility of adverse reaction had been given. Most staff in clinical transfusion practice act as *suppliers* of products and are therefore not themselves liable unless they transfuse inappropriately, modify products or fail to convey warning material which should accompany the products. It is, however, essential to keep adequate records of the sources of blood products that have been supplied in order to maintain this exemption.

REFERENCES

1 Code for Good Laboratory Practice in Haematology Laboratories (Including Hospital Blood Banks) (1991). In: Roberts, B. (ed.), *Standard Haematology Practice*, pp. 1–22. Oxford: Blackwell Scientific.
2 Voak, D. and Napier, J.A.F. (1990) Quality assurance in the hospital transfusion laboratory: quality control in blood group serology. In: Cavill, I. (ed.), *Quality Control*, 2nd edn, pp. 129–153. Edinburgh: Churchill Livingstone.
3 Lewis, S.M. (1990) Quality assessment schemes. In: Cavill, I. (ed.), *Quality Control*, 2nd edn, pp. 14–30. Edinburgh: Churchill Livingstone.
4 Grindon, A.J., Tomasulo, P.S., Bergin, J.J., Klein, H.G., Miller, J.D. and Mintz, P.D. (1985) The hospital transfusion committee: guidelines for improving practice. *JAMA*, **253**: 540–543.
5 Blumberg, N. (1990) Beyond ABO and D antigen matching: how far and for whom? (Editorial.) *Transfusion*, **30**: 482–484.
6 Garratty, G. (1979) *Clinically Significant and Insignificant Antibodies*. Bethesda, MD: American Association of Blood Banks.
7 *Standards for Blood Banks and Transfusion Services* (1981) 10th edn. Bethesda, MD: American Association of Blood Banks.
8 Farr, A.D. (1980) Selection of procedures for compatibility testing of blood. *Med. Lab. Sci.*, **37**: 105–106.
9 Sosler, S.D. (1982) A list of 25 LISS scores. *Am. J. Clin. Pathol.*, **77**: 231–232.
10 Merry, A.H., Thomson, E.E., Lagar, J. *et al.* (1984) Quantitation of antibody binding to erythrocytes in LISS. *Vox Sang.*, **47**: 125–132.
11 Moltham, L. and Strohm, P.L. (1981) Hemolytic transfusion reaction due to anti-Kell undetectable in low-ionic strength solutions. *Am. J. Clin. Pathol.*, **75**: 629–631.
12 Voak, D., Downie, M., Haigh, T. and Cook, N. (1982) Improved antiglobulin tests to detect difficult antibodies: detection of anti-Kell by LISS. *Med. Lab. Sci.*, **39**: 363–370.
13 Wright, M.S. and Issitt, P.D. (1979) Anticomplement and the indirect antiglobulin test. *Transfusion*, **19**: 688–694.
14 Howell, P. and Giles, C.M. (1983) A detailed serological study of five anti-Jk[a] sera reacting by the antiglobulin technique. *Vox Sang.*, **45**: 129–138.
15 Howard, J.E., Winn, L.C., Gottlieb, C.E., Grumet, F.C., Garratty, G. and Petz, L.D. (1982) Clinical significance of the anti-complement component of antiglobulin antisera. *Transfusion*, **22**: 692–272.
16 Voak, D., Downie, D.M., Moore, B.P.L. and Engelfriet, C.P. (1986) Anti-human globulin reagent specifications; the European and ISBT/ICSH View. *Biotest Bull.*, **1**: 7–22.

17 Voak, D., Downie, D.M., Moore, B.P.L., Ford, D.S., Engelfriet, C.P. and Case, J. (1988)
    Replicate tests for the detection and correction of errors in anti-human globulin (AHG)
    tests: optimum conditions and quality control. *Haematologia,* **21**: 3–16.
18 Issitt, P.D., Combs, M.R., Bredehoeft, S.J. *et al.* (1993) Lack of clinical significance of
    'enzyme-only' red cell alloantibodies. *Transfusion,* **33**: 284–293.
19 Judd, W.J., Barnes, B.A. *et al.* (1986) The evaluation of a positive direct antiglobulin test
    (autocontrol) in pretransfusion testing revisited. *Transfusion,* **26**: 220–224.
20 Wildmann, F.K. (1993) Too much pretransfusion testing? *Transfusion,* **33**: 186–188.
21 Shulman, I.A., Nelson, J.M. and Nakayama, R. (1990) When should antibody screening
    tests be done for recently transfused patients? *Transfusion,* **30**: 39–41.
22 Perkins, J.T., Arruza, M., Fong, K., Sosler, S.D. and Saporito, C. (1990) The relative
    utility of the autologous control and the antiglobulin test phase of the crossmatch.
    Transfusion, **30**: 503–507.
23 Meyer, E.A. and Shulman, I.A. (1989) The sensitivity and specificity of the immediate-
    spin crossmatch. *Transfusion,* **29**: 99–102.
24 Judd, W.J., Steiner, E.A., O'Donnell, D.B. and Oberman, H.A. (1988) Discrepancies in
    reverse ABO typing due to prozone: how safe is the immediate-spin crossmatch? *Trans-
    fusion,* **28**: 334–338.
25 Judd, W.J., Steiner, E.A., Oberman, H.A. and Nance, S.J. (1992) Can the reading for
    serologic reactivity following 37 °C incubation be omitted? *Transfusion,* **32**: 304–308.
26 Trudeau, L.R., Judd, W.J., Butch, S.H. and Oberman, H.A. (1983) Is a room-temperature
    crossmatch necessary for the detection of ABO errors? *Transfusion,* **23**: 237.
27 Pohl, B.A. (1985) Correspondence. *Transfusion,* **25**: 588–589.
28 Oberman, H.A. (1992) The present and future crossmatch. (Editorial.) *Transfusion,* **32**:
    794–795.
29 de la Rubia, J., Sempere, A., Arriaga, F., Lopez, F. and Marty, M.L. (1992) Safety of
    the antibody screening test as the sole method of pretransfusion testing. *Vox Sang.,* **63**:
    141.
30 Napier, J.A.F. (1991) Clinical annotation: the crossmatch. *Br. J. Haematol.,* **78**: 1–4.
31 Judd, W.J. (1991) Are there better ways than the crossmatch to demonstrate ABO
    incompatibility? (Editorial.) *Transfusion,* **31**: 192–194.
32 Garratty, G. (1986) Abbreviated pretransfusion testing. *Transfusion,* **26**: 217–219.
33 Heddle, N.M., O'Hoski, P., Singer, J. *et al.* (1992) A prospective study to determine the
    safety of omitting the antiglobulin crossmatch from pretransfusion testing. *Br. J. Haema-
    tol.,* **81**: 579–584.
34 Pinkerton, P.H., Coovadia, A.S. and Goldstein, J. (1992) Frequency of delayed hemolytic
    transfusion reactions following antibody screening and immediate-spin crossmatching.
    Transfusion, **32**: 814–817.
35 *Standards for Blood Banks and Transfusion Services,* 15th edn. (1993) Bethesda, MD: Amer-
    ican Association of Blood Banks.
36 Pinkerton, P.H., Zuber, E.D., Wood, D.E., Holburn, A.M. and Prior, D. (1985) Proficiency
    testing in immunohaematology in Ontario, Canada, and in the United Kingdom: a com-
    parative study. *J. Clin. Pathol.,* **38**: 570–574.
37 Holburn, A.M. and Prior, D. (1986) The UK National External Quality Assessment
    Scheme in Blood Group Serology: ABO and D grouping and antibody screening 1982–
    1983. *Clin. Lab. Haematol.,* **8**: 243–256.
38 Shulman, I.A., Nelson, J.M., Saxena, S. *et al.* (1984) Experience with the routine use of an
    abbreviated cross-match. *Am. J. Clin. Pathol.,* **82**: 178–181.
39 BCSH (1990) Guidelines for microplate techniques in liquid phase blood grouping and
    antibody screening. *Clin. Lab. Haematol.,* **12**: 437–460.
40 Scott, L.M. (1991) The principles and applications of solid phase blood group serology.
    Trans. Med. Rev., **1**: 60–72.
41 Plapp, F.V., Sinor, L.T., Rachel, J.M. *et al.* (1984) A solid phase antibody screen. *Am. J.
    Clin. Pathol.,* **82**: 719.
42 Lapierre, Y., Rigel, D., Adams, J. *et al.* (1990) The gel-test: a new way to detect red cell
    antigens–antibody reactions. *Transfusion,* **30**: 109–113.

43 Editorial (1992) Validation of new technology for antibody detection by antiglobulin tests. *Transfusion Med.*, **2**: 177–179.
44 Pinkerton, P.H., Ward, J., Chan, R. and Coovadia, A.S. (1993) An evaluation of a gel technique for antibody screening compared with a conventional tube method. *Transfusion Med.*, **3**: 201–205.
45 British Committee for Standards in Haematology (1991) Hospital blood bank documentation and procedures. In: Roberts, B.E. (ed.), *Standard Haematology Practice*, pp. 128–138. Oxford: Blackwell Scientific.
46 Wood, J.K., Nolan, S.L., Blecher, T.E. *et al.* (1990) The M1 Kegworth aircraft disaster: experience in three hospital blood transfusion laboratories and the regional transfusion centre. *Clin. Lab. Haematol.*, **12**: 1–7.
47 Mintz, P.E., Nordine, R.B., Henry, J.B. and Webb, W.R. (1976) Expected hemotherapy in elective surgery. *NY State J. Med.*, **76**: 532–537.
48 Napier, J.A.F., Biffin, A.H. and Lay, D. (1985) Efficiency of use of blood for surgery in South and Mid Wales. *Br. Med. J.*, **291**: 299–301.
49 Camann, W.R. and Datta, S. (1991) Red cell use during cesarean delivery. *Transfusion*, **31**: 12–15.
50 Roualt, C. and Gruenhagen, J. (1978) Reorganisation of blood ordering practices. *Transfusion*, **18**: 448–453.
51 Stehling, L.C., Ellison, N., Faust, R.J., Grotta, A.W. and Moyers, J.R. (1987) A survey of transfusion practices among anesthesiologists. *Vox Sang.*, **52**: 60–62.
52 Coffin, C., Matz, K. and Rich, E. (1989) Algorithms for evaluating the appropriateness of blood transfusion. *Transfusion*, **29**: 298–303.
53 Hume, H.A., Ali, A.M., Decary, F. and Blajchman, M.A. (1991) Evaluation of pediatric transfusion practice using criteria maps. *Transfusion*, **31**: 52–58.
54 Rosen, N.R., Bates, L.H. and Herod, G. (1993) Transfusion therapy: improved patient care and resource utlization. *Transfusion*, **33**: 341–347.
55 Giovanetti, A.M., Parravicini, A. *et al.* (1988) Quality assessment of transfusion practice in elective surgery. *Transfusion*, **28**: 166–169.
56 Mozes, B., Epstein, M., Ben-Bassat, I., Modan, B. and Halkin, H. (1989) Evaluation of the appropriateness of blood and blood product transfusion using present criteria. *Transfusion*, **29**: 473–476.
57 Lepage, E.F., Gardner, R.M., Laub, R.M. and Golubjatnikov, O.K. (1992) Improving blood transfusion practice: role of a computerized hospital information system. *Transfusion*, **32**: 253–259.
58 Silver, H., Tahnan, H.R., Anderson, J. and Lachman, M. (1992) A non-computer-dependent prospective review of blood and blood component utilization. *Transfusion*, **32**: 260–265.
59 Baldwin, M.L., Ness, P.M., Barrasso, C. *et al.* (1985) In vivo studies of the long-term 51Cr red cell survival of serologically incompatible red cell units. *Transfusion*, **25**: 34–38.
60 Holt, J.T., Spitalnik, S.L., McMican, A.E., Wilson, G. and Blumberg, N. (1983) A technetium-99m red cell survival technique for in vivo compatibility testing. *Transfusion*, **23**: 148–151.
61 Mollison, P.L. (1983) *Blood Transfusion in Clinical Medicine*, 7th edn. Oxford: Blackwell Scientific.
62 *Guidelines for the Blood Transfusion Service* (1993) London: HMSO.
63 Linden, J.V. and Kaplan, H.S. (1994) Transfusion errors: causes and effects. *Transfusion Med. Rev.*, **3**: 169–183.

Further Reading: Medicolegal Aspects

Bernstein, A.H. (1 August 1981) Legal Implication of Administering Blood. *Law in Brief Hospitals*. Bristol: Family Law.

Brazier, M. (1992) *Medicine, Patients and the Law*, 2nd edn. Harmondsworth, UK: Penguin Books.

Diamond, A.L. and Laurence, D.R. (1985) Product liability in respect of drugs. *Br. Med. J.*, **290**: 365–368.

Farndale, W.A.J. (1979) *Law on Hospital Consent Forms. Studies in Law and Practice for Health Service Management*, Vol. 8. Beckenham, UK: Ravenswood Publications.

Grubb, A. and Pearl, D.S. (1990) *Blood Testing, AIDS and DNA Profiling*. Bristol: Family Law.

Jacob J. (1978) *Speller's Law Relating to Hospitals and Kindred Institutions*, 6th eds, pp. 186–197, London: H.K. Lewis.

Treatment without consent: emergency (1985) *Br. Med. J.*, **290**: 1505–1506.

Treatment without consent: intervention by the court (1985) *Br. Med. J.*, **290**: 1408–1409.

Whincup, M.H. (1982) *Legal Aspects of Medical and Nursing Service: Studies in Law and Practice for Health Service Management*, Vol. 5, 3rd edn, pp. 106–109. Beckenham, UK: Ravenswood Publications.

Appendix A

RARE DONOR REGISTRIES

American Association of Blood Banks Register of Rare Blood, Memorial Blood Center of Minneapolis, 2304 Park Avenue, Minneapolis, MN 55404, USA. (Tel: 612 8713300)

European Bank of Frozen Blood, Netherlands Red Cross Blood Transfusion Service, Plesmanlaan 125, PO Box 9190, 1006 AD Amsterdam, The Netherlands. (Tel: 20-512 3377 Fax: 20-512 9222)

National Reference Laboratory for Blood Group Serology. American Red Cross, 15601 Crabbs Branch Way, Rockville, MD 20855-2743, USA. (Tel: 0101 3017380532)

UK National Frozen Blood Bank, West Midlands Regional Blood Transfusion Service, Vincent Drive, Edgbaston Birmingham, UK. (Tel: 0121 4141155)

WHO International Donor File. Held at the International Blood Group Reference Laboratory, Southmead Road, Bristol, UK. (Tel: 01272 507777. Fax: 01272 591660)

TRANSPLANT DONOR PANELS/COORDINATING AGENCIES

Most countries have established their own bone marrow donor register and solid organ transport support services. Within the UK facilities are provided from:

Anthony Nolan Bone Marrow Appeal, Anthony Nolan Research Trust, Royal Free Hospital, Pond Street, Hampstead, London NW3 2QG, UK. (Tel: 0171 2841234. Fax: 0171 284 8226)

United Kingdom Transplant Support Service Authority, Fox Den Road, Stoke Gifford, Bristol, UK. (Tel: 01272 757575 Fax: 01272 757577)

SOCIETIES FOR THE PROMOTION OF BLOOD TRANSFUSION

American Association of Blood Bank, 8101 Glenbrook Road, Bethesda, MD 20814, USA.

British Blood Transfusion Society, Plymouth Grove, Manchester, UK. (Tel: 0161 2737181)

International Society of Blood Transfusion (ISBT) Central Office, National Directorate, Gateway House, Piccadilly South, Manchester, UK.

Societies for the promotion and development of Blood Transfusion Service are being established in many other countries throughout the world.

FURTHER READING

American Association of Blood Banks Standards for Blood Banks and Transfusion Services. 16th edn (1994) Beckenham, UK: S. Kanger.

Gibbs, W.N. and Britten, A.F.H. (eds) (1992) *Guidelines for the Organization of a Blood Transfusion Service*. London: World Health Organization.

Handbook of Transfusion Medicine (1989) United Kingdom Blood Transfusion Services. London: HMSO.

Hollan, S.R., Wagstaff, W., Leikola, J. and Lothe, F. (eds) (1990) *Management of Blood Transfusion Services*. Geneva: World Health Organization.

Roberts, B. (ed.) (1991) *Standard Haematology Practice*, Vol. I. Oxford: Blackwell Scientific.

Roberts, B. (ed.) (1995) *Standard Haematology Practice*, Vol. II. Oxford: Blackwell Scientific (in press).

Appendix B

Department of Health and Social Security Blood Transfusion Record Keeping and Stock Control Arrangement HC(84)7.

Medicines Act (UK) 1968 and Health Service Circular HS(IS)149 1975. Application of Medicines Act 1968 to Health Authorities: Blood Transfusion Service.

Index

Note: Page references in *italics* refer to Figures; those in **bold** refer to Tables

Index compiled by Annette J. Musker